D1223138

TOXICOLOGY AND THE NEWBORN

TOXICOLOGY AND THE NEWBORN

edited by

Sam Kacew and Mark J. Reasor

with a Foreword by

Gabriel L. Plaa

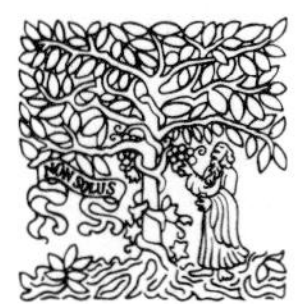

ELSEVIER
AMSTERDAM – NEW YORK – OXFORD – 1984

© 1984 ELSEVIER SCIENCE PUBLISHERS B.V.

All rights reserved. No part of this publication may be reproduced, stored in a retrieval system, or transmitted, in any form or by any means, electronic, mechanical, photocopying, recording or otherwise, without the prior permission of the copyright owner. However, this book has been registered with the Copyright Clearance Center, Inc. Consent is given for copying pages for personal or internal use of specific clients. This consent is given on the condition that the copier pay through the Center the per page fee stated below for copying beyond that permitted by the U.S. Copyright Law.

The appropriate fee should be forwarded with a copy of front and back of the title page of the book to the Copyright Clearance Center, Salem, MA 01970. This consent does not extend to other kinds of copying, such as for general distribution, resale, advertising and promotional purposes, or for creating new works. Special written permission must be obtained from the publisher for such copying.

The per page fee code for this book is 0-444-80598-2:84/\$ + .80.

ISBN 0-444-80598-2

Published by:

Elsevier Science Publishers B.V.
PO Box 211
1000 AE Amsterdam
The Netherlands

Sole distributors for the USA and Canada:

Elsevier Science Publishing Company, Inc.
52 Vanderbilt Avenue
New York, NY 10017
USA

Library of Congress Cataloging in Publication Data

Main entry under title:

Toxicology and the newborn.

Bibliography: p.
Includes index.
1. Pediatric toxicology. 2. Infants (Newborn)—Diseases. 3. Infants (Newborn)—Physiology. I. Kacew, Sam. II. Reasor, Mark J. [DNLM: 1. Infant, Newborn, Diseases—chemically induced. 2. Drugs—adverse effects. 3. Fetal Diseases—chemically induced. WS 420 T755]
RA1225.T69 1984 618.92 84-13572
ISBN 0-444-80598-2

PRINTED IN THE NETHERLANDS

Foreword

The potentially adverse effect of chemical substances on the fetus and the newborn is of major concern in today's society. In the last 30 or so years, a number of drugs have been shown to be particularly toxic in immature or developing organisms. The thalidomide tragedy of the 1960s emphasized the marked susceptibility of the human fetus to exposure to certain types of chemical agents. Exposure of the fetus to diethylstilbestrol (DES) and the subsequent appearance of neoplasms in female children of women given DES is another example. The field of teratology has expanded tremendously in the last 20 years, with the result that much knowledge has been acquired of the development of the fetus. This interest in the developing fetus has followed its natural course. In the 1980s we see a newly emerging field, developmental toxicology, which follows development well beyond the fetus, through maturity, and even into senescence.

Newborn animals generally are more susceptible than adults of the same species, although some exceptions do exist. Newborn rats have been found to be 0.1 to 20 times more susceptible than adult rats to the lethal effects of drugs. The newborn infant also can be particularly susceptible to chemical agents. Many of these exaggerated responses, particularly with drugs, can be explained by altered pharmacokinetics (absorption, distribution, biotransformation, elimination) in the newborn. Chloramphenicol toxicity in the newborn is characterized by cardiovascular collapse, coma and cyanosis (grey syndrome). The neonate cannot glucuronidate this antibiotic adequately, resulting in high and prolonged plasma concentrations of chloramphenicol. Now that the mechanism is known (impaired biotransformation), this adverse reaction can be avoided by adjustment of the dosages of chloramphenicol administered to infants.

Membrane permeability can affect drug response markedly. The blood-brain barrier is not developed fully in the human neonate, and this characteristic is the explanation for the appearance of neonatal kernicterus sometimes observed following sulfonamide therapy in the newborn infant. Normally unconjugated bilirubin is bound highly to plasma protein; sulfonamides can displace the bilirubin from the binding sites, and the unbound bilirubin passes through the immature blood-brain barrier into the central nervous system. This adverse reaction is now avoided by not administering drugs that can displace bilirubin from plasma proteins.

Drugs are not the only chemicals that can affect the newborn. During the last decade, society has become keenly aware of the numerous chemical substances present in the environment. Chemical contamination of waterways, air or soil is of major concern. A number of these substances are highly persistent. Furthermore, some may enter into the food chain because they can bioaccumulate. The potential impact of these agents on the newborn is not well known, and society rightfully is demanding that toxicologists address the issue. The questions are clear: What are the toxic manifestations in the newborn? Do they differ from those observed in mature organisms? Is the newborn at higher risk than the adult? What biological mechanisms are involved? Can the effects be predicted? What are the short- and long-term consequences? How can the effects be prevented?

The modern toxicologist must be informed about these problems. The present monograph is a welcome addition to the toxicology literature. A number of specific chemical substances are treated in detail. Furthermore, experimental approaches and their interpretation are described. This monograph will surely enhance our knowledge of toxicology and the newborn.

Gabriel L. Plaa

List of Contributors

JOHN U. BELL, Ph.D., *Associate Professor, Departments of Preventive Medicine and of Pharmacology and Therapeutics, University of Florida, Gainesville, FL 32610, U.S.A.*

LOUIS W. CHANG, Ph.D., *Director, Experimental Pathology Program and Professor, Department of Pathology, University of Arkansas for Medical Sciences, Little Rock, AR 72205, U.S.A.*

DONALD J. ECOBICHON, Ph.D., *Professor, Department of Pharmacology and Therapeutics, McIntyre Medical Sciences Building, McGill University, Montreal, Quebec, H3G 1Y6, Canada.*

LAURENCE D. FECHTER, Ph.D., *Assistant Professor, Department of Environmental Health Sciences, The Johns Hopkins University School of Hygiene and Public Health, Baltimore, MD 21205, U.S.A.*

LEE FRANK, M.D., Ph.D., *Assistant Professor, Department of Medicine, Pulmonary Division, University of Miami, School of Medicine, Miami, FL 33101, U.S.A.*

PETER A. FRIED, Ph.D., *Professor, Department of Psychology, Carleton University, Ottawa, Ontario, K1S 5B6, Canada.*

BRYAN D. HARDIN, *Research Biologist, Acute and Subchronic Toxicology Section, Experimental Toxicology Branch, National Institute of Occupational Safety and Health, Cincinnati, OH 45226, U.S.A.*

SAM KACEW, Ph.D., *Associate Professor, Department of Pharmacology, University of Ottawa, Ottawa, Ontario, K1H 8M5, Canada.*

CAROLE A. KIMMEL, Ph.D., *US Environmental Protection Agency, RD 689, Reproductive Effects Assessment Group, Washington, DC 20460, U.S.A.*

JAMES B. LaBORDE, *Division of Teratogenesis Research, National Center for Toxicology Research, Jefferson, AR 72079, U.S.A.*

NADIA Z. MIKHAEL, M.D., *Head, Pharmacology Pathology Unit, and Associate Professor, Department of Pathology, University of Ottawa, Ottawa, Ontario, K1H 8M5, Canada.*

DENNIS V. PARKE, D.Sc., F.R.C. Pathol., *Professor and Head, Department of Biochemistry, University of Surrey, Guildford, Surrey, GU2 5XH, U.K.*

HAROLD W. PEEL, Ph.D., *Scientific Advisor — Toxicology, Science and Technology Advisory Group, Royal Canadian Mounted Police, Ottawa, Ontario, K1A 0R2, Canada.*

GABRIEL L. PLAA, Ph. D., *Vice Dean of Graduate Studies and Professor, Department of Pharmacology, University of Montreal, Montreal, Quebec, H3C 3J7, Canada.*

MARK J. REASOR, Ph.D., *Professor, Department of Pharmacology and Toxicology, West Virginia University, Morgantown, WV 26506, U.S.A.*

ROBERT J. ROBERTS, M.D., Ph.D., *Professor, Departments of Pediatrics and of Pharmacology, University of Iowa, Iowa City, IA 52242, U.S.A.*

DEBRA L. THOMA-LAURIE, Ph.D., *Department of Toxicology, Syntex, Inc., Palo Alto, CA 94304, U.S.A.*

JOHN A. THOMAS, Ph.D., *Vice President, Life Sciences, Travenol Laboratories, Inc., Morton Grove, IL 60053, U.S.A.*

MICHAEL J. THOMAS, *Department of Pharmacology and Toxicology, West Virginia University, Morgantown, WV 26506, U.S.A.*

BRUCE B. VIRGO, Ph.D., *Associate Professor, Department of Biology, University of Windsor, Windsor, Ontario, N9B 3P4, Canada.*

DANIEL WIERDA, Ph.D., *Assistant Professor, Department of Pharmacology and Toxicology, West Virginia University, Morgantown, WV 26506, U.S.A.*

Contents

S. Kacew and M.J. Reasor (eds), *Toxicology and the Newborn*
© 1984 Elsevier Science Publishers B.V.

Chapter 1

Development of Detoxication Mechanisms in the Neonate

DENNIS V. PARKE

Department of Biochemistry, University of Surrey, Guildford, Surrey, U.K.

CONTENTS

I. INTRODUCTION

It is well known that the foetus and neonate are particularly susceptible to the toxic effects of drugs and other chemical substances. The treatment of infants with the newly discovered antibiotic chloramphenicol in the 1946–1947 European epidemic of infantile diarrhoea is believed to have contributed largely to the high mortality of that tragic catastrophe (Lischner et al., 1961) and confirmed the widely held opinion that infants were especially vulnerable to the toxic side-effects of drugs. Nearly 20 years later, this view was reaffirmed by the thalidomide disaster, in which thousands of babies were born deformed by foetal malformations induced as the result of the mother taking the tranquillizing drug thalidomide, which had been especially noted for its freedom from toxic side-effects in adults (Lenz, 1965). More recently, it was found that the synthetic oestrogenic drug diethylstilbestrol, given in high dosage to pregnant women to maintain their pregnancies in threatened spontaneous abortion, has been the cause of adenocarcinoma of the vagina occurring in their female offspring on reaching sexual maturity (Herbst et al.,1975). The antiseptic hexachlorophene, widely used in the bathing of young babies, had to be restricted in its use since it was found to be associated with the occurrence of convulsions and brain damage (Kimbrough, 1973); and infants exposed to polychlorinated biphenyls present as contaminants in their mother's breast milk exhibited muscular weakness and apathy (Kuwabara et al., 1979). Infant mortality, teratogenesis, transplacental carcinogenesis and infant ill-health may thus be the occasional tragic results of drug administration to neonates or the results of incautious taking of drugs, or exposure to toxic environmental chemicals, during pregnancy, the puerperium or the postnatal period of lactation. These clinical aspects of developmental pharmacology and toxicology have recently been reviewed in detail (Aranda and Stern, 1983).

Research during the past few decades has elucidated some of the reasons why the foetus and neonate are particularly vulnerable to the toxic effects of drugs and environmental chemicals. Accumulated scientific evidence has shown that the deactivation and detoxication of drugs and other chemicals are undeveloped in the foetus, and that drugs may cross the placenta from the maternal blood into the foetus, effecting damage that may result in the death or maldevelopment of the unborn infant or give rise to latent malignancy. Furthermore, it has been shown that the neonate has only limited detoxication ability, and therefore little natural protection against the toxic effects of the drugs and chemicals, which may reach the child not only by direct administration but also indirectly through secretion in the mother's milk.

II. MAMMALIAN METABOLISM OF XENOBIOTICS

When environmental chemicals, or xenobiotics, are ingested by the mammalian organism they may be rapidly excreted, if they are polar, non-lipophilic materials. If they are lipophilic, they generally undergo metabolism into more polar, water-soluble

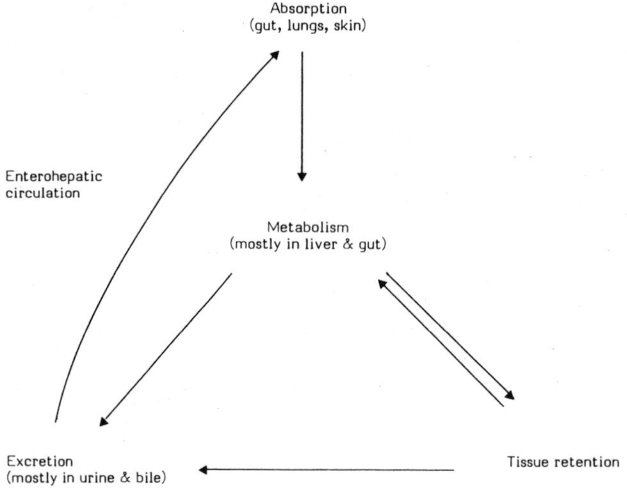

Figure 1. Disposition of xenobiotic chemicals in mammals.

compounds, which are then excreted more readily. The original chemical, or any of its metabolities, may be distributed into the tissues or excreted from the body (see Fig. 1). In this way lipophilic chemicals are made more polar and are eventually eliminated in the urine or bile. Many compounds which are excreted into the bile may undergo further metabolism in the gastrointestinal tract, be absorbed, then excreted once again in either the urine or bile, a process known as enterohepatic circulation.

However, increasing numbers of synthetic chemicals, especially halogenated compounds, are metabolised with difficulty by mammals, and only very slowly by micro-organisms, despite their being highly lipophilic. These chemicals, for example, hexachlorobenzene, hexabromobiphenyl and tetrachlorodibenzodioxin (TCDD), are thus characterized by their environmental persistence, their very long biological half-lives, and their progressive accumulation in the fatty tissues of animals exposed to these chemicals.

1. Absorption, distribution and excretion

The absorption and excretion of xenobiotic chemicals involves transfer of these compounds across the various barrier membranes of the body, such as the gastrointestinal epithelium, renal tubular epithelium, hepatic parenchyma, the skin and placental membranes. This transfer of substances across biological membranes may occur by four different mechanisms, namely: simple diffusion, filtration through aqueous pores in the lipoprotein membrane, active transport by carrier mechanisms (usually limited to nutrients), and pinocytosis. In the transfer of xenobiotics by simple diffusion only lipophilic non-ionized molecules readily pass through the membranes, so that non-electrolytes are transferred according to their lipid solubility and electrolytes according to their degree of ionization and the lipid-solubility of the non-ionized molecules.

(a) Absorption

Absorption of xenobiotics may occur through all the body's external surfaces, including the mouth, the gastrointestinal tract, the lungs and skin, and mostly involves only simple diffusion.

Substances absorbed from the mouth are not exposed to gastrointestinal secretions, microflora or intestinal drug-metabolising enzymes, and are not so rapidly metabolised, as they are not transported directly to the liver, where most drug metabolism takes place. Absorption from the stomach depends on the pH of the gastric contents, and the dissociation constant (pK) and lipid solubility of the environmental chemical; low gastric acidity, as occurs in neonates, also predisposes to microbial overgrowth, which may lead to reductive metabolism of xenobiotics and reduction of ingested nitrate to nitrite, with the formation of nitrosamines in situ. Absorption from the intestines occurs readily for non-ionized, lipophilic chemicals and for weak acids and bases, but highly ionized compounds are absorbed only slowly.

Absorption through the skin depends on age, as the main barrier to the absorption of environmental chemicals is the keratinized outer layer, the stratum corneum, which tends to thicken with age; absorption is much greater through abraded skin and human skin is less permeable than that of most fur-covered laboratory animals. Absorption from the lungs occurs readily for lipid-soluble gases, and for lipophilic compounds with high vapour pressures, e.g., *p*-dichlorobenzene.

(b) Distribution

Once absorbed, xenobiotic chemicals may be distributed to other tissues, first to the liver when absorbed from the gastrointestinal tract, and to fat depots if highly lipophilic. The blood–brain and blood–cerebrospinal barriers are typical lipoprotein membranes and are permeable to non-ionized or ionized lipophilic molecules. The placenta similarly is permeable to lipophilic molecules, but polar molecules are transferred with difficulty.

Certain chemicals have affinity for specific tissues, e.g., tetracycline antibiotics have an affinity for bones and teeth; the herbicide, paraquat, and the toxin of mouldy sweet potatoes, 4-ipomeanol, become concentrated in lung tissue; alkylmercury and alkyllead compounds are found in high concentrations in the brain; the toxic metal, cadmium, accumulates in the kidney, and arsenic, selenium and other metals accumulate in the hair (Parke, 1982).

(c) Excretion

Excretion of xenobiotics by the kidney comprises three distinct processes, namely: glomerular filtration, passive tubular transfer (of lipophilic non-ionized molecules), and active tubular transport (secretion of highly ionized acids and bases, e.g., glucuronides, sulphate esters and tetra-alkylammonium compounds). Binding of compounds to plasma proteins markedly impairs their renal excretion, but leads to their excretion in the bile; the rates of biliary excretion of a number of azo dyes have been shown to be functions of their binding to plasma and liver proteins (Parke, 1982).

The biliary excretion of xenobiotic chemicals varies with species and is dependent on molecular size, being negligible for compounds of a molecular weight of less than 300, e.g., 4-hydroxybiphenyl glucuronide (molecular weight, 346) is readily excreted in the bile of rats, but 4-aminophenyl glucuronide (molecular weight, 285) is not. As the molecular weight of the excretion product increases above a value of around 300, biliary excretion progressively increases, and urihary excretion correspondingly decreases. Chemicals are excreted in the bile mostly as conjugates, which may be hydrolysed by enzymes (β-glucuronidases, sulphatases, etc.) present in the bile, or subsequently by enzymes of the intestinal microflora. Biliary excreted conjugates of xenobiotics, being polar, are not reabsorbed from the gastrointestinal tract, but their hydrolysis products, if non-polar, may be reabsorbed, transported to the liver, re-conjugated, and excreted again in the bile, a process known as enterohepatic circulation.

Other routes of excretion are relatively minor, and include the secretion of bases into the stomach, the excretion of acids into the pancreatic juice and into the lumen of the intestine, the elimination of volatile compounds in the expired air, and the secretion of lipophilic materials, such as polychlorinated biphenyls and hexachlorobenzene, into the milk (Bailey et al., 1980).

2. *Metabolism*

Xenobiotic chemicals are metabolised in mammals by mammalian enzymes, which are most active in the liver and gastrointestinal tract, and also by the microbial enzymes of the gastrointestinal microflora. The mammalian enzymes have been classified into (a) phase I reactions (biotransformations) and (b) phase II reactions (conjugations).

These biotransformation and conjugation reactions may lead either to the detoxication of the chemical and the excretion of its metabolites, or to activation of the chemical into reactive intermediates, which subsequently may be detoxicated by interaction with glutathione, or may react with tissue proteins, enzymes, RNA or DNA, to result in toxic reactions (see Fig. 2). The major types of biotransformation reactions are oxidations (oxygenations), reductions, and hydrolyses, catalysed mostly by the mammalian enzymes of the endoplasmic reticulum (microsomal enzymes), and by non-microsomal enzymes of the cell cytosol, mitochondria, or of the blood plasma, and reductions and hydrolyses (but not oxidations) catalysed by enzymes of the microflora present in the gastrointestinal tract (see Table 1). The major types of conjugation reactions are glucuronylations, sulphations, methylations, acetylations, and peptide conjugations with glutathione and various amino acids (see Table 2).

The major sites of metabolism by mammalian enzymes are the liver and gastrointestinal tract, with lesser activity present in the lungs, kidneys and the skin. The xenobiotic-metabolizing enzymes of the intestine are similar to those of the liver,

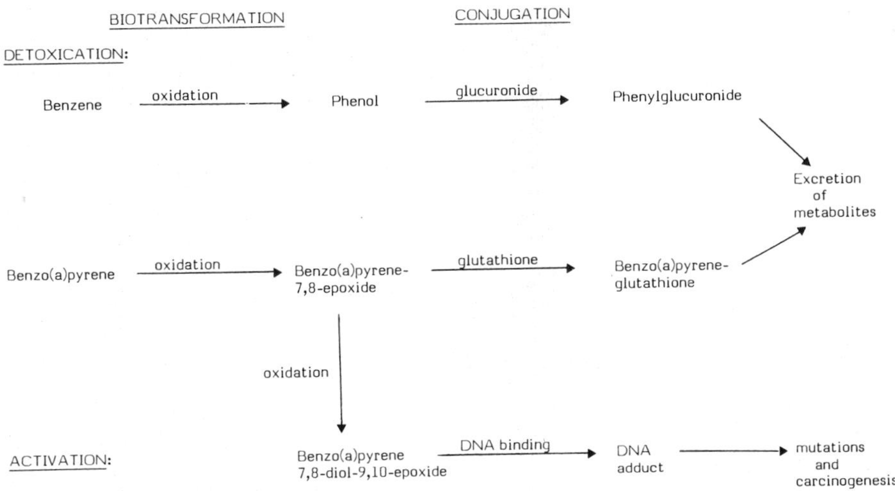

Figure 2. The roles of metabolism in the detoxication and activation of carcinogens and toxic chemicals.

except that in general they give rise to lower rates of metabolism (Chhabra, 1979). The extrahepatic metabolism of xenobiotics has recently been reviewed (Vainio and Hietanen, 1980).

(a) Biotransformation

The phase I reactions of oxidations, reduction and hydrolysis are catalysed by enzymes of the endoplasmic reticulum (microsomes) and of the cell cytosol. The microsomal mixed-function oxidases of the endoplasmic reticulum of liver and other tissues catalyse numerous oxidations of xenobiotics, including aromatic and aliphatic hydroxylation, epoxidation, *N*-oxidation, *S*-oxidation, dealkylation and deamination (see Table 1).

These mixed-function oxidations are mostly catalysed by an enzyme system consisting of the terminal oxygen transferase, cytochrome *P*-450, coupled to cytochrome *P*-450 reductase (a flavoprotein containing both FAD and FMN) and linked to a source of electrons from NADPH (see Fig. 3) (Hodgson, 1979).

Recent studies of this membrane-bound cytochrome *P*-450 system have enabled the enzyme to be solubilized, separated and purified, and have thus revealed that cytochrome *P*-450 and cytochrome *P*-450 reductase both exist in multiple forms, and that lipid, especially phosphatidylcholine, is essential for enzymic activity (Guengerich, 1979). These multiple cytochromes *P*-450 are regarded as isoenzymes, or enzyme variants with overlapping substrate specificities, and have been shown to have identical or very similar active sites (Dus, 1982). Further structural and kinetic studies have shown that, in contrast, the active site of cytochrome(s) *P*-448 is different to that of cytochrome *P*-450 (Dus, 1982; Phillipson et al., 1982). The different tissue distribution (*P*-448 predominates in extrahepatic, placental, foetal, neonatal and neoplastic tissues; *P*-450 predominates in the gut and liver) and the

TABLE 1

MAMMALIAN BIOTRANSFORMATION REACTIONS OF XENOBIOTICS

Microsomal Mixed Function Oxidations

Aliphatic oxidation:	$R\text{-}CH_3 \longrightarrow R\text{-}CH_2OH$
Aromatic oxidation:	⌬ $\longrightarrow$ ⌬-OH
Epoxidation:	$R\text{-}CH{=}CH_2 \longrightarrow R\text{-}CH\text{-}CH_2$ (with O bridging the two carbons)
Oxidative deamination:	$R\text{-}CH(NH_2)(CH_3) \longrightarrow [R\text{-}C(OH)(NH_2)(CH_3)] \longrightarrow R\text{-}C(=O)\text{-}CH_3 + NH_3$
N-Dealkylation:	$R\text{-}N(CH_3)(CH_3) \longrightarrow [R\text{-}N(CH_2OH)(CH_3)] \longrightarrow R\text{-}N(H)(CH_3) + HCHO$
O-Dealkylation:	$R\text{-}O\text{-}CH_3 \longrightarrow R\text{-}OH + HCHO$
S-Dealkylation:	$R\text{-}S\text{-}CH_3 \longrightarrow R\text{-}SH + HCHO$
N-Oxidation:	$R_3{\geqq}N \longrightarrow R_3{\geqq}N{\rightarrow}O$
N-Hydroxylation	⌬-$NH_2 \longrightarrow$ ⌬-NHOH
Sulphoxidation:	$R_2{>}S \longrightarrow R_2{>}S{\rightarrow}O \longrightarrow R_2{>}S{=}O$
Desulphuration:	$R_2{>}C{=}S \longrightarrow R_2{>}C{=}O$
Dehalogenation:	$R\text{-}CH_2Cl \longrightarrow R\text{-}CH_2OH$

Non-microsomal Oxidations

Monoamine and diamine oxidation:	$R\text{-}CH_2NH_2 \xrightarrow{O_2} R\text{-}CH{=}NH \xrightarrow{H_2O} R\text{-}CHO + NH_3$
Alcohol dehydrogenation:	$R\text{-}CH_2OH \longrightarrow R\text{-}CHO$
Aldehyde dehydrogenation:	$R\text{-}CHO \longrightarrow R\text{-}COOH$

Microsomal Reductions

Nitro reduction:	$R\text{-}NO_2 \longrightarrow R\text{-}NO \longrightarrow R\text{-}NHOH \longrightarrow R\text{-}NH_2$
Azo reduction:	$RN{=}NR^1 \longrightarrow RNH\text{-}NHR^1 \longrightarrow R\text{-}NH_2 + R^1\text{-}NH_2$
Reductive dehalogenation:	$R\text{-}CCl_3 \longrightarrow R\text{-}CHCl_2$

TABLE 1 (continued)

Non-microsomal Reductions			
Aldehyde reduction:	$R_2C{=}O$	→	R_2CHOH
Hydrolyses			
Ester hydrolysis:	$RCO\text{-}OR^1$	$\xrightarrow{H_2O}$	$RCOOH + R^1OH$
Amide hydrolysis:	$RCO\text{-}NH_2$	$\xrightarrow{H_2O}$	$RCOOH + NH_3$
Epoxide hydration:	$RCH\text{-}CH_2$ (epoxide, O bridge)	$\xrightarrow{H_2O}$	$RCH(OH)CH_2OH$

TABLE 2

MAMMALIAN CONJUGATION REACTIONS OF XENOBIOTICS

UDPGA-mediated Glucuronylations			
Ether glucuronide:	ROH	→	$RO\text{-}C_6H_9O_6$
Ester glucuronide:	RCOOH	→	$RCOO\text{-}C_6H_9O_6$
N-Glucuronide:	RNH_2	→	$RNH\text{-}C_6H_9O_6$
S-Glucuronide:	RSH	→	$RS\text{-}C_6H_9O_6$
PAPS-mediated Sulphate Ester Formation			
Alkyl or aryl sulphate:	ROH	→	$RO\text{-}SO_3H$
Sulphamate:	RNH_2	→	$RNH\text{-}SO_3H$
S-Adenosylmethione-mediated Methylations			
O-Methylation:	ROH	→	$RO\text{-}CH_3$
N-Methylation:	RNH_2	→	$RNH\text{-}CH_3$
S-Methylation:	RSH	→	$RS\text{-}CH_3$
Acetylations	RNH_2	$\xrightarrow{\text{acetyl CoA}}$	$RNH\text{-}COCH_3$
Peptide Conjugations	RCOOH	$\xrightarrow{\text{CoA + glycine}}$	$RCO\text{-}NHCH_2COOH$
	$RCH\text{-}CH_2$ (epoxide, O bridge)	$\xrightarrow{GSH}$	$RCHOH.CH_2\text{-}SG$

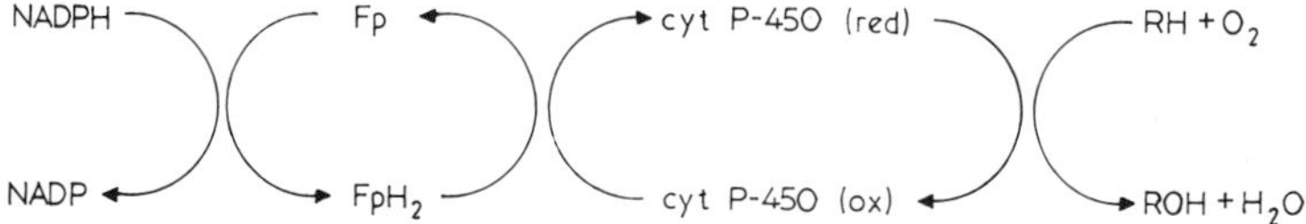

Figure 3. The microsomal cytochrome *P*-450-dependent mixed-function oxidase system. A simplified version in which both electrons are provided by the NADPH-dependent cytochrome *P*-450 reductase (Fp), to oxygenate the substrate (RH) to the metabolite (ROH).

different types of enzyme induction (*P*-450 only is induced by phenobarbitone and certain drugs; *P*-448 only is induced by carcinogenic polycyclic hydrocarbons) indicate that the cytochromes *P*-450 and *P*-448 are two different classes of enzyme, the products of two different genomes, and under different mechanisms of regulation. The physiological roles of these two classes of cytochrome also appear to differ, with the cytochromes *P*-450 being mostly concerned with the detoxication of xenobiotics and the cytochromes *P*-448 with the biogenesis of the steroid hormones. This is of importance in the perinatal development of these cytochromes, as the appearance of cytochrome(s) *P*-448 seems to precede the appearance of the cytochromes *P*-450. Lack of appreciation of these differences, and especially of the different physiological functions of these two groups of enzymes, has previously confused many aspects of the perinatal development of detoxication mechanisms.

Cytochrome *P*-450 may also catalyse the reduction of certain xenobiotics as it has a low redox potential; aromatic nitro compounds, tertiary amine oxides, polycyclic hydrocarbon epoxides and polychlorinated alkanes have all been shown to be reduced by cytochrome *P*-450 (Harada and Omura, 1980).

Xenobiotic oxidations, especially *N*-oxidations and *S*-oxidations (Hajjar and Hodgson, 1980; Hlavica and Hülsmann, 1979), may also be catalysed by microsomal flavoprotein oxidoreductases.

Phase I reactions catalysed by enzymes of the cytosol include oxidations by alcohol dehydrogenase, aldehyde oxidase and monoamine and diamine oxidases, enzymic reductions involving nitro-reductase, azo-reductase and reductive dehalogenation, and the hydrolysis of epoxides, esters and amides (see Table 1). Epoxide hydrase, which with the glutathione *S*-tranferases is responsible for the detoxication of the potentially toxic and mutagenic epoxides, may be considered as a phase I (hydrolysis) or a phase II (conjugation with water) enzyme. Its importance, relative to the glutathione *S*-transferases, in the detoxication of xenobiotics, is greatest in humans and the higher primates (Parke, 1982).

(b) Conjugations

In the phase II conjugation reactions the xenobiotic chemical or its active metabolites are coupled with various endogenous moieties to make them more polar and more readily excretable. These endogenous moieties may be sugars (glucuronic acid), acids (sulphuric), alkyl groups (methyl), or amino acid and peptides (glutathione), and some of the more important conjugation mechanisms are listed in

Table 2. These conjugation reactions are associated with enzymes found in the endoplasmic reticulum (UDPglucuronyltransferases), or in the cytosol (sulphotransferases), and the enzymic mechanisms have been reviewed fully by Hirom and Millburn (1979).

(c) Detoxication or activation

Environmental chemicals may be metabolised by several different reactions simultaneously, some resulting in detoxication and others in activation, and complex drugs such as chlorpromazine may give rise to more than a hundred chemically different metabolites. The different oxygenases and reductases (isoenzymes of cytochromes *P*-450 and *P*-448, and the flavoprotein oxidoreductases) yield many different phase I metabolites, and the different conjugating enzymes may further metabolise these to an almost infinite variety of different metabolites.

It has been shown that, in general, xenobiotic chemicals are activated by oxidative metabolism to yield epoxides, quinones, semiquinones and other free radicals as highly electrophilic 'reactive intermediates', which interact with nucleophilic biological macromolecules (enzymes, membranes, DNA) to cause cellular damage, mutations or carcinogenesis (Parke and Ioannides, 1982). Furthermore, it has been established that the oxygenations that activate toxic chemicals are catalysed mostly by cytochrome *P*-448 or the flavoprotein oxidases, and not by the cytochromes *P*-450, which usually catalyse oxygenations which result in detoxication (Ioannides et al., 1984). The reason for this is that the cytochromes *P*-448, but not the *P*-450s, have an active site which is able to accommodate large molecules and to effect their oxygenation in conformationally hindered positions to form reactive intermediates; these reactive intermediates, because of the conformationally hindered oxygenation, do not appear to be readily acceptable substrates for the phase II conjugation enzymes, and hence are not readily detoxicated, so react non-enzymically with intracellular macromolecules such as enzymic proteins or DNA.

The metabolic activation of toxic chemicals has, in a few instances, also been associated with conjugation reactions. The proximate carcinogen, *N*-hydroxy-2-acetamidofluorene, is considered to require further activation by sulphate conjugation to form the ultimate carcinogen, and various vicinal dihalogen compounds, such as 1,2-dichloroethane, are converted into mutagens by conjugation with glutathione, which yields β-halogen thioethers or sulphur mustards (Van Bladeren et al., 1979).

(d) Enzyme induction

Repeated dosing with certain xenobiotic chemicals leads to increased activity of the microsomal mixed-function oxidases and certain other associated enzymes, as a result of increased de novo enzyme synthesis. It is possible that saturation of the enzyme active site by substrate, resulting in reversible inhibition, is responsible for the increased enzymic activity. Hence, environmental chemicals which are metabolised only slowly or are metabolised with difficulty (e.g., phenobarbital, DDT, polycyclic hydrocarbons, polychlorobiphenyls, TCDD) are generally found to be the most potent enzyme-inducing agents. Three major classes of inducing agent have been recognised:

(i) 'Drugs' (phenobarbital) — which increase the activity of cytochrome(s) *P*-450, the coupled *P*-450 reductase, UDPglucuronyltransferases and other conjugating enzymes.

(ii) 'Carcinogenic polycyclic hydrocarbons' (3-methylcholanthrene) — which increase the activity of the cytochrome(s) *P*-448, but not of the reductase.

(iii) 'Catatoxic steroids' (pregnenolone-16α-carbonitrile) — which give no major increase in the cytochromes *P*-450/*P*-448, but result in a substantial increase in NADPH-cytochrome *c* reductase.

As metabolism of xenobiotic chemicals by cytochrome(s) *P*-450 generally leads to ultimate detoxication, induction of these enzymes by 'drugs' generally will enhance this process, thereby constituting a protective feed-back mechanism. In contrast, as metabolism by cytochrome(s) *P*-448 generally leads to activation of carcinogens and toxic chemicals, induction of these enzymes generally will result in the increased likelihood of toxicity, mutagenicity and carcinogenicity. One possible explanation for this suicidal mechanism of regulation is that the normal biological role of the cytochromes *P*-448 is the metabolism of endogenous substrates vital to the existence of the organism, such as the biogenesis of the steroid hormones. The metabolic activation of certain chemical carcinogens by this enzyme system is probably purely fortuitous, because they happen to have a similar molecular size and conformation to cholesterol, which can be accommodated in the active site(s) of the cytochromes *P*-448, and thereby are oxygenated.

III. DETOXICATION IN THE FOETO-PLACENTAL UNIT

1. *Placental transfer of xenobiotics*

The placenta is a highly complex tissue with a unique metabolic pattern but, with respect to drugs and xenobiotics, it behaves similarly to a semipermeable filter which readily allows the passage of lipid-soluble molecules of quite large dimension. Consequently, it can be penetrated by numerous drugs and environmental chemicals, which then find their way into the tissues of the foetus. Indeed, no longer is the foremost consideration whether or not a drug may cross the placenta, but rather at what rate it does so and how much is transferred into the foetus (Moya and Thorndike, 1962).

The transport of substances across the placenta may involve the following mechanisms: (1) ultrafiltration, (2) simple and facilitated diffusion, (3) active transport, (4) pinocytosis, and (5) breaks in the placental villi, and the most important as far as drugs and xenobiotic chemicals are concerned is 'simple diffusion'.

The concept of the placenta as a simple lipoid barrier has been widely accepted as a criterion of the permeability of the placenta to drugs and chemicals. Therefore, compounds that are highly dissociated into lipid-insoluble ionic forms at physiologi cal pH or that in their non-ionized forms are relatively lipid-insoluble (such as succinylcholine) will penetrate the placenta to only a minor degree, whereas highly lipid-soluble compounds, such as antipyrine and polychlorinated biphenyls, will cross this barrier readily. The rate of transfer is also dependent on the molecular weight of the chemical, and on the concentration gradient, that is, essentially the concentration in the maternal blood. In general, the lower the molecular weight, the greater the diffusibility, so that drugs of a molecular weight of less than 600 are transferred readily, if sufficiently lipid-soluble, whereas at a molecular weight of over 1,000 diffusion becomes almost impossible. However, if administered at sufficiently high dosage, even the relatively lipid-insoluble succinylcholine will cross the placenta in amounts sufficient to be demonstrable in the foetal blood. Other factors that may modify this concept of simple diffusion across a lipoid barrier are: (1) binding to the plasma proteins of the mother and to the proteins of the placenta, (2) the kinetics of maternal plasma concentration, determined by the rates of maternal absorption, metabolism and excretion, and (3) the possibility of placental metabolism.

Two comprehensive reviews of this field, (Moya and Thorndike, 1962; Moya and Smith, 1965) have shown that numerous drugs, including most of those used in obstetrics, with the possible exception of the muscle relaxants, cross the placenta to some degree. The barbiturates, chlorpromazine, diazepam (Idänpään-Heikkilä et al., 1971) and other tranquilizers, the gaseous anesthetics, such as trichlorethylene, halothane and nitrous oxide, diphenylhydantoin (Waddell and Mirkin, 1972), digoxin (Rodgers et al., 1972), nortriptyline (Sjoqvist et al., 1972), a variety of sulphonamides and antibiotics, and the chlorinated hydrocarbon pesticides, DDT, gammexane (BHC) and dieldrin (Curley et al., 1969), all readily cross the placenta into the foetus.

Most narcotics are capable of crossing the placenta, and infants born to mothers addicted to morphine or heroin are now a major social problem and are often reported to show symptoms of withdrawal (Perlmutter, 1967). Nicotine has been shown to cross the placenta in several different animal species; in the rat, nicotine and its metabolites rapidly attain high levels in the foetus, which for unchanged nicotine are higher in the foetal than in the maternal circulation (Mosier and Jansons, 1972).

2. *Placental metabolism of xenobiotics*

The role of the placenta in the metabolism and development of the foetus has been likened to the role of the liver in the adult animal, and it has been suggested that in the same way that the liver is responsible for the detoxication of drugs and toxic chemicals in the adult, the placenta might similarly be responsible for the detoxication of drugs and xenobiotics in the foeto-placental unit. Consequently, there has been considerable interest in the possible metabolism of drugs and foreign compounds in placental tissues (Juchau, 1972).

Placental tissue has significant quantities of smooth endoplasmic reticulum in the trophoblastic cells, and a carbon monoxide-binding cytochrome *P*-450 is present in both the microsomes and mitochondria (Meigs and Ryan, 1968). However, conflicting results have been reported, both for the amount of cytochrome *P*-450 present in placental tissues and for the placental metabolism of drugs and other foreign compounds, but these discrepancies may be explained in terms of species differences or gestational age, or both of these. Homogenates of human placental tissue, of 9–12 weeks' gestation, exhibited minimal activity for the *N*-demethylation of aminopyrine, *p*-hydroxylation of aniline, oxidative deamination of amphetamine, sulphoxidation of chlorpromazine, and hydroxylation of benzo(*a*)pyrene and zoxazolamine (Juchau et al., 1968b), but no measurable *N*-demethylation of 3-methyl-4-monomethylaminoazobenzene was observed except where the placentas were obtained from mothers with histories of regular cigarette smoking (Welch et al., 1969). However, other investigators have reported the absence of drug hydroxylations in the human placenta, and Juchau and Symms (1972) showed that human placental trophoblasts per se were extremely low in, or possibly devoid of, aniline *p*-hydroxylating activity, and that the observed *p*-hydroxylation of aniline in human placental tissue was probably catalysed by haemoglobin. In an extensive survey of the situation, Creaven and Parke (1965) found no oxidative metabolism of coumarin or biphenyl in placentas of several different animal species.

Benzo(*a*)pyrene hydroxylase (also known as aryl hydrocarbon hydroxylase), a cytochrome *P*-450-dependent enzyme, has been widely studied in human placental tissue (Nebert et al., 1969; Welch et al., 1969). Little or no aryl hydrocarbon hydroxylase was found in human placentas from nonsmokers, but this enzymic activity was found in significant amounts in placentas obtained from women who smoked 10–40 cigarettes a day (Pelkonen et al., 1972). Placental benzo(*a*)pyrene hydroxylase, zoxazolamine hydroxylation and phenacetin *O*-deethylase are all induced in experimental animals by polycyclic aromatic hydrocarbons, but not by phenobarbitone or other drugs, thus indicating the presence of cytochrome *P*-448 (Nebert et al., 1969; Juchau et al., 1973). Steroids synthesized in the human placenta (β-oestradiol, oestrone and progesterone) markedly inhibited the placental-catalyzed hydroxylation of benzo(*a*)pyrene, and the low drug-metabolising activities of placental tissue might be attributable to the high placental concentration of these steroids, which may be endogenous substrates of this enzyme.

Unlike the cytochrome *P*-450 system, the microsomal flavoprotein monooxygenase shows increasing activity (dimethylaniline *N*-oxidation) in the placenta of mice during pregnancy (0.3 nmol/min per mg microsomal protein at day 12 increases to 1.4 nmol at day 18), probably because the flavoprotein enzyme system is not inhibited by high concentrations of progestational steroids (Osimitz and Kulkarni, 1982).

The reduction of a wide variety of drugs and other substrates has been shown to be catalysed by placental subcellular fractions, and reduction of *p*-nitrobenzoic acid proceeds via both enzymic and non-enzymic pathways involving NADPH- and NADH-generating systems (Juchau, 1969). Human placenta also contains a soluble NADPH-dependent system capable of reducing the azo linkage of neoprontosil to form sulphanilamide, a different enzyme from the azo-reductase system(s) present in hepatic tissues (Juchau et al., 1968a).

The placenta is largely deficient in its capacity for conjugating drugs and other chemicals. Glucuronide conjugation in the placenta of rabbit has been reported for oxazepam (Berté et al., 1969), but many other workers have been unable to find any glucuronyltransferase activity. Glycine conjugation is catalysed in the presence of human placental mitochondria (Juchau and Yaffe, 1969), but the major conjugation present in the placenta seems to be with sulphate (Troen et al., 1966). Glutathione conjugation of styrene oxide has been demonstrated in placentas of humans (Pacifici and Rane, 1981) and of naphthalene epoxide in monkeys (Juchau and Namkung, 1974). Epoxide hydrolase has similarly been demonstrated in human and monkey placentas (Pacifici and Rane, 1983a; Juchau and Namkung, 1974). It may be that, by having a limited ability to form conjugates with drugs and other xenobiotics, the placenta functions protectively by allowing these chemicals and endogenous substrates, such as oestrogens and bilirubin, to pass from the foetus and placenta back into the maternal circulation, where they are conjugated and are thus unable to return to the foetoplacental unit.

In the light of this very limited ability of the placenta to biotransform and conjugate drugs and other xenobiotics, particularly the very limited ability to hydroxylate drugs, it is surprising to find that the placenta has a very high level of aromatase activity, the monooxygenase system responsible for the biosynthesis of oestrogens. This biosynthesis of oestrogens in the placenta, involving the aromatization of ring A of the C_{19} steroids, requires three separate oxygenations of the molecule and one or more of these may be mediated by a form of cytochrome *P*-450 (Akhtar and Skinner, 1968). In view of the many different known forms of cytochrome *P*-450, it is probable that the cytochrome(s) found in placentas are one or more forms of cytochrome *P*-448, the enzyme(s) catalysing steroid hydroxylations, which also show selective hydroxylation of certain xenobiotics, including benzo(*a*)pyrene, and the drugs phenacetin and zoxazolamine.

3. *Foetal metabolism of xenobiotics*

Although much of the published evidence is equivocal and somewhat confused, it is generally considered that the liver and other tissues of the mammalian foetuses, except possibly human, have only a very limited ability to metabolize drugs and other chemicals. However, most of the studies have been carried out on foetal tissues of rodents and other non-primate species. Rabbit foetal liver preparations were able to metabolize chlorpromazine only to the sulphoxide (Bhatnagar, 1971), a reaction catalysed by flavoprotein oxidoreductases (Fig.4). Nevertheless, treatment of pregnant rabbits or rats near full-term with inducing agents of the liver microsomal drug-metabolising enzyme system can result in some increase of these enzymes and in the metabolism of drugs such as pentobarbital and meperidine (Pantuck et al., 1968). Undoubtedly, the enzymes that detoxicate drugs and chemicals begin to develop very late in the foetuses of most animals, and are present only at low levels in foetal tissue at full-term. However, there is considerable evidence of an earlier and greater ability to hydroxylate steroids and to conjugate with sulphate, so it is possible that cytochrome(s) *P*-448 predominate and are largely saturated with endogenous steroid

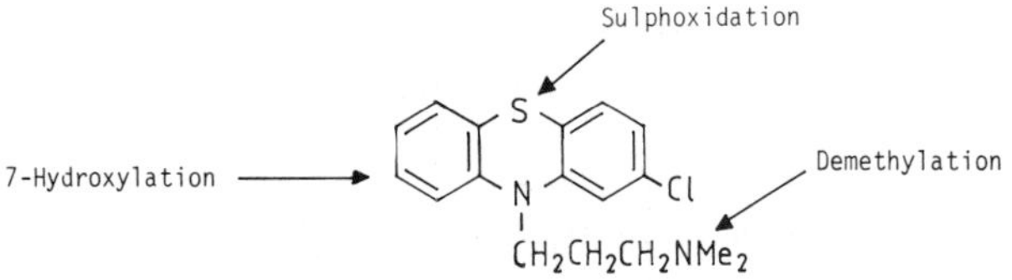

Sulphoxidation

7-Hydroxylation

Demethylation

$CH_2CH_2CH_2NMe_2$

Figure 4. The development of chlorpromazine (CP) metabolism in the rabbit. Metabolites formed from liver preparations in vitro were as follows: foetus, CP-sulphoxide; neonate (3 days old), CP-sulphoxide, 7-hydroxy-CP and desmethyl-CP; adult, CP-sulphoxide, 7-hydroxy-CP, desmethyl-CP, desdimethyl-CP, desmethyl-CP-sulphoxide, desmethyl-7-hydroxy-CP, 7-hydroxy-CP-sulphoxide, desdimethyl-CP-sulphoxide, desdimethyl-7-hydroxy-CP and desmethyl-7-hydroxy-CP-sulphoxide.

substrates, thereby inhibiting the metabolism of added exogenous foreign compounds.

(a) Biotransformations

In contrast to the foetuses of rodents, livers from human foetuses and from the foetuses of non-human primates, such as the stump-tailed macaque, do have relatively well-developed oxidative, hydrolytic and conjugative detoxicating mechanisms early in gestation (Dvorchik and Hartman, 1982). Studies with human foetuses showed that the concentrations of microsomal cytochromes and NADPH-cytochrome *c* reductase in foetal liver were similar to those found in adult human liver. The reason for this may lie in the fact that the cells of human foetal liver are resistant to homogenisation, so that the enzymic activity remains located in the cell debris, instead of in the microsomal fraction (Ackerman et al., 1972). This may account for the low levels of drug-metabolising enzymes found in foetal liver microsomal preparations in vitro, but would not explain the decreased activities observed in vivo. The pattern of perinatal hepatocellular differentiation in humans also differs from that in rodents, and the human foetal hepatocyte has been shown to contain smooth endoplasmic reticulum, indicative of the presence of the cytochrome *P*-450-dependent monooxygenase system, as early as the 6th week of gestation (Short et al., 1976). This tends to confirm the foetal appearance of the cytochrome *P*-450 system in human, and possibly also in the higher primates. The metabolism of chlorpromazine, hexobarbital, meperidine, *N*-methylaniline and benzo(*a*)pyrene in the human foetus have all been observed, but at much slower rates than in the adult; these metabolic reactions all involve hydroxylations, catalysed by cytochrome *P*-450, the presence of which has been demonstrated in human foetal liver by several other workers (Yaffe et al., 1970; Pelkonen and Karki, 1971). Similar anomalies in the preparation of liver microsomes from foetal and neonatal rats have been observed, and much higher enzyme activities were obtained by refinement of the usual techniques for microsomal preparation; nevertheless, the cytochrome *P*-450 content was much lower in foetuses than in neonates, and very much less than in adult rats (see Table 3) (Cresteil et al., 1979).

Foetal tissues are able to catalyse the reduction of nitro groups in drugs, and this activity develops in human foetuses at around 12 weeks of gestation. Nitroreductase

TABLE 3

DEVELOPMENT OF CYTOCHROME *P*-450 IN RAT LIVER

Age	Untreated	Phenobarbital-treated	3-Methylcholanthrene-treated
Foetus			
20 days	1.0	1.2	1.8
22 days	2.3	2.3	3.2
Neonates			
12 hours	4.8	6.1	5.9
5 days	10.4	–	–
Adults (male)	32.6	109	62

Data are from Cresteil et al. (1979). Values are nmol cytochrome *P*-450/g liver (wet weight).

activity is present in human foetal liver, adrenal and lung, but the requirement of high coenzyme levels for maximal enzyme activity in vitro indicates that the activity in vivo may be slow (Juchau, 1971).

(b) Conjugations

Glucuronylation occurs to only a limited extent in the foetal livers of most animal species studied, but this varies with species and with substrate. For example, in rat, foetal liver glucuronyltransferase activity towards *p*-nitrophenol is above the adult value, but towards bilirubin it is less than 10% of the adult level, indicating the development of two distinct groups of enzymes, corresponding to the 'late-foetal' and neonatal clusters described by Greengard (1971). In man, foetal levels of glucuronyltransferase activities are low for all substrates.

In contrast, sulphate conjugation occurs much more readily. The human foetus has high levels of steroid sulphotransferase activities, with some approaching adult levels in the foetal liver just prior to birth. The phenol sulphotransferases develop less rapidly in the foetus, but for some substrates may approach adult levels at birth (Yaffe et al., 1968).

Glutathione-*S*-transferase activities are low in the foetal livers of most animal species except man; in human foetal liver this activity may reach adult levels (Chasseaud, 1973).

Epoxide hydrase activity (styrene oxide as substrate) was present in human foetal livers at about 40% of the activities found in adult liver (Pacifici and Rane, 1983b).

IV. NEONATAL METABOLISM OF XENOBIOTICS

Considerable evidence has accumulated that drugs are metabolised only slowly in newborn animals and that the activities of many of the drug-metabolising enzymes of the neonate are considerably less than in the adult. The liver microsomes of newborn rats, rabbits, mice and guinea pigs either are lacking in certain hepatic drug-metabolizing enzyme activities or exhibit low levels of these enzymes (Fouts and Adamson, 1959; Jondorf et al., 1959). However, these enzyme activities develop rapidly after birth and eventually achieve adult levels, at various times, depending on the particular enzyme concerned and the animal species studied. The initial low activities at birth have been attributed to the presence of inhibitory substances in the neonate (Fouts and Adamson, 1959), or to the lack of stimulation of enzyme biosynthesis (Fouts and Hart, 1965).

Studies of newborn human infants have shown a slow rate of excretion of metabolites of the drug phenylbutazone, a slower rate of appearance of acetanilide metabolites in the blood plasma, and prolonged plasma half-lives of sulphobromophthalein, *p*-aminobenzoic acid and bilirubin, which probably reflect deficiencies of the conjugating systems (Rane and Sjoqvist, 1972). Antibiotics, known not to be metabolised but excreted unchanged, have been shown to have longer plasma half-lives in neonates than in adults, which has been attributed to undeveloped renal glomerular filtration and tubular secretion, which do not reach maturity until 3 months of age.

1. Neonatal development of biotransformations

In most mammalian species studied, except human in which there is some foetal development of the monooxygenase system, the enzymes that catalyze the biotransformation of xenobiotic chemicals by oxidations or reductions have low activities at birth and increase progressively with age, to reach adult levels within a few weeks. The drugs hexobarbital, pentobarbital, meprobamate, carisoprodol and strychnine were all metabolised in the newborn rat at rates of less than 10% of adult values, but the rates of metabolism increased rapidly with development of the neonates, reaching normal adult levels at 30 days after birth (Kato et al., 1964). Basu et al. (1971) found that the liver mixed-function oxidase activity developed maximally in neonatal rats at 24 days for biphenyl 4-hydroxylase (cytochrome *P*-450) and at 21 days for biphenyl 2-hydroxylase (cytochrome *P*-448); however, whereas the 4-hydroxylase activity, like cytochrome *P*-450 (see Fig. 5), remained at moderately high levels throughout adult life, the 2-hydroxylase activity (*P*-448) continuously decreased and disappeared completely at 70 days after birth (Fig. 6). This varying ontogenesis of the different isoenzymes of cytochromes *P*-450 and *P*-448 has been noted by several other workers, and might have been expected from the different physiological functions of these various cytochromes.

In a study in rabbits of the development of the different oxidation enzymes involved in the in vitro metabolism of the tranquillizer, chlorpromazine, only sulphoxidation was found to occur in the foetus, whereas the 3-day-old neonate was able to effect sulphoxidation, *N*-demethylation and aromatic hydroxylation, and the adult animals were able to catalyze *N*-didemethylation also, indicating different rates of development of the various oxidation enzymes (see Fig. 4) (Bhatnagar, 1971).

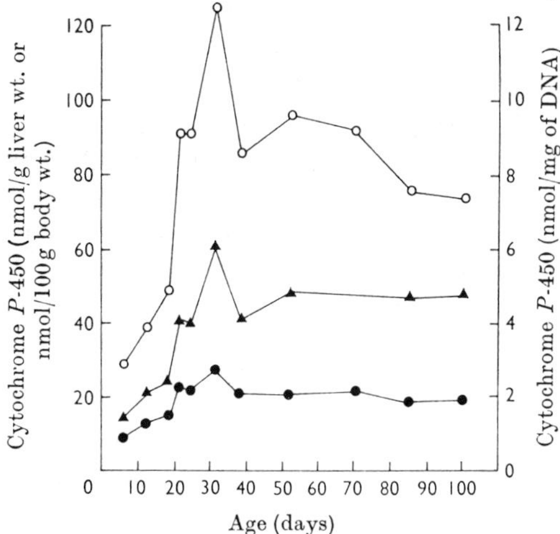

Figure 5. Development of cytochrome *P*-450 in neonatal rat liver. The concentration of cytochrome *P*-450 is expressed as nmol per 100 g bodyweight (o), per g liver weight (●), and per mg of DNA (▲). (From Basu et al., 1971.)

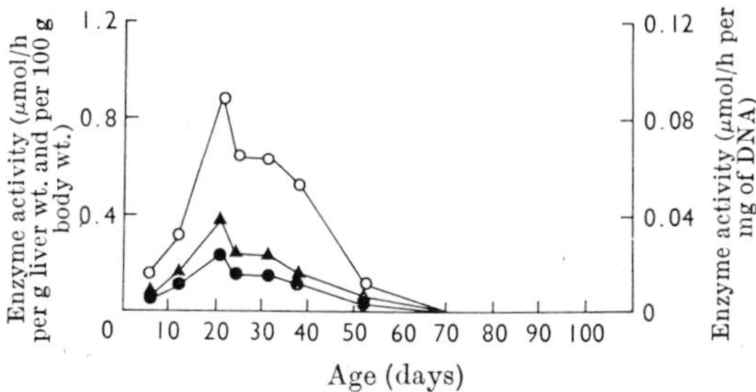

Figure 6. Development of biphenyl 2-hydroxylase activity in neonatal rat liver. The enzyme activity is expressed as nmol of product formed/hour per 100 g bodyweight (o), per g liver weight (●) and per mg of DNA (▲). (From Basu et al., 1971.)

The newborn ferret, like other neonatal animals, has very low levels of liver microsomal drug-metabolizing enzymes, which increase rapidly with time and are still increasing even at 8 weeks of age. NADPH-cytochrome *c* reductase and biphenyl 4-hydroxylase reach adult levels at about 2 weeks after birth, but cytochrome *P*-450, cytochrome *P*-450 reductase, ethylmorphine *N*-demethylase and nitrobenzoate reductase do not attain maximum development until 8 weeks of age, or later (Ioannides and Parke, 1975).

(a) The cytochrome P-450-dependent oxygenase system

The impaired neonatal hydroxylation of drugs and environmental chemicals has been correlated with low levels of the components of the liver mixed-function oxidase system. In the neonatal rat liver, cytochrome *P*-450 and cytochrome *P*-450 reductase are about 10%, and NADPH-cytochrome *c* reductase is 30–40%, of normal adult levels at birth, and reach adult levels at about 4–5 weeks of age (Basu et al., 1971; McLeod et al., 1972). The neonatal rabbit has similar low levels of these components, with liver concentrations of cytochrome *P*-450 at 20%, and NADPH-cytochrome *c* reductase 60% of normal adult levels, and lung concentrations of 30% for cytochrome *P*-450 and 50% for NADPH-cytochrome *c* reductase, with all components reaching adult levels at 30 days after birth (Fouts and Devereux, 1972). Therefore, neonatal impairment of mixed-function oxidation is not limited to the liver, and probably also involves extrahepatic tissues. The development of the cytochrome *P*-450 system is under glucocorticoid control, but requires an additional 'trigger' (possibly xenobiotic substrates) to initiate enzyme synthesis. Administration of dexamethasone to neonatal rats causes precocious development of liver cytochromes *P*-450; adult liver is less responsive, but foetal liver shows no response at all (Leakey and Fouts, 1979). Developmental aspects of the liver cytochrome *P*-450 system, with particular reference to drug metabolism in man (Neims et al., 1976), and hepatocellular morphology (Short et al., 1976) have been very fully reviewed.

The low levels of activity of the mixed-function oxidases in neonatal and foetal animals may also be due to the inhibitory activities of progesterone metabolites, namely, 5α- and 5β-pregnanediol, pregnanolone and 5α isomers of pregnanedione, which are very high in maternal tissues in pregnancy and are also present in foetal and neonatal tissues and in milk. When these reduced progesterone metabolites were administered to newborn rats the hydroxylation of drugs by liver preparations were inhibited by 20–60%, and the premature weaning of neonatal rats increased the liver drug-metabolising enzyme activities by as much as 120%, which was reversed by administration of the reduced progesterone derivatives (Kardish and Feuer, 1972). In the human, as in other animal species, the levels of these progesterone metabolites are high in maternal, foetal and neonatal tissues and in milk, and probably would similarly inhibit the mixed-function oxidase system, but they have not been shown, in either humans or laboratory animals, to impair the development of any of the components of the cytochrome *P*-450 system.

Treatment of pregnant rats or rabbits at full-term with phenobarbitone, polychlorinated biphenyls or other inducing agents of the mixed-function oxidase system results in increases of these enzyme activities in the foetus or neonate (Hart et al., 1962; Pantuck et al., 1968; Inoue et al., 1981), and treatment of neonatal animals with these enzyme-inducing agents similarly increases the development of the components of the cytochrome *P*-450 system and enhances the rates of mixed-function oxidations (Basu et al., 1971).

In the guinea pig, liver cytochrome *P*-450 levels and cytochrome *P*-450 reductase, benzo(*a*)pyrene hydroxylase, 4-chloro-*N*-methylaniline demethylase and chlorcyclizine demethylase activities developed slowly in the foetus, but very rapidly after birth, attaining adult levels, or even higher, at 24–72 hours post-partum (Kuenzig et al., 1975). Mitchell (1983) has recently reviewed the anomalous early development of the detoxication enzymes in the neonatal guinea pig (all these enzymes, with the exception of glucuronyltransferases, develop rapidly after birth), and has associated this with the relatively long gestation of the guinea pig (68 days, in contrast to the 20–30 days usual for rodents and lagomorphs) and its high degree of physiological development at birth (solid food is eaten on the first day after birth).

(b) Flavoprotein monooxygenases

In contrast to the somewhat slow development of the cytochrome *P*-450 mixed-function oxidase system in the rat and other rodents, the flavoprotein-mediated *N*-oxidation of *N,N*-dimethylaniline and *N*-methylaniline reaches maximal levels in the neonatal rat at 2–3 days after birth (Uehleke et al., 1971).

(c) Microsomal reductions

The reduction of *p*-nitrobenzoate by neonatal rat liver microsomal preparations is maximal at about 30–40 days after birth, and tends to follow the postnatal development of cytochrome *P*-450, which probably is the enzyme concerned (Basu et al., 1971).

The flavin-dependent NADPH-cytochrome *c* reductase develops earlier, and is maximal in the rat at 2–3 days after birth (30 days for *P*-450) (Uehleke et al., 1971), and is maximal in ferret at 2 weeks (8 weeks for *P*-450) (Ioannides and Parke, 1975).

2. Neonatal development of conjugations

The phase 2 metabolism of drugs, xenobiotics and their metabolites to form the more polar conjugates is effected by the mechanisms of glucuronylation, other glycosylations, sulphation, acetylation, conjugation with amino acids, conjugation with glutathione and methylation, most of which are deficient or absent in the foetus, and develop perinatally.

(a) Glucuronylation

Excretion of glucuronides by neonates is well documented (Yaffe and Juchau, 1974); urinary glucuronide excretion is generally low at birth but increases rapidly afterwards, dependent on substrate and species (Dutton, 1978). The deficiency is probably due to progressive development of the activities of the UDPglucuronyltransferases. Alternatively, there may be a defective uptake of drugs and xenobiotics by the liver, due to deficiencies of organic anion-binding proteins, which have been shown to be deficient in foetal and neonatal guinea pigs (Levi et al., 1969). A number of endogenous substances, such as the steroids, progesterone and pregnanediol, are known inhibitors of the UDPglucuronyltransferases, and the low levels of UDPglucuronyltransferase activities in neonates may also be attributed to high tissue levels of these steroids transferred from the placenta and maternal tissues before birth and in the milk during lactation (Hsia et al., 1964). Pregnanediol glucuronide is an even more effective inhibitor of glucuronide excretion and possibly exerts its inhibitory action by interfering with the glucuronide secretory mechanisms.

The perinatal development of the different UDPglucuronyltransferases show individual variations in any given animal species (Dutton, 1966); furthermore, any one of these enzymes may also show different patterns of development in different species, and in a few instances may exhibit the highest activity at birth. UDPglucuronyltransferases of rat liver have been classified into two groups, namely, the 'late-foetal-developing' group, with 2-aminophenol as typical substrate, and the 'neonatal-developing' group, with bilirubin as substrate. The UDPglucuronyltransferase activities towards both 2-aminophenol and bilirubin develop neonatally in humans; they are low in human neonatal liver and develop slowly, reaching adult values at 3 months after birth (Onishi et al., 1979). The mechanisms of the development of the UDPglucuronyltransferases have been reviewed very fully (Dutton, 1978).

This deficiency in glucuronide conjugation in the neonate may affect the glucuronide conjugation of bilirubin, giving rise to high serum bilirubin levels in newborn infants, leading to kernicterus. This impairment may be exacerbated by drugs such as chloramphenicol, which compete with bilirubin for glucuronide conjugation and biliary excretion, and with drugs such as the sulphonamides, which are highly bound to plasma proteins and competitively displace bilirubin from these binding sites.

(b) Other glycosylations

Perinatal glycosylation is low, similar to glucuronylation, and develops at a similar rate (Dutton and Burchell, 1976). The three UDPglycosyltransferases (glycosyl-, xylosyl- and glucuronyl-) responsible for bilirubin conjugation in rat develop at different rates (Vaisman et al., 1976).

(c) Sulphation

Excretion of sulphate conjugates are almost as high in the neonate as in the adult, and normal levels of the sulphotransferases are attained during foetal life, very early in the case of steroid conjugations (Roy, 1971). Drugs and xenobiotics tend to be excreted preferentially as sulphates by neonates, which confirms that the sulphotransferases develop earlier than the glucuronyltransferases. The phenol sulphotransferases develop later than the steroid sulphotransferases, although for some substrates these may attain adult levels at birth (Yaffe et al., 1968); some of the steroid sulphotransferases may have overlapping specificity towards xenobiotics. Phenolsulphotransferase has been shown to be inhibited by a non-dialysable inhibitor present in neonatal gut homogenate supernatants, which may account for a spurious decrease in the early-developing enzyme (Dodgson, 1977).

(d) Acetylation

Premature infants acetylated sulphonamides less readily than did normal newborn, and both effected the conjugations at lower rates than did adults (Fichter and Curtis, 1955). The *N*-acetyltransferase for isonicotinic hydrazide in rabbits increases from low levels at 6 days after birth to 15–20% of adult values at 2 weeks, and attains adult levels at 3–4 weeks of age; different forms of the enzyme may exist at different stages during development (Cohen et al., 1973).

(e) Conjugation with amino acids

Conjugation with glycine in rats and humans, at least for the substrate benzoic acid, appears to increase steadily during perinatal development (Vest and Rossier, 1963; Brandt, 1966) although more recently it has been claimed that human neonates conjugated salicylate with glycine more readily than do adults (Levy, 1975).

(f) Conjugations with glutathione

Bromsulphophthalein conjugation with glutathione (GSH) in neonatal animals slowly increases over several weeks after birth (Klaassen, 1975), and GSH conjugation of aryl epoxides reaches adult levels in rats, rabbits and guinea pigs at about 20 days after birth (Mukhtar and Bresnick, 1976; James et al., 1977). Maturation of GSH *S*-transferases probably occurs earlier in human, as this activity was present at adult levels in human foetal liver (Chasseaud, 1973), and with naphthalene-1,2-epoxide as substrate the enzymic activity in many human foetal and placental tissues was higher than in adult rat liver (Juchau and Namkung, 1974).

In several animals and man, GSH sulphotransferase B (ligandin) is absent in the foetuses, but reaches adult levels during the first week of life (Arias et al., 1976). Liver GSH levels in rats are about 30% of adult levels at birth and increase in the neonate to reach adult levels at about 10 days of age (Lambert and Thorgeirsson, 1976). Ligandin develops precociously in the livers of foetal Gunn rats (impaired glucuronide conjugation of bilirubin) (Foliot et al., 1973) and in a strain of mice that lack many microsomal enzymes (Gatmaitan et al., 1977), indicating that bilirubin and other substrates metabolised by the microsomal enzymes may act as inducers of this enzyme.

(g) Epoxide hydrase

The activity of epoxide hydrase with naphthalene 1,2-epoxide as substrate was low in monkey and human placentas, but in monkey and human foetal liver was highly developed and greater than the activities present in adult rat or rabbit livers (Juchau and Namkung, 1974; Pacifici and Rane, 1983b). Therefore, epoxide hydrase appears to develop in the foetus in man and primates, and in the neonate in rodents.

(h) Methylation

Catechol *O*-methyltransferase is low in foetal and neonatal liver of both rat and man and increases slowly in the neonate over a period of several weeks (Agathopoulos et al., 1971). Phenylethanolamine *N*-methyltransferase requires glucocorticoids for development (Margolis et al., 1966).

3. Effects of enzyme-inducing agents

Administration of drugs during late pregnancy may greatly enhance the low levels of the drug-metabolising enzymes found in the foetus and neonate and increase the rate of their development (Hart et al., 1962). Similarly, neonatal animals treated with phenobarbitone and other enzyme-inducing chemicals have enhanced rates of development of the cytochrome *P*-450 system, the glucuronyltransferases and certain other conjugating enzyme systems, and increased rates of detoxication of xenobiotics (Pantuck et al., 1968). The administration of phenobarbitone to pregnant women, or to young babies, to increase the neonatal glucuronyltransferase activities, and thereby to enhance the biliary excretion of bilirubin, has been used in the treatment of neonatal hyperbilirubinaemia (Yeung and Field, 1969).

It is possible that the enzyme-inducing action of the xenobiotics occurring naturally in the diet, and also at low concentration in the maternal milk, comprises the physiological mechanism by which cytochrome *P*-450 and the other detoxication enzyme systems undergo neonatal development.

V. IMPAIRED DETOXICATION AND PERINATAL TOXICOLOGY

1. *Chemical-induced teratogenesis*

Despite much public concern over the teratogenic potential of drugs, it is likely that medicines account for only a very small percentage of the total burden of human developmental defects and, apart from thalidomide, few drugs have been shown to have teratogenic potential in man. Most teratogens probably exert their toxic action because of the particular vulnerability of the developing foetus, rather than because of any impairment of detoxication, and modes of action of teratogens include: (i) direct toxicity to the foetus, (ii) indirect toxicity to the foetus, (iii) effects on the foeto-placental unit, (iv) effects on the mother, and (v) possibly effects on the sperm. Thalidomide, cytotoxic drugs and tetracyclines have a direct toxic effect on the foetus; folic acid antagonists such as methotrexate and diphenylhydantoin probably act indirectly by affecting foetal nutrition and metabolism; catecholamines probably cause the loss of foetal limbs through production of foetal vasospasm and the resulting gangrenous necrosis; and steroids and hypoglycaemic drugs probably result in congenital abnormalities because of interference with foetal hormonal balance. In the foeto-placental unit, serotonin may adversely affect placental blood flow, depriving the foetus of adequate nutrition and causing all types of congenital malformations; cortisone causes cleft palate in some species (mouse and rabbit), probably by reducing the volume of amniotic fluid, which causes flexion of the foetal head so that the tongue prevents closure of the palate. Drugs such as the monoamine oxidase inhibitors, which alter the hormonal status of the mother, or drugs which affect maternal nutrition may consequently lead to foetal malformations.

The most serious example of drug-induced teratogenicity is that of thalidomide; an estimated 10,000 babies born with rudimentary stumps instead of normal limbs are the sad testimony of the relationship between the maternal use of this drug and foetal malformations (Lenz and Knapp, 1962). The incidence of malformation was nearly 100% when the drug was taken between the 34th and 45th day after the last menstrual period, even if taken only in small doses or for short periods of time (Lenz and Knapp, 1962). The malformations were very varied in type, involving abnormalities of the limbs, the heart, the gastrointestinal and urinogenital systems, and sensory organs (Sutherland and Light, 1965). They have been produced in a variety of animal species, including rat, mouse, rabbit, monkey and chicken. Furthermore, [^{14}C]-thalidomide, together with a number of its spontaneous hydrolysis products, has been demonstrated to occur in the blastocyst of the rabbit after oral administration to the pregnant doe (Fabro et al., 1964).

The anticonvulsant phenytoin has been shown to be highly teratogenic to mice even in single doses, producing cleft palate, skeletal abnormalities and other deformities (Harbison and Becker, 1969); this toxicity is dose-dependent, is affected by the extent of maternal metabolism of the drug, and is also influenced by the timing of administration of the drug in relation to the pregnancy. Phenytoin has been shown to cross the placental barrier in rats and mice and foetal distribution studies in these animals have indicated that the teratology may be due to interference with folate utilization (Gabler and Falace, 1970) or with steroid hormone metabolism (Waddell and Mirkin, 1972). Placental transfer of the drug has also been demonstrated in human subjects (Mirkin, 1971), and several cases have been reported of babies with skeletal and other abnormalities born to mothers taking phenytoin and phenobarbitone throughout their pregnancy (Loughnan et al., 1973).

The chlorinated weed killers 2,4-dichlorophenoxyacetic acid (2,4-D) and 2,4,5-trichlorophenoxyacetic acid (2,4,5-T) have been associated with allegations of teratogenic effects in humans, and they have been shown to be teratogenic to hamsters when administered at high dosage. However, the incidence of developmental abnormalities, mostly associated with foetal head development, were markedly increased when the content of an impurity, 2,3,7,8-tetrachlorodibenzo-*p*-dioxin (TCDD), was increased and the teratogenicity is now attributed to this dioxin, which is a highly potent inducing agent of cytochrome *P*-448. Similarly, the insecticides DDT and carbaryl (Sevin) have been shown to be embryopathic and teratogenic at very high dosage to experimental animals; tissue accumulation of DDT is greater in intrauterine life than in the neonate, but it is concluded that normal human exposure constitutes only a very low level of risk of embryotoxicity (Khera and Clegg, 1969).

2. *Chemical-induced foetotoxicity*

Drugs given after the first trimester of pregnancy are unlikely to be teratogenic but, nevertheless, they may adversely affect the growth or function of the tissues or organs of the foetus. Tetracyclines form chelate complexes with calcium and, as a consequence, become concentrated in foetal bones and teeth, producing yellow discolouration and enamel hypoplasia of the teeth and reversible impairment of skeletal growth. Chloramphenicol can be toxic to the foetus in late pregnancy, as it is to the neonate, because of the inability of the foetus to conjugate the antibiotic. Sulphonamides administered to the mother in late pregnancy will be transferred to the foetus where, because of their displacement of plasma protein-bound bilirubin, they may give rise to jaundice and kernicterus in the neonate.

Women who smoke heavily during pregnancy experience a higher incidence than nonsmokers of abortion, premature births, delayed delivery, low infant birth weight, and loss of birth weight with decreased survival potential. These observations have been confirmed by studies of the effects of acute doses of nicotine to rats, when adverse effects similar to smoking were observed in pregnancy and in neonates (Becker and King, 1966). Cigarette smoking also markedly increases the cytochrome *P*-448 content of the placenta, but the significance of this is still unknown (Pelkonen et al., 1972).

A rare form of foetal drug toxicity is the transplacental carcinogenicity associated with the administration of diethylstilbestrol during pregnancy (Greenwald et al., 1971). Similar transplacental carcinogenesis has been demonstrated in experimental animals treated with urethane and other carcinogens (Druckrey, 1973; Nomura and Okamoto, 1973). A single injection of urethane to mice administered on the 9th day of gestation gave rise to lung and tail deformities and malignant teratomas, to hepatomas when administered after day 11, and to lung tumours after day 13, showing a correlation between organogenesis and development of xenobiotic-metabolizing enzymes with teratogenesis and carcinogenesis (Nomura and Okamoto, 1973). Druckrey (1973) has similarly shown a correlation between transplacental carcinogenesis and teratogenesis induced by nitrosamines and triazenes, with the development of foetal drug-metabolising enzymes.

3. *Chemical toxicity in neonates*

Newborn infants and other neonatal animals, especially if premature, are particularly sensitive to the toxic actions of drugs and other chemicals, primarily because the hepatic and intestinal enzymes that are concerned with the metabolic deactivation of these compounds are insufficiently developed. Impaired renal excretion, because of the incomplete development of glomerular filtration and tubular secretion mechanisms at birth, exacerbates the situation, with the consequence that drugs are slowly excreted, with resultant increases in toxicity.

Hyperbilirubinaemia and kernicterus may be produced by several drugs by: (1) competitive displacement of bilirubin from plasma protein-binding sites, (2) competition with the bilirubin for hepatic conjugation with glucuronic acid and with bilirubin glucuronide for biliary excretion, (3) non-competitive inhibition of the hepatic enzymes which form the bilirubin glucuronide, viz., the glucuronyltransferases, and (4) oxidation of haemoglobin to methaemoglobin, with the consequent haemolysis of the erythrocyte and excessive formation of bilirubin. Sulphonamides and many nonsteroidal anti-inflammatory drugs affect the protein-binding of bilirubin; paracetamol and salicylates are competitive inhibitors, and novobiocin and vitamin K non-competitive inhibitors, of bilirubin glucuronyltransferase; nitrofurantoin, phenacetin and nitrites may cause methaemoglobinaemia. Moreover, glucuronyltransferase activities in the neonate are suboptimal because of slow development, or through inhibition by progestational steroids, and the impaired ability to synthesize glucuronide conjugates undoubtedly results in the enhanced toxicity to the neonate of chloramphenicol, paracetamol, salicylates and many other drugs (Yeary et al., 1966).

Administration of chloramphenicol to newborn infants gives rise to the 'grey syndrome', consisting of cyanosis, vomiting and vascular collapse, and was one of the major contributory causes of thousands of infant deaths which occurred in the epidemics of infantile diarrhoea that spread across Europe immediately following World War II (Lischner et al., 1961). Impaired glucuronide conjugation and possible impairment of other metabolic pathways of this antibiotic no doubt contribute greatly to its high toxicity to the neonate.

Hexachlorophene (2,2′-methylene bis[3,4,6-trichlorophenol]), an antiseptic widely used in the bathing of babies to prevent nursery staphylococcus infections and also contained in soaps and baby toilet powders, has been reported to lead to convulsions in neonates. Hexachlorophene is absorbed through the normal skin of humans and rats, and at high concentrations may affect the central nervous systems of both species, giving rise to oedema of the white matter or 'status spongiosus' (Kimbrough, 1973). It may also produce paralysis in rats, rabbits, cats and pigs and blindness in sheep and, both in vivo and in vitro, stimulates mitochondrial respiration, followed by inhibition of respiration, indicative that uncoupling of oxidative phosphorylation may be the primary biochemical lesion (Caldwell et al., 1972). Hexachlorophene in rats is excreted almost entirely in the bile, as the monoglucuronide conjugate, but in the neonate because of impaired glucuronide conjugation elimination is greatly delayed and the plasma half-life is increased from 4.5 (adult) to 27 hours (neonate), with probable tissue accumulation; adult-type conjugation and elimination occur in rats at about 2 weeks after birth (Neims et al., 1975).

Most organophosphate insecticides are more toxic to weanling animals than to adults, because of the delayed development of the carboxylesterase enzyme system, which detoxicates phosphothionate and phosphate insecticides such as malathion and malaoxon (Brodeur and Dubois, 1967). Similarly, weanling rats are more susceptible than adults to the toxicity of parathion, and both parathion and its more toxic metabolite paraoxon are metabolised less effectively by weanling animals (Gagné and Brodeur, 1972).

4. *Drugs and lactation*

Drugs and chemicals that are present in the circulating blood of the mother will pass into the alveolar cells of the mammary gland and will be excreted into the milk. Drugs that are present in the maternal blood in high concentration for long periods of time will be secreted in the milk in the most significant amounts. Lipid-soluble drugs are secreted in association with the fatty components of the milk and aqueous-soluble drugs may be bound to lactalbumin, casein and other proteins of milk. Nevertheless, the mammary gland is, on the whole, a relatively unimportant route for the excretion of drugs.

Alcohol is secreted in breast milk in only very small amounts, but infant intoxication following the excessive consumption of alcohol by the mother has been recorded. Anticoagulants may be secreted in the milk, and a case has been reported of an infant developing a huge haematoma following the repair of an inguinal hernia when the mother was breast feeding while taking phenindione (Eckstein and Jack, 1970). The secretion into milk of drugs which are the inducers of the hepatic microsomal drug-metabolising enzymes, e.g. phenobarbitone, may result in substantial increases in these enzymes in the suckling offspring and enhances the rates of metabolism of drugs in the neonate (Darby, 1971). The occurrence of other drugs and environmental chemicals in milk, and the clinical and biological consequences of these, have been reviewed (Welch and Findlay, 1981).

VI. CONCLUSIONS

The absence, or very low levels, of detoxication enzymes in the foetus and placenta is biologically protective, since the metabolism of lipophilic chemicals to more polar metabolites and conjugates in the the placenta or foetal tissues would lead to their retention in the allantoic fluid instead of facilitating their reverse placental transfer to the mother, with subsequent maternal excretion. Indeed, the lack of metabolism in the foetus and placenta accelerates the elimination of the lipid-soluble chemical from the foeto-placental unit, by equilibration with the decreasing maternal plasma concentration. The presence of cytochrome *P*-448 in the placenta and the active sulphotransferases in the placenta and foetus are primarily concerned with the biogenesis, transport and metabolism of the steroid hormones, and any involvement with drugs and xenobiotics is fortuitous and is likely to lead to activation in preference to detoxication, as cytochrome *P*-448 has been shown to result in the activation of toxic chemicals and carcinogens.

The progressive development of the detoxication enzymes in the neonate tends to parallel the need for a chemical defence system in the young animal. For, while the neonate is being suckled, exposure to environmental chemicals is minimal, even though certain drugs and xenobiotics can be secreted in breast milk. Then, as the dietary intake of xenobiotic chemicals increases during weaning, the detoxicating cytochrome *P*-450-dependent mixed-function oxidase system, the glucuronyltransferases and the various other conjugases develop in their activities, possibly induced by the increasing dietary intake of xenobiotics, until they attain normal adult levels. However, because of the slow development of the cytochrome *P*-450 system, the glucuronyltransferases and other conjugases, and the earlier development of cytochrome(s) *P*-448 and the sulphotransferases, the foetus and neonate are particularly vulnerable to the toxic actions of drugs and xenobiotic chemicals, which will be detoxicated more slowly and possibly activated to greater extents than in the normal adult animal.

VII. REFERENCES

Ackerman, E., Rane, A. and Ericsson, J.L.E. (1972) Clin. Pharmacol. Ther. 13, 652–662.

Agathopoulos, A., Nicolopolous, D., Matsaniotis, N. and Papadatos, C. (1971) Pediatrics 47, 125–128.

Akhtar, M. and Skinner, S.J.M. (1968) Biochem. J. 109, 318–321.

Aranda, J.V. and Stern, L. (1983) Pharmacol. Ther. 20, 1–51.

Arias, I.M., Fleischner, G., Kirsch, R., Miskkin, S. and Gatmaitan, Z. (1976) in Glutathione — Metabolism and Function (Arias, I.M. and Jakoby, W.B., eds.), pp. 175–188, Raven Press, New York.
Bailey, J., Knauf, V., Mueller, W. and Hobson, W. (1980) Environ. Res. 21, 190–196.
Basu, T.K., Dickerson, J.W.T. and Parke, D.V. (1971) Biochem. J. 124, 19–24.
Becker, R.F. and King, J.E. (1966) Am. J. Obstet. Gynecol. 95, 515–522.
Berté, F., Manzo, L., De Bernardi, M. and Benzi, G. (1969) Arch. Int. Pharmacodyn. Ther. 182, 182–185.
Bhatnagar, S.P. (1971) Can. J. Physiol. Pharmacol. 49, 649–656.
Brandt, K. (1966) Biochem. Pharmacol. 15, 994–995.
Brodeur, J. and Dubois, K.P. (1967) Can. J. Physiol. Pharmacol. 45, 621–631.
Caldwell, R.S., Nakaue, H.S. and Buhler, D.R. (1972) Biochem. Pharmacol. 21, 2425–2441.
Chasseaud, L.F. (1973) Biochem. J. 131, 765–769.
Chhabra, R.S. (1979) Environ. Hlth. Persp. 33, 61–69.
Cohen, S.N., Baumgartner, R., Steinberg, M.S. and Weber, W.W. (1973) Biochim. Biophys. Acta 304, 473–481.
Creaven, P.J. and Parke, D.V. (1965) Fed. Eur. Biochem. Soc. Sec. Meet. Abstr. 128, 88.
Cresteil, T., Flinois, J.P., Pfister, A. and Leroux, J.P. (1979) Biochem. Pharmacol. 28, 2057–2063.
Curley, A., Copeland, F. and Kimbrough, R.D. (1969) Arch. Environ. Health 19, 628–632.
Darby, F.J. (1971) Biochem. J. 122, 41–47.
Dodgson, K.S. (1977) in Drug Metabolism from Microbe to Man (Parke, D. V. and Smith, R.L., eds.), pp. 91–104, Taylor and Francis, London.
Druckrey, H. (1973) Xenobiotica 3, 271–303.
Dus, K. (1982) Xenobiotica 12, 745–772.
Dutton, G.J. (1966) Biochem. Pharmacol. 15, 947–951.
Dutton, G.J. (1978) Annu. Rev. Pharmacol. Toxicol. 18, 17–35.
Dutton, G.J. and Burchell, B. (1976) in Progress in Drug Metabolism (Bridges, J.W. and Chasseaud, L.F., eds.), Vol.2, pp. 1–70, Wiley, London.
Dvorchik, B.H. and Hartman, R.D. (1982) Biochem. Pharmacol. 31, 1150–1153.
Eckstein, H.B. and Jack, B. (1970) Lancet 1, 672–673.
Fabro, S., Schumacher, H., Smith, R.L. and Williams, R.T. (1964) Nature 201, 1125–1126.
Fichter, E.G. and Curtis, J.A. (1955) Am. J. Dis. Child. 90, 596–597.
Foliot, A., Housset, E., Ploussard, J.P., Petite, J.P. and Infante, R. (1973) Biomedicine 19, 488–491.
Fouts, J.R. and Adamson, R.H. (1959) Science 129, 897–898.
Fouts, J.R. and Devereux, T.E. (1972) J. Pharmacol. Exp. Ther. 183, 458–468.
Fouts, J.R. and Hart, L.G. (1965) Ann. N.Y. Acad. Sci. 123, 245–251.
Gabler, W.L. and Falace, D. (1970) Arch. Int. Pharmacodyn. Ther. 184, 45–58.
Gagné, J. and Brodeur, J. (1972) Can. J. Physiol. Pharmacol. 50, 902–915.
Gatmaitan, Z., Lewis, S., Turchin, H. and Arias, I.M. (1977) Biochem. Biophys. Res. Commun. 75, 337–341.
Greengard, O. (1971) Essays Biochem. 7, 159–205.
Greenwald, P., Barlow, J.J., Nasca, P.C. and Burnett, W.S. (1971) N. Engl. J. Med. 285, 390–393.
Guengerich, F.P. (1979) Pharmacol. Ther. 6, 99–121.
Hajjar, N.P. and Hodgson, E. (1980) Science 209, 1134–1136.
Harada, N. and Omura, T. (1980) J. Biochem. 87, 1539–1554.
Harbison, R.D. and Becker, B.A. (1969) Teratology 2, 305–311.
Hart, L.G., Adamson, R.H., Dixon, R.L. and Fouts, J.R. (1962) J. Pharmacol. Exp. Ther. 137, 103–106.
Herbst, A.L., Poskanzer, D.C., Robboy, S.J., Friedlander, L. and Soulby, R.E. (1975) N. Engl. J. Med. 292, 334–339.
Hirom, P.C. and Millburn, P. (1979) in Foreign Compounds Metabolism in Mammals (Hathaway, D.E., ed.), Vol.5, pp. 132–158, Chemical Society, London.
Hlavica, P. and Hülsmann, S. (1979) Biochem. J. 182, 109–116.
Hodgson, E. (1979) Drug Metab. Rev. 10, 15–33.
Hsia, D.Y.Y., Dowben, R.M. and Riabov, S. (1964) Ann. N.Y. Acad. Sci. 111, 326–336.

Idänpään-Heikkilä, J.E., Jouppila, P.U., Puolakka, J.O. and Vorne, M.S. (1971) Am. J. Obstet. Gynecol. 109, 1011–1016.

Inoue, K., Takanaka, A., Mizokami, K., Fujimori, K., Sunouchi, M., Kasuya, Y. and Omori, Y. (1981) Toxicol. Appl. Pharmacol. 59, 540–547.

Ioannides, C. and Parke, D.V. (1975) in Basic and Therapeutic Aspects of Perinatal Pharmacology, (Morselli, P.L., Garattini, S. and Sereni, F., eds.), pp. 245–264, Raven Press, New York.

Ioannides, C., Lum, P. and Parke, D.V. (1984) Xenobiotica 14, 235–247.

James, M.O., Bend, J.R., Foureman, F.C., Law, F.C. and Bend, J. (1977) Drug Metab. Dispos. 5, 19–28.

Jondorf, W.R., Maickel, R.R. and Brodie, B.B. (1959) Biochem. Pharmacol. 1, 352–354.

Juchau, M.R. (1969) J. Pharmacol. Exp. Ther. 165, 1–8.

Juchau, M.R. (1971) Arch. Int. Pharmacodyn. Ther. 194, 346–358.

Juchau, M.R. (1972) Fed. Proc. 31, 48–52.

Juchau, M.R. and Namkung, M.J. (1974) Drug Metab. Dispos. 2, 380–385.

Juchau, M.R. and Symms, K.G. (1972) Biochem. Pharmacol. 21, 2053–2064.

Juchau, M.R. and Yaffe, S.J. (1969) in Foeto-Placental Unit (Pecile, A. and Finzi, C., eds.), p. 260, Excerpta Medica Foundation, Amsterdam.

Juchau, M.R., Krasner, J. and Yaffe, S.J. (1968a) Biochem. Pharmacol. 17, 1969–1979.

Juchau, M.R., Niswander, K.R. and Yaffe, S.J. (1968b) Am. J. Obstet. Gynecol. 100, 348–356.

Juchau, M.R., Pederson, M.G., Fantel, A.G. and Shepard, T.H. (1973) Clin. Pharmacol. Ther. 14, 673–679.

Kardish, R. and Feuer, G. (1972) Biol. Neonate 20, 58–67.

Kato, R., Vassanelli, P., Frontino, G. and Chiesara, E. (1964) Biochem. Pharmacol. 13, 1037–1051.

Khera, K.S. and Clegg, D.J. (1969) Can. Med. Assoc. J. 100, 167–172.

Kimbrough, R.D. (1973) Pediatrics 51, 391–394.

Klaassen, C.D. (1975) J. Pharmacol. Exp. Ther. 195, 366–375.

Kuenzig, W., Kamm, J.J., Boublik, M. and Burns, J.J. (1975) in Basic and Therapeutic Aspects of Perinatal Pharmacology (Morselli, P.L., Garattini, S. and Sereni, F., eds.), pp. 289–300, Raven Press, New York.

Kuwabara, K., Yakushiji, T., Watanabe, I., Yoshida, A., Koyama, K. and Kunita, N. (1979) Bull. Envir. Contam. Toxicol. 21, 458–462.

Lambert, G.H. and Thorgeirsson, S.S. (1976) Biochem. Pharmacol. 25, 1777–1781.

Leakey, J.E.A. and Fouts, J.R. (1979) Biochem. J. 182, 233–235.

Lenz, W. (1965) Ann. N.Y. Acad. Sci. 123, 228–236.

Lenz, W. and Knapp, K. (1962) Arch. Environ. Hlth. 5, 100–105.

Levi, A.J., Gatmaitan, Z. and Arias, I.M. (1969) Lancet 2, 139–140.

Levy, G. (1975) in Basic and Therapeutic Aspects of Perinatal Pharmacology (Morselli, P.L., Garattini, S. and Sereni, F., eds.), pp. 319–330, Raven Press, New York.

Lischner, H., Seligman, S.J., Krammer, A. and Parmelee, A.H. Jr. (1961) J. Pediatr. 59, 21–34.

Loughnan, P.M., Gold, H. and Vance, J.C. (1973) Lancet 1, 70–72.

Margolis, R.F., Roffi, J. and Jost, A. (1966) Science 154, 275–276.

McLeod, S.M., Renton, K.W. and Eade, N.R. (1972) J. Pharmacol. Exp. Ther. 183, 489–498.

Meigs, R.A. and Ryan, K.J. (1968) Biochim. Biophys. Acta 165, 476–482.

Mirkin, B.L. (1971) J. Pediatr. 78, 329–337.

Mitchell, S.C. (1983) Xenobiotica 13, 453–460.

Mosier, H.D., Jr. and Jansons, R.A. (1972) Teratology 6, 303–311.

Moya, F. and Smith, B.E. (1965) Anesthesiology 26, 465–476.

Moya, F. and Thorndike, V. (1962) Am. J. Obstet. Gynecol. 84, 1778–1798.

Mukhtar, H. and Bresnick, E. (1976) Cancer Res. 36, 937–940.

Nebert, D.W., Winker, J. and Gelboin, H.V. (1969) Cancer Res. 29, 1762–1769.

Neims, A.H., Warner, M., Yang, G., Hales, B., Chung, L.W.K. and East, D.S.R. (1975) in Basic and Therapeutic Aspects of Perinatal Pharmacology (Morselli, P.L., Garattini, S. and Sereni, F.,eds.), pp. 177–190, Raven Press, New York.

Neims, A.H., Warner, M., Loughman, P.M. and Aranda, J.V. (1976) Annu. Rev. Pharmacol. Toxicol. 16, 427–445.
Nomura, T. and Okamoto, E. (1973) Gann. 63, 731–742.
Onishi, S., Kawade, N., Itoh, S., Isobe, K. and Sugiyama, S. (1979) Biochem. J. 184, 705–707.
Osimitz, T.G. and Kulkarni, A.P. (1982) Biochem. Biophys. Res. Commun. 109, 1164–1171.
Pacifici, G.M. and Rane, A. (1981) Drug Metab. Dispos. 9, 472–475
Pacifici, G.M. and Rane, A. (1983a) Devel. Pharmacol. Therap. 6, 83–93.
Pacifici, G.M. and Rane, A. (1983b) Pharmacology 26, 241–248.
Pantuck, E., Conney, A.H. and Kuntzman, R. (1968) Biochem. Pharmacol. 17, 1441–1447.
Parke, D.V. (1982) in The Handbook of Environmental Chemistry, Vol. 2, Part B, Reactions and Processes (Hutzinger, O., ed.), pp.141–178, Springer-Verlag, Berlin.
Parke, D.V. and Ioannides, C. (1982) in Biological Reactive Intermmediates II, Part A (Snyder, R., Parke, D.V., Kocsis, J.J., Jollow, D.J., Gibson, G.G. and Witmer, C.M., eds.), pp. 23–38, Plenum Press, New York.
Pelkonen, O. and Karki, N.T. (1971) Acta Pharmacol. Toxicol. 30, 158–160.
Pelkonen, O., Jouppila, P. and Karki, N.T. (1972) Toxicol. Appl. Pharmacol. 23, 399–407.
Perlmutter, J.F. (1967) Am. J. Obstet. Gynecol. 99, 569–572.
Phillipson, C., Ioannides, C. and Parke, D.V. (1982) Biochem. J. 207, 51–56.
Rane, A. and Sjoqvist, F. (1972) Pediatr. Clin. North Am. 19, 37–48.
Rogers, M.C., Willerson, J.T., Goldblatt, A. and Smith T.W. (1972) N. Engl. J. Med. 287, 1010–1013.
Roy, A.B. (1971) Handb. Exp. Pharmacol. 28, 536–563.
Short, C.R., Kinden, D.A. and Stith, R. (1976) Drug Metab. Rev. 5, 1–42.
Sjoqvist, F., Bergfors, P.G., Borga, O., Lind, M. and Ygge, H. (1972) J. Pediatr. 80, 496–500.
Sutherland, J.M. and Light, I.J. (1965) Pediatr. Clin. North Am. 12, 781–806.
Troen, P., De Miguel, M. and Alonso, C. (1966) Biochemistry 5, 332–337.
Uehleke, H., Reiner, O. and Hellmer, K.H. (1971)) Res. Commun. Chem. Pathol. Pharmacol. 2, 793–805.
Vainio, H. and Hietanen, E. (1980) in Concepts in Drug Metabolism (Jenner, P. and Testa, B., eds.), pp. 251–284, Dekker, New York.
Vaisman, S.L., Lee, K.S. and Gartner, L.M. (1976) Pediatr. Res. 10, 967–971.
Van Bladeren, P.J., Van der Gen, A., Breimer, D.D. and Mohn, G.R. (1979) Biochem. Pharmacol. 28, 2521–2524.
Vest, M.F. and Rossier, R. (1963) Ann. N.Y. Acad. Sci. 111, 183–198.
Waddell, W.J. and Mirkin, B.C. (1972) Biochem. Pharmacol. 21, 547–552.
Welch, R.H., Harrison, Y.E., Gommi, B.W., Poppers, P.J., Finster, M. and Conney, A.H. (1969) Clin. Pharmacol. Therap. 10, 100–109.
Welch, R.M. and Findlay, J.W.A. (1981) Drug Metab. Rev. 12, 261–277.
Yaffe, S.J. and Juchau, M.R. (1974) Annu. Rev. Pharmacol. 14, 219–238.
Yaffe, S.J., Krasner, J. and Catz, C.S. (1968) Ann. N.Y. Acad. Sci. 151, 887–899.
Yaffe, S.J., Rane, A., Sjoqvist, F., Boreus, L.D. and Orrenius, S. (1970) Life Sci. 9, 1189–1200.
Yeary, R.A., Benish, R.A. and Finkelstein, M. (1966) J. Pediatr. 69, 663–667.
Yeung, C.Y. and Field, C.E. (1969) Lancet 2, 135–139.

S. Kacew and M.J. Reasor (eds), *Toxicology and the Newborn*
© 1984 Elsevier Science Publishers B.V.

Chapter 2

The Perinatal Guinea Pig as a Model for Toxicological Studies

D.J. ECOBICHON

McGill University, Department of Pharmacology and Therapeutics, McIntyre Medical Sciences Building, Montreal, Quebec, H3G 1Y6, Canada

CONTENTS

I. INTRODUCTION

The cavy, guinea pig, meerschweinchen (little sea pig), cochon de mer, lapin de Barbarie, is one of the most interesting species of research animals available and is a welcome alternate species to the laboratory rat. It has been used extensively in research projects in bacteriology, pathology and parasitology, the bioassay of drugs, vaccination procedures, anaphylaxis and toxicity testing. It is my hope that, in this chapter, I can extol its virtues and usefulness as a fetal-maternal-neonatal model for toxicological studies and, drawing on my own research, that of my former graduate students and the studies of other colleagues, demonstrate the versatility of the animal.

II. ORIGIN OF THE SPECIES

Taxonomically, the guinea pig belongs to the chordata (phylum), craniata (subphylum), mammalian (class), theira (subclass), eutheria (infraclass — placental mammals), rodentia (order), hystricomorpha (suborder), cavioidae (superfamily), caviidae (family) and caviinae (subfamily) (Wagner, 1976). The name of the genus underwent a number of changes over a period of time, being described as the *Aperea braziliensibus* or *Cavia cobaya* in 1648 by Marcgrave; the *Mus cobaya* in 1747 and *Mus braziliensis* in 1754 by Linneaus; with the term *Cavia* as a generic name in 1766 with the trivial name *porcellus* (little pig) appearing in the 10th edition of Linneaus' Systema Naturae in 1758. The binomial form *Cavia porcellus* was first used by Erxleben in 1777 (Weir, 1974).

While the origins of the guinea pig are obscured in history, it is apparent that several related types of cavy were indigenous to Peru, Argentina, Paraguay and parts of Brazil (Weir, 1974). Following an extensive study of mummified remains, Hückinghaus (1961) suggested that domestication first occurred in the region of Lake Titicaca (Peru and Bolivia), though Muñoz (1970) presented evidence of simultaneous domestication in Peru, Columbia and Ecuador about 1000 B.C. At the time of the Spanish invasion of Peru in 1532, guinea pigs had been domesticated by the Incas as a source of food and for religious sacrifices, but it appears that domestication preceded this era by some 500–1000 years since ceramic figures of guinea pigs are known from the pre-Inca period (Schmidt, 1929). Invariably, early descriptions of the species noted the multi-coloured appearance of the coat, and such animals are still raised in some parts of Andean South America as a food delicacy.

Synonyms for the cavy all have some connotation of the ocean. Within reason, a date of 1580, some 50 years after the 'discovery' of Peru by the conquistadors, has been established as the time of importation into Europe by Spanish or Dutch sailors. It spread rapidly throughout Europe, acquiring a variety of common names, including Indian little pig coney, cobaye, cochon d'Inde d'Angora, conejillo de Indias, porcello de India and Indianach varken in addition to those mentioned earlier (Wagner, 1976). The animal was not adopted as a food source except, perhaps, by seamen but individuals began to raise them as a fancy or as pets. While the name cavy has been used exclusively by breeders, scientists have consistently utilized the rather absurd name of guinea pig, the origin of which is quite obscure. The name guinea may have derived from the fact that the animals arrived on ships that had stopped at Guiana, geographically in the same general region as Brazil. The term may have arisen in the English-speaking world when the animal arrived by slave ships via the coast of Guinea, West Africa. It may also have been derived from the fact that in England in the 17th century one could be purchased for a coin, the guinea. The name pig may have been derived from the manner in which it was prepared for cooking, by scalding and scraping off the fur before roasting whole as one does a suckling pig.

A number of fancy strains of cavy have been cultivated since its importation into Europe, including the Abyssinian wire-haired strain, the long silky-haired Peruvian and a variety of single colour coated strains including the albino. The white hair of the guinea pig is a trait of domestication in that it, along with pink eyes, breeds true. Any cavy with white in its pelage may have domestic blood (Castle and Wright, 1916). Many laboratory strains of guinea pigs derive from a strain established in 1926 by Dunkin et al. (1930). A number of inbred strains of guinea pigs were developed by Wright (1960) during a lifetime study of their genetics

III. REPRODUCTIVE PHYSIOLOGY

When choosing an animal model for toxicity studies, one generally attempts to select a species which will mimic man closely in the manner of the absorption, distribution, biotransformation (both rate and route of detoxification) and elimination of the agent and its degradation products. Frequently, these are almost impossible constraints on an investigation. In the area of perinatal toxicology, an additional constraint centers around the similarity in the development of the fetal animal and the human fetus. In this, the characteristics of the guinea pig pregnancy, including a trimester-type gestational period, hormonal changes, the type of placentation and the relatively precocious development of fetal tissues during the latter part of gestation, all contribute to make this species significantly different from most of the laboratory mammals used in perinatal toxicological studies.

1. Reproduction

Domesticated guinea pigs are polyestrous, non-seasonal breeders with a prolonged estrous cycle, spontaneous ovulation and an actively secreting corpus luteum (Reed and Hounslow, 1971). The female guinea pig pup matures early, at approximately 33 days of age. Young et al. (1939), in an extensive study of 617 females, reported a mean age at first heat of 67.8 ± 21.5 (S.D.) days, with a range of 33–134 days. Male animals reached sexual maturity at a much slower rate and, though they demonstrated sexual activity early, fertile matings did not usually occur until they were 60–80 days old (Lane-Petter and Porter, 1963).

The estrous cycle of the guinea pig has been estimated in several studies to range from 13 to 20 days for different strains. Stockard and Papanicolaou (1917) recorded a mean estrous cycle length of 15.7 days (range of 15–17 days) while Young et al. (1935) reported a mean length of 16.25 days, with a range of 13–21.5 days. Some variability in the length of the cycle may arise from the fact that the average lengths of the first two cycles of a given animal are shorter than subsequent cycles (Young et al., 1939). With an estrous cycle this long, the duration of various stages within the cycle have been estimated at 1.0–1.5 days for proestrus, 9–11 hours for estrus and 2.5–3.0 days for metestrus (Ishii, 1920). Variability has been observed in the length of estrus, with a time of 24 hours being estimated on the basis of distinct characteristics of vaginal fluids (Stockard and Papanicolaou, 1917), 8.2 ± 0.07 hours (range of 1–18 hours) on the basis of sexual receptivity (Young et al., 1935) or 6–11 hours on the basis of sexual receptivity (Ishii, 1920). Ovulation occurs within 10 hours of the onset of estrus and occurs usually within 1.5–2.0 hours of the end of estrus (Blandau and Young, 1939; Young et al., 1935). Characteristic behavioral patterns accompany the proestrous and estrous intervals, and these will be discussed below.

2. *Breeding*

An almost foolproof method of obtaining successful matings in guinea pigs is associated with the postpartum estrus and ovulation observed within 12–15 hours of the delivery of a litter. The length of the postpartum estrus is short, approximately 3.5 hours, occurring within 2–10 hours of parturition (Boling et al., 1939). Placing a proven fertile male with a sow about to deliver will ensure approximately a 74–80% success rate in pregnancy in postpartum matings (Bruce and Parkes, 1948; Rowlands, 1949). While the postpartum ovulation-mating technique is best in studies where timed embryological age is desired, the usual practice is to allow the sexes of appropriate age (3.5–4.5 months for females and 6 months for males) to mix freely and mate at will. The optimum proportions of numbers appear to be 12 females with each male, this type of breeding program resulting in an efficient breeding group with a high proportion of successful postpartum matings (Lane-Petter and Porter, 1963). With this size of operation, it is possible to breed the same female approximately five times in a year and to obtain some 15–20 young per female. If smaller groups are dictated by the nature of the research, then a group of four or five females may be placed with one male, removing those ascertained to be pregnant and replacing them with new females.

If one wishes to treat the timed-pregnant females during selected stages of gestation or during the postpartum development of the young, thereby eliminating the possibility of the postpartum ovulatory cycle, one will have to rely on other signs of estrus to co-ordinate the breeding schedule for timed-pregnant animals. This requires close daily observation and time-consuming handling of each female. The onset of estrus and its duration can be detected by the behavior of the female guinea pig. In the proestrous phase, increased activity, pursuit of cage mates, a swaying motion of the hindquarters and a gutteral cooing sound will be observed in the female (Sisk, 1976). Mounting behavior may occur before estrus but will be vigorous only during the 10 hours before estrus (Young et al., 1935). The most dependable sign of estrus is the copulatory reflex (opisthotonus), an arching and straightening of the back and a raising of the posterior with dilatation of the pudendum (Young et al., 1935). This behaviour is more marked at the beginning of estrus and decreases with time.

Normally, the vaginal opening is sealed with an epithelial membrane but, preceding estrus, the membrane opens for approximately 2–5 days in the mature female (Sisk, 1976). This physiological event may be used to indicate the onset of estrus in mature animals, but, in younger animals, the length of opening is frequently prolonged: 11.2 days in the first and 5 days in the second cycle (Harned and Casida, 1972). Closure of the vaginal membrane does not occur until after ovulation (Ford and Young, 1953).

The vaginal smear may be used as a more definitive indicator of the onset of estrus. Stockard and Papanicolaou (1917) used the guinea pig to establish that the composition of vaginal fluids changed with different stages of the estrous cycle. A description of the appearance of the smears is presented in Table 1. The histology of the vaginal smear has been studied by Donovan and Lockhart (1972) who showed that, in proestrus, the smears contained epithelial cells, cornified cells and leukocytes. As estrus approached, the number of leukocytes diminished and large numbers of brightly stained, rounded, cornified cells were found. With the end of estrus and at the time of ovulation, increased numbers of leukocytes were found in the vaginal smear again.

With these short and highly critical time intervals, it is essential to place the nearly receptive female with a male of proven breeding ability at the appropriate time. In addition to the fact that the time period of estrus is only 50 hours, the ovulated ovum can be fertilized in the fallopian tube and undergo normal development for only a very short time span of some 20 hours (Hunter et al., 1969). While the exact time of fertilization has not been determined for the guinea pig, estimates as low as 1–2 hours or as high as 6–15 hours postcoitus have been reported (Blandau, 1949; Sisk, 1976). If fertilized, the ova enter the uterine horns some 72 hours after ovulation in the 8–12-

TABLE 1

DESCRIPTION OF THE VAGINAL SMEARS OF GUINEA PIGS IN ESTRUS

Stage	Time interval (hours)	Description
I	6–12	Mucous fluid plus masses of pyknotic squamous cells, few elongated cornified cells.
II	2–4	Cheese-like consistency, large numbers of cells of healthy squamous architecture.
III	4–6	Liquefaction of the cheesy mass, less numerous epithelial cells but polymorphonuclear leukocytes in a thin fluid discharge.
IV	1–2	Characterized by varying numbers of erythrocytes, large numbers of leukocytes and desquamated epithelial cells. Not consistently seen in all individuals.

Data are from Stockard and Papanicolaou (1917).

cell state of development, with implantation occurring some 6.0–7.5 days postcoitus (Blandau, 1949; Deanesly, 1960; Hunter et al., 1969).

How does one know when an animal has been receptive and has bred? Daily examination of the vaginal opening of each female should reveal the presence or remnants of a rigid white plug, the bouchon vaginal, filling the lumen of the vagina and cervix when mating has occurred. The plug is formed from a portion of the male ejaculate secreted by the seminal vesicles and the coagulation is catalyzed by an enzyme secreted by the anterior lobe of the prostate gland (Stockard and Papanicolaou, 1919). This plug persists for only a few hours after its formation, necessitating examination of the animals at least twice a day.

How does one know when an animal is pregnant? It is exceedingly difficult to palpate the developing fetus until approximately 45 days of gestation. However, by 35–40 days of gestation, the symphysis pubis begins to separate so that the birth canal through the pelvic girdle is larger. This separation, of approximately 6–8 mm, can be felt by placing a finger on the pelvis (Hisaw et al., 1944; Sisk, 1976). Shortly thereafter, one should see a sharp increase in body weight as fetuses become significantly larger. The total conceptus weight (fetus, membranes, placenta) may represent as much as 30% of the total maternal body weight (Fuchs, 1952).

3. *Placentation*

Placental development requires an increase in uterine blood flow. Studies have shown that there are regional variations and fluctuations in uterine blood flow during early pregnancy in the guinea pig, most likely governed by ovarian steroids recognized to be both vasoactive and uterotrophic (Marcus, 1974; Einer-Jensen et al., 1975; Garris, 1980; Garris and Whitehead, 1981). Estradiol-induced uterine hyperemia in the guinea pig has been measured concomitantly with a postovulatory increase in circulating levels of this steroid between days 5 and 7 (Einer-Jensen et al., 1975; Garris, 1980; Garris and Whitehead, 1981). In a recent paper, Garris et al. (1983), using guinea pigs with three pregnancy sites per horn, demonstrated a significant change in uterine blood flow through the uterine artery between days 4 and 8 of pregnancy, the flow changing from basal levels of 1.3 ± 0.3 ml/minute on day 4 to a peak level of 3.0 ± 0.3 ml/minute on day 6, corresponding to the time of implantation, and followed by a return to basal levels at day 8. In conjunction with the flow changes, these same authors reported regional differences in uterine blood flow which they postulated might be associated with pregnancy site selection in the guinea pig. Regional differences in uterine blood flow were noted between days 10 and 20 of gestation, the tubal and cervical thirds of the uterus consistently exhibiting a greater flow rate than did the middle uterine zone. These results confirmed earlier suggestions that localized hyperemic areas of the uterus are best suited to support nidation and fetal-placental viability (Emrys-Roberts, 1909; Garris and Whitehead, 1981). Fetal-placental growth may be impaired in ischemic uterine zones, thereby providing adequate space for the development of the relatively large guinea pig fetus.

The placenta of the guinea pig is unique among the rodents in that it bears a striking similarity to the human placenta. While the mouse, rat and hamster have a hemotrichorial type of placenta with three distinct layers of trophoblasts separating the maternal blood spaces from the fetal blood vessels and the rabbit has a hemodichorial (two trophoblast layers) placenta, the guinea pig and man show only a single trophoblast layer, hence the term hemomonochorial given to the placental type (Amoroso, 1961; Enders, 1965; Hendrickx and Houston, 1970). In the hemochorial placentae, the fetal trophoblasts are in direct contact with the maternal bloodstream, the maternal blood circulating in a meshwork of trophoblastic septae carrying fetal capillaries (Amoroso, 1961; Enders, 1965; Hendrickx and Houston, 1970).

The guinea pig placenta appears to be quite efficient at gas exchange, the oxygen tension being 10 mmHg higher in fetal guinea pig arteries than in the uterine vein (Bartels et al., 1967). The trophoblast layer in the chorioallantoic placenta is an important barrier to the maternal-fetal passage of proteins whereas the visceral yolk sac of the guinea pig is a major route of acquisition of antibodies and serum proteins (King and Enders, 1971). Extensive studies of the transplacental transfer of iron (Wong and Morgan, 1973), amino acids (Dancis et al., 1968), fatty acids (Hershfeld and Nemeth, 1968), thyroid hormones (London et al., 1963) and various chemicals, to be discussed below, have demonstrated that the guinea pig placenta is efficient. Transplacental transport of agents is accomplished by simple diffusion, the movement of molecules from a region of high concentration to a lower concentration, possibly the most important mechanism (Miller and Berndt, 1975). Active transport systems, in which considerable energy is expended, are essential for the acquisition of needed nutrients, etc., by the developing fetus (Dancis, 1964). Minor processes, phagocytosis (engulfing of food) and pinocytosis (engulfing of water), are also contributory to the transplacental transfer of agents from the maternal circulation to the fetus. Water is transferred from the mother to the fetal guinea pig, the rate increasing steadily throughout pregnancy. This does not appear to be a process of simple osmosis since the water moves against a higher maternal osmotic pressure and protein concentration, resulting in a fetal hemodilution, a physiologic anemia of pregnancy (Hendrickx and Houston, 1970).

Much has been made of the importance of the anatomical differences in the number of membrane layers in the placentae of experimental animal species in governing the rate of transplacental passage of foreign chemicals. In my opinion, this concern is not justified since most investigators have found that the placenta is not an effective barrier to any chemical toxicant. While it is possible that the rate of passage might be affected slightly, ultimately most agents will be acquired by the fetus in a qualitative and quantitative manner without excessive delay. Only in short-term, acute, prepartum exposures can I see that placental complexity might exert an influence on the rate of fetal acquisition of a chemical.

4. *Gestation*

The gestation period of the guinea pig is approximately 68 days, depending upon the strain being used and the litter size, in the latter case the length being inversely related to the number of fetuses (Goy et al., 1957; Sisk, 1976). Values ranging from 63 to 71 days have been reported by various investigators (Lane-Petter and Porter, 1963). In a recent study of 34 timed-pregnant albino Hartley strain sows, the gestational period was found to be 67 ± 3 days (mean $\pm$ S.D.) (Ecobichon et al., 1978). The shorter the gestational period, the higher the incidence of fetal mortality (Goy et. al., 1957). This long gestational period is particularly useful in teratogenic studies as one can separate the toxic or teratogenic effects on the embryo from those upon the fetus, where differential effects may be observed depending upon the stage(s) of development (Hoar, 1976; Sisk, 1976).

The gestational period of the guinea pig can be subdivided into three distinct periods, the trimester characteristics being linked to the changing steroidal pattern, which is similar to that observed in the human. The plasma levels of progesterone begin to increase rapidly after day 15 postcoitus, reaching peak levels during days 30–45, with a decrease between days 45–60, followed by a modest increase just before parturition (Heap and Deanesly, 1966; Bedford et al., 1972; Sisk, 1976). Challis et al. (1971) suggested that the midgestational lowering of plasma progesterone may reflect the fact that the placenta now becomes the primary producer of this hormone rather than the ovary. Detectable levels of unconjugated estrogen (17α- and 17β-estradiol, 16α-epiestriol and an estrone-like hormone) appear in the plasma at day 20 of gestation and begin to increase dramatically, reaching peak levels at day 60, just prior to parturition. Estrone was found to constitute 35–45% of the total plasma estrogens, while 17β-estradiol accounted for approximately 10% (Challis et al., 1971).

The factor that initiates parturition in the guinea pig is not known. It does not appear that progesterone is the regulator of myometrial activity in the guinea pig, unlike the situation found in other species. Progesterone did not block uterine contractions and did not prolong gestation (Porter, 1971b). There was no precipitous decrease in progesterone levels immediately before birth. The hormone relaxin, present in ovarian extracts (Releasin powder — Warner Chilcott Laboratories), was first detected in guinea pig blood plasma on day 21 of gestation, reaching peak levels by day 28 and remaining relatively constant until day 63, when concentrations began to decline, followed by a sharp decrease at parturition (Zarrow, 1947). Porter (1971a) demonstrated that injections of relaxin inhibited uterine contraction, and other experiments suggested that this agent might be responsible for the control of uterine muscle activity, parturition being precipitated concomitantly with the sharp decline in plasma relaxin levels (Porter, 1971a, b, 1972).

5. *Lactation*

As one might expect, the composition of the milk from mammalian species is strikingly different, as is shown in Table 2, which lists the major chemical components of milk from various laboratory species, the cow and the human. The marked differences in fat and protein content could pose significant problems of toxicant bioavailability due to liposolubility of agents, with sequestration into the mammary

TABLE 2

COMPOSITION OF MILK OBTAINED FROM DIFFERENT MAMMALS

Species	Water	Fat	Protein	Lactose	Ash
Human	88.1	3.8	0.9	7.0	0.2
Cow	87.4	3.7	3.4	4.8	0.7
Rat	68–72.5	12.6–15.0	9.2–12.0	3.0–3.3	1.4
Rabbit	71.3	13.1	12.3	1.9	2.3
Guinea pig	81.9	3.9	8.1	3.02	0.85
Cat	81.6	6.3	10.1	4.4	0.75
Dog	76.3	9.5	9.3	3.0	1.2

Values are in g per 100 g whole milk. Data are derived from Nelson et al. (1951), Spector (1956) and Wilson et al. (1980).

tissue during milk synthesis, and due to protein binding. These species variations should be taken into consideration when an animal model is chosen for perinatal studies. The significant difference between guinea pig and human milk is the 9-fold higher protein content of the former, though the fat content is similar. While the lactose concentration in human milk is 2-fold greater than in guinea pig milk, this should not present problems in the pharmacokinetics of agent transport via the milk, as would variations in lipid and protein content. It should be noted that the milk of all the laboratory species contained at least 9-fold higher protein content than did the human.

In contrast to the usual prolonged postpartum nursing period of 21–28 days seen in most laboratory species, the guinea pig sow has a short lactational period and weans its young by day 10–15 after birth. In our own studies, we have observed that most sows wean their young by day 7 (Ecobichon et al., 1978). In fact, we found it difficult to obtain uncontaminated stomach milk samples in pups at 4 days of age since, by that time, they were eating the food provided for the dam. Guinea pig pups, being born in an advanced state of maturity, are not dependent upon the mother's milk for nutrition and can quickly adapt to solid food within a day or so of birth, without any untoward effects being observed other than hunger and some body weight loss for 2–3 days (Ecobichon, unpublished results). Linzell (1971) showed that 50% of the litters born to mammectomized females survived without ever receiving milk, an observation that reflects our experiences.

In a detailed study of the yield and composition of guinea pig milk, Mepham and Beck (1973) demonstrated that peak production (70 g/day) was achieved by day 7 after birth, with a gradual tailing-off of production between days 7 and 13. The levels of lactose (4.0–5.0 g/100 ml) and protein (6.0–7.0 g/100 ml) remained quite constant throughout lactation, until day 10, when the former decreased transiently and the latter increased sharply. Gradual changes in potassium (decrease) and sodium (increase) levels were seen during the lactational period. Sows with large litters gave the best milk yield, the rate of pup growth being directly related to the milk yield of the dam (Linzell, 1972). Sows ceased to lactate if the young were removed for longer than 24 hours (Nelson et al., 1951). Histologically, retrogressive changes in the mammary gland appeared after 21 days of lactation or shortly after the pups have been weaned (Hesselberg and Loeb, 1937).

Milk can be collected easily from the lactating sow by a capillary tube collecting device, maximum volumes of 5.0 ml being obtained at a single milking, adequate for most residue analyses by sensitive gas or liquid chromatographic techniques following extraction. Since the nursing guinea pig is very sensitive to the biological effects of oxytocin, the injection of small amounts of this hormone can enhance the yield of milk markedly. Elaborate vacuum devices have been employed to collect milk, the best of these possibly being the apparatus described by Nelson et al. (1951).

IV. PERINATAL DEVELOPMENT

1. Growth

Fetal development begins with the fertilization of the ovum and ends with the expulsion of the fetus at parturition. Following fertilization within 3–8 hours after ovulation, the ovum migrates down the fallopian tubes and by 3 days post coitum is an 8-cell zygote in the uterus, and by day 8 post coitum has become a blastocyst (Blandau, 1949, 1961). By 7 days after fertilization, the blastocyst becomes attached to the uterine epithelium (Blandau, 1949). The cellular changes in the blastocyst at implantation are described by Roberts and Perry (1974). The embryo in a 10-day ovum is too small to be isolated and weighed, but by day 17 of gestation this can be accomplished with considerable care. Studies of fetal guinea pig development are few and one must consult the classical study of Draper (1920) for the most detailed description of this aspect. Figure 1 shows the curve, plotted from the data in Draper's tables, of the embryo weight in relationship to age. The first indication of a dramatic weight change occurs at 28 days, explained by the fact that the weight of the embryo from day to day is not great enough in relation to the age and the lack of ability to measure small changes. An embryo of 40 days weighs approximately 10 g while at 50 and 60 days gestation the body weights are approximately 35 and 65 g, respectively. The birth weight of a term guinea pig is of the order of 80–100 g. The crown–rump lengths of the embryos were measured by calipers, having fixed the embryos in formalin, the results of these measurements being presented in Figure 1. Considerable variability was observed, particularly toward the end of gestation, when, because of the size of the littermates and crowding in the abdomen, maximum growth can be affected. In my own experience, I have not found the crown–rump length measurement to be a useful index of gestational age. It is not impossible to have two fetuses of 90–100 mm in length with a littermate of 75–80 mm in length. The larger the litter, the more variability will be observed in both length and body weight (McKeown and MacMahon, 1956).

Figure 2 shows the percent increases in embryo weights per day, a true rate of

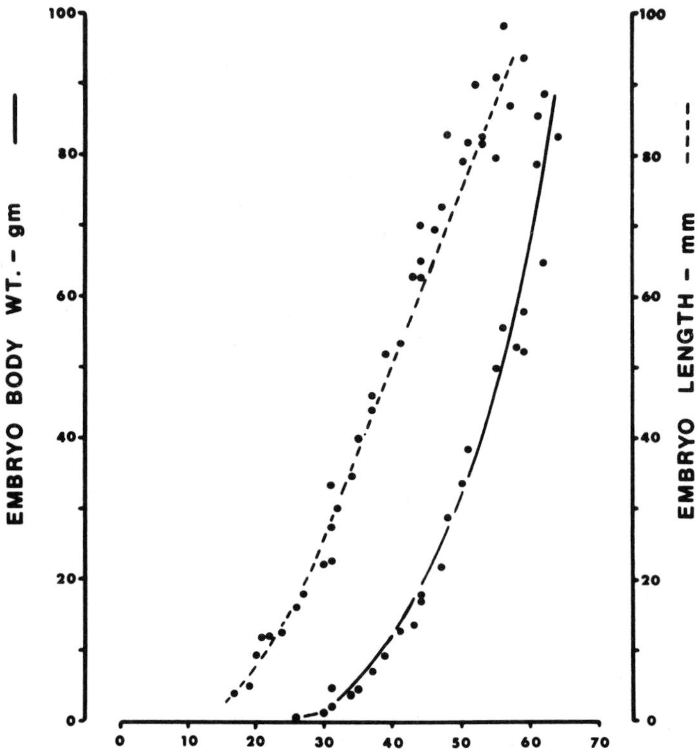

Figure 1. The relationship between embryonic weight or length and the corresponding gestational age of fetal guinea pigs. The data are derived from the studies of Draper (1920).

growth, the data being drawn from the observations of Draper (1920). A tremendous increase in the rate of growth is observed in the early stages of development. At the end of the 17th day of gestation, the daily percentage is 200%, but by day 20 it has dropped to 20% followed by a rise to 35% around day 40 and a subsequent gradual decline to 10% at the end of 64 days.

Litter size is dependent upon the number of follicles ovulating and being fertilized, the percentage implantation and the percentage surviving early fetal death (Sisk, 1976). The litter size has been found to affect markedly the incidence of stillbirth but not of abortion. As the litter size increased, stillbirth and neonatal mortality increased (Haines, 1931). The larger the litter, the greater the possibility of early parturition and death of the immature newborn. The lowest incidence of neonatal mortality was observed among litters born on day 69 (Goy et al., 1957). The main cause of death at birth has been reported to be asphyxia from fetal membranes (Rowlands, 1949). Our own experience has been that, even in caesarean sections with rapid removal of the membranes and manipulation of the pups to assist them in initiating respiration, approximately one pup in four is sluggish and often cannot maintain voluntary respiration.

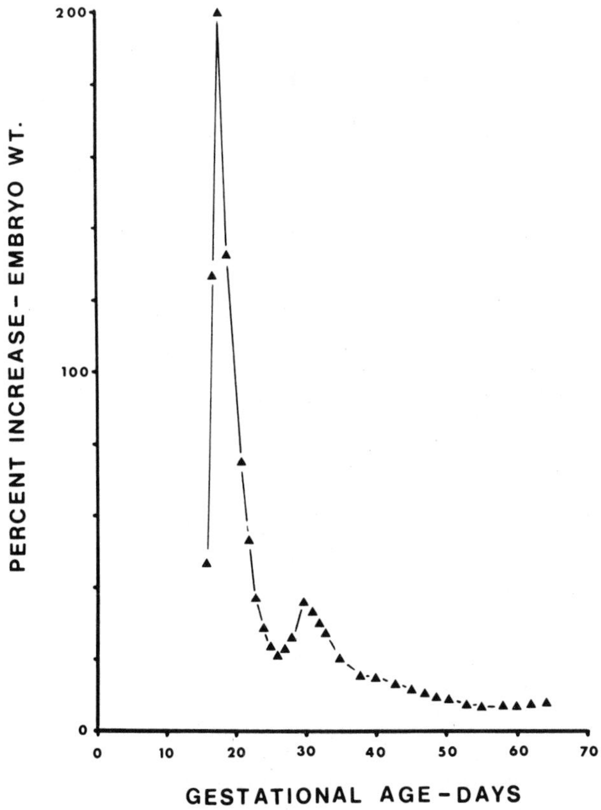

Figure 2. A representation of the daily percentage increase in embryonic body weight in relation to the corresponding gestational age of fetal guinea pigs. The graph demonstrates the tremendous increase in the rate of growth in the early stages of development compared to that at later stages. The data are derived and redrawn from the studies of Draper (1920).

We have noted that, in dams carrying large litters, there is a tendency toward toxemia of pregnancy, not unlike the eclamptic state found in humans, with death of the dam occurring before the expected parturition date or death of all of the fetuses at birth. While no in-depth study was conducted, we did find that a dilute (2.5–5.0%) glucose solution appeared to have some protective role in averting mortality. If one could consistently produce large litters in fecund females, this might prove to be an interesting animal model in which to study eclampsia and methods of minimizing the risk to the dam and the newborn pups.

At birth, in a study of 1032 young from 292 litters, the mean weight at birth was 93.4 g, and there is frequently an inverse relationship between litter size and birth weight (Dunkin et al., 1930; McKeown and MacMahon, 1956). Guinea pig pups grow rapidly following parturition (Ecobichon et al., 1978). Between birth and 2 days of age there was a slight decrease in body weight, possibly due to starvation and mobilization of body adipose tissue, but this decrease in weight was regained by 4 days of age. From day 4 until day 14 of age, the animals gained approximately 10 g of body weight/day. From day 14, the rate of growth was more rapid.

2. *Liver*

Being the major metabolic organ of the body, the development of the liver in the perinatal animal is of particular interest. Studies of most nonprimate fetal liver preparations have revealed little biological activity comparable to that found in the human fetal liver at midgestation, a subject that has been the topic of many reviews (Short et al., 1976; Neims et al., 1976). A small but definite increase in such activities as monooxygenase or carboxylesterase, glutathione *S*-aryltransferase, etc., can be measured near term but, unlike the enzymes of the human fetal liver, there is little or no tissue response following the exposure of the fetus to chemicals which can induce a variety of drug-metabolizing enzymes. By contrast, the fetal guinea pig will respond to such agents, thereby reflecting the more mature status of the liver.

Beginning with fetuses at 58–60 days gestation, little change was observed until 64 days gestation, when a slight increase in liver weight was measured. A sharp transient drop in liver weight occurred at 2 days of age, but by 4–7 days of age this loss had been regained. From day 2 until day 14 the increase in liver weight was approximately linear at a rate of 0.3 g/day. From day 14 onward, the increase in tissue weight was more pronounced.

The hepatocellular DNA (per g of tissue wet weight) was extremely high prior to birth, reflecting the large proportion of cells of the hematopoietic cell lines compared to hepatocytes, an observation confirmed by electron microscopy (Ecobichon et al., 1978). Hepatocytes represented about 30% of the liver volume at midgestation, this increasing to 70–80% by term in the guinea pig (Faulkner and Jones, 1979). By parturition, the fetal hepatic DNA had dropped sharply to a level comparable to that found in adult liver, and no significant changes were measured subsequently. A similar pattern was observed for hepatic RNA, the high prenatal concentrations decreasing sharply at birth but, in contrast to the DNA, rising just as rapidly following parturition. After 2 days postpartum, significant changes in RNA were not observed on direct measurement but, expressing the RNA content in terms of the cellular DNA, a steady increase in the ratio was observed from 63 days of gestation onward, reaching a peak at 21 days of age and then declining slowly (Ecobichon et al., 1978).

Hepatic glycogen, ascorbic acid and glutathione (GSH), three important hepatocellular constituents, show a similar development in the perinatal guinea pig liver, as is shown in Figure 3 (Ecobichon, unpublished data). At 58 days of gestation, the glycogen and ascorbic levels were 4.55 ± 1.02 mg/g and 73 ± 5.0 mmol/g, respectively. By 5 days before birth, these concentrations had increased by 30%, and by 4 days after birth the hepatic glycogen and ascorbic acid was almost 50% of those concentrations found in adult liver in the case of glycogen and in excess of the adult level for ascorbic acid. A gradual increase in hepatic glycogen to adult levels occurred

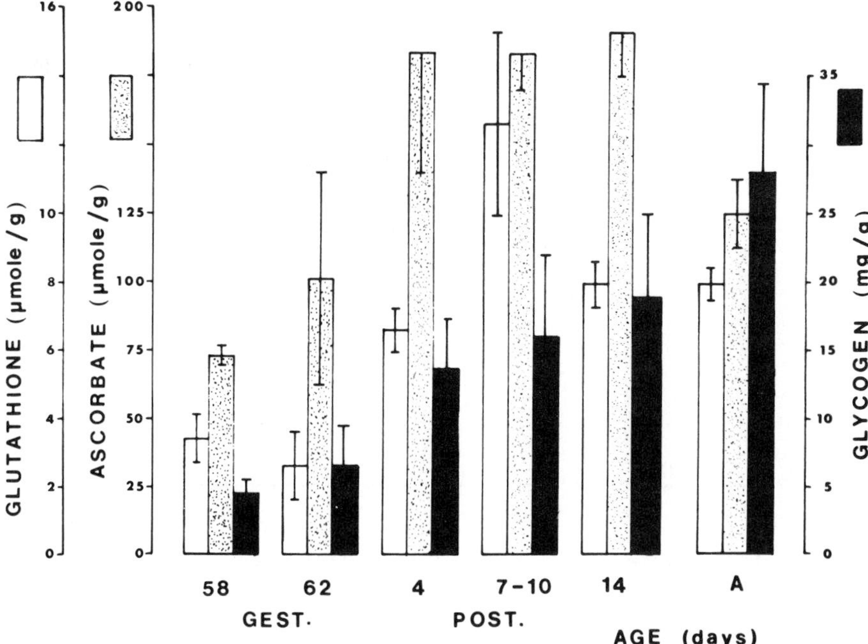

Figure 3. The hepatocellular concentrations of glutathione, ascorbic acid and glycogen measured in homogenates of fresh perinatal guinea pig liver from 9 days prior to birth until 14 days of age and compared with concentrations measured in adult female animals (Ecobichon, unpublished data).

slowly in the older pups. GSH was found to increase rapidly between the prenatal intervals studied and 4 days of age, when it was found to be only slightly lower than concentrations measured in adult liver. While considerable variability was noted, a GSH peak was measured at 7–10 days of age, which subsequently decreased to 'adult' levels.

Several studies have correlated enzymatic changes with morphological alterations in the hepatic tissues of developing perinatal animals (Short et al., 1976; Bell et al., 1975, 1976; Kuenzig et al., 1974; Lucier et al., 1977; Ecobichon et al., 1978). In most species, hepatic microsomal monooxygenase activities have been associated with the subcellular smooth endoplasmic reticulum (SER) and the fetal hepatocytes of most species have been devoid of SER, with little or no drug-metabolizing activity being detected. In the fetal guinea pig, in contrast to the fetal rat, considerably more SER was visible, and low but measurable enzymatic activities were detectable prior to birth (Kuenzig et al., 1974; Ecobichon et al., 1978). Figure 4 illustrates the ontogeny of two hepatic microsomal monooxygenases, *p*-nitroanisole *O*-demethylase (OD) and aniline hydroxylase (AH), in the perinatal guinea pig, showing the maximum activities detected at different pre- and postnatal ages (Ecobichon et al., 1978). The *O*-demethylase activity was just above the limit of detection at 58 days of gestation. Between 4 days prior to and 4 days after birth, an approximate 10-fold increase in

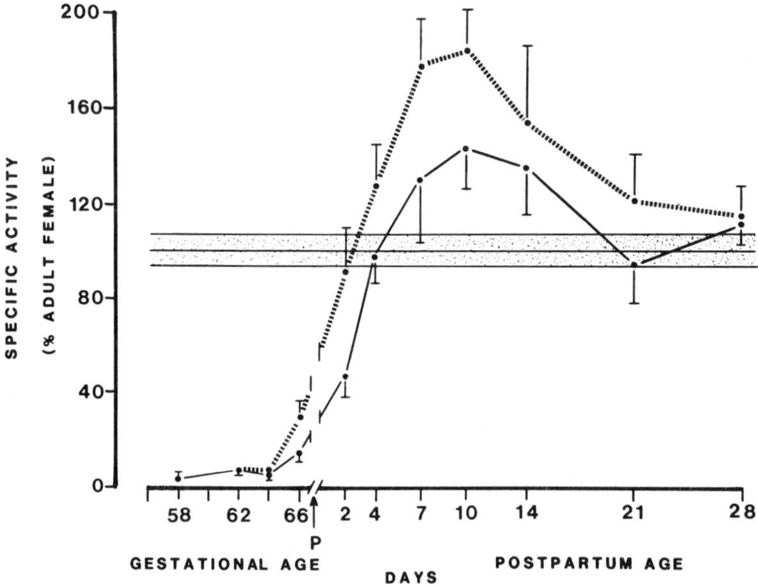

Figure 4. The perinatal development of guinea pig hepatic microsomal *p*-nitroanisole *O*-demethylase (——) and aniline hydroxylase (----) activities from 9 days prior to birth until 28 days of age. The values are presented in terms of specific activity (nmol per minute per mg) and compared as a percent of the activities measured in adult female guinea pigs. Bars show standard error of the mean. Adapted from Ecobichon et al. (1978).

both activities was observed. Maximum 20- and 30-fold increases in activity were observed by 7–10 days of age for OD and AH, respectively. By 28 days of age, the hepatic monooxygenases had declined to levels comparable to those measured in adult liver.

In Figure 5, the activities of microsomal uridine diphosphoglucuronate β-glucuronosyltransferase (GT) and nonspecific carboxylesterase (CE) are shown over the time span of perinatal development studied (Ecobichon et al., 1978). Considerably more enzymatic activity was detected for both enzymes in fetal liver as early as 58 days of gestation, and these activities increased steadily as parturition approached. A slower postnatal development of GT and CE occurred, adult levels of activity being attained by 14–21 days after birth, with little subsequent change being observed.

The ontogeny of a variety of enzymatic activities in the perinatal guinea pig has been studied. The enzymes involved in hepatic gluconeogenesis have been studied by Jones and Ashton (1976), by Robinson (1976) and by Raghunathan and Arinze (1977), dramatic changes being seen in the first 24 hours of postnatal life, with peak activities being attained by 7–10 days of age. The ontogeny of blood plasma pseudocholinesterase and CE as well as of hepatic and renal CE has been studied in the guinea pig (Chow and Ecobichon, 1975). The plasma pseudocholinesterase made its appearance between 56 and 60 days of gestation whereas the plasma CE activity was quite low until parturition, whereupon it increased rapidly some 4-fold by 20

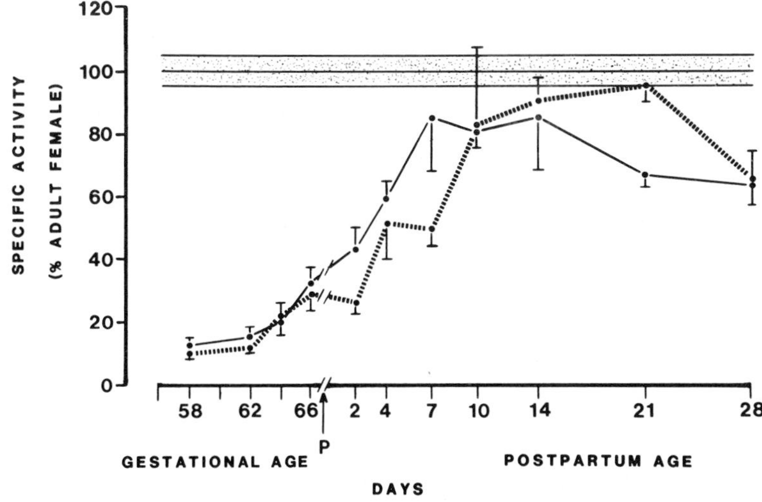

Figure 5. The perinatal development of guinea pig hepatic microsomal nonspecific carboxylesterase (----) and UDPGglucuronosyltransferase (——) (aglycone acceptor = α-naphthol) activities from 9 days prior to birth until 28 days of age. The values are presented in terms of specific activity (μmol or nmol per minute per mg) and compared as a percent of the activities measured in adult female guinea pigs. Bars show standard error of the mean. Adapted from Ecobichon et al. (1978).

days of age. While the hepatic CE activity was detectable prior to parturition, only in the postnatal period was a marked increase in activity measured. Fetal as well as neonatal guinea pigs are capable of enzymatic *N*-acetylation, the peak hepatic and lung activities occurring between 3 and 8 days after birth (Sonawane, 1982).

3. *Brain*

The brain of the perinatal guinea pig has been noted for its high degree of neurological maturity at birth, in contrast to that of other rodents. It has been suggested that the period of fastest brain growth, the 'brain growth spurt', is one of particular vulnerability to nutritional deficiency, physiological changes and perhaps even to toxicants, such events causing permanent deficits in brain size, cell numbers and myelination, with little chance of rehabilitation in later stages (Dobbing, 1968a, b). The rat was characterized as a postnatal brain developer, the guinea pig as a prenatal developer and the pig as a perinatal developer with the human considered to be similar to the pig (Dobbing and Sands, 1973).

In a study of the rate of development of the guinea pig brain from 29 days of gestation until adulthood, Dobbing and Sands (1970) demonstrated that the fastest rate of increase in brain weight occurred between 45 and 53 days of gestation, in the last trimester of pregnancy. This increased growth was closely followed by an increased rate of DNA synthesis. The observed decline in DNA content with increasing age, in spite of an absolute increase in cell numbers, was due to the increasing cell size and the synthesis of non-cellular myelin. The time of the fastest multiplication of glial cells just preceded the increased accumulation of cholesterol, which achieved peak levels just before birth. Histologically, the period of myelination was analogous to the period of cholesterol accumulation in the guinea pig brain (Wender and Waligora, 1961, 1964).

With a survey of the literature, Dobbing and Sands (1970) showed that major developmental events occurred in the guinea pig brain before 50 days of gestation. Such parameters as Nissl body accumulation, increases in the number and maturity of nerve processes, maturation of neuronal nucleoli, changes in cerebral enzymes, appearance of ground substance and appearance of electrical activity in the cortex all occurred at the end of the second or at the beginning of the third trimester (41–50 days of gestation). Other events, such as continuous electrical activity, glial cell multiplication, myelination, etc., occurred between 50 and 63 days of gestation.

While the 'brain growth spurt' in the guinea pig occurs primarily in the last trimester of pregnancy, this is different from what is found in the human, where the growth spurt was found to be much more postnatal than was previously supposed (Dobbing and Sands, 1973). According to these investigators, at least five-sixths of the human brain growth appeared postnatally, all the parameters measured (weight, nucleic acid, cholesterol, etc.) continuing to increase following parturition. These developmental differences may play an important role in modifying tissue responses following exposure to toxic agents, though this target organ may be quite sensitive at earlier stages, i.e., for neuronal migration, as will be discussed in a later section for one neurotoxin.

4. *Other tissues*

Few studies have examined the ontogeny of drug-metabolizing enzymes of tissues other than the liver in the perinatal guinea pig. Chow and Ecobichon (1975), studying the development of renal CE, showed that at 32, 37 and 45 days of gestation the levels of activity were exceedingly low but detectable. By 60 days of gestational age, the renal activity was comparable to that measured in adult tissue, and by birth the activity was in excess of that of the adult kidney. In an extensive study of the development of microsomal epoxide hydrase and cytosolic glutathione *S*-epoxydetransferase and glutathione *S*-aryltransferase in liver, lung, kidney and small intestine of the perinatal guinea pig, James et al. (1977) demonstrated that the rate(s) of maturation in extrahepatic tissues differed considerably from that in the liver. Both cytosolic glutathione *S*-transferases showed very similar development profiles in any one organ and were always comparable to adult levels before birth. While the development of the hepatic microsomal epoxide hydrase was similar to that observed in Figure 4, a small 'spurt' in activity observed just prior to birth and a rapid development to adult levels within 8 days of parturition, the activity of the epoxide hydrase in intestinal microsomes was very low, and by 27 days of age was still only 30% of adult activity levels. No epoxide hydrase data was presented for pulmonary or renal microsomes because the specific activities were below the level of detection (James et al., 1977).

With early interest in sulfobromophthalein (BSP) as a test of liver function, particularly the conjugation with GSH and subsequent biliary secretion, the excretion of this agent and the conjugated product was examined in fetal and neonatal guinea pigs (Goldstein et al., 1965; Schenker et al., 1965). In the fetal guinea pig, the rate of delivery of both BSP and the product was markedly reduced, the biliary excretion of unconjugated BSP being so disproportionately depressed as to suggest impairment of the conjugating mechanism. The excretion of conjugated BSP into bile was also impaired. The nature of this impairment was later identified as a combination of decreased transport of the dye from hepatocytes into bile and decreased ability to conjugate BSP (Whelan et al., 1970). In young newborn guinea pigs, injected conjugated BSP was secreted into the bile as readily as in the adult animal, indicating that the transport mechanism had developed fully by birth. The excretion of conjugated BSP into the bile, indicative of the ontogeny of the *S*-transferase necessary for the conjugating mechanism, revealed that excretion of the product was slow in the 1-day-old animal, but by 5–12 days after birth the rate of biliary elimination of conjugated BSP (formed in vivo) was comparable to adult rates (Goldstein et al., 1965). Measurement of hepatic levels of GSH and the enzyme that catalyzes BSP conjugation with GSH revealed low levels of each in the tissue of newborn animals.

From the above research, there is ample evidence that the development of the fetal guinea pig advances to a more mature state in utero than do the young of other laboratory species. Evidence, both morphological and physiological as well as biochemical, suggests that the tissues of the young of this species are more precocious near the time of parturition, and therefore may respond, as does the fetal human, to transplacentally acquired toxic agents. In this respect, the guinea pig maternal-fetal unit may serve as a useful surrogate model for the human maternal-fetal unit. In the postnatal period of development, there are less distinctive differences between the neonatal guinea pig and other neonatal rodents in that rapid development of tissue drug-metabolizing enzymes occurs in most species and the tissues are exceedingly responsive to foreign chemicals and toxicants.

V. TOXICOLOGICAL STUDIES

The degree and/or rate of placental transfer of chemicals is dependent upon physical properties of the agents, such as lipid solubility, degree of ionization, plasma protein binding and the molecular weight of the agents, in conjunction with physiological factors associated with the placenta, including blood circulation, surface area, lipid content, age and diseases (Mirkin, 1974). The relationship between drug levels in maternal blood and concentrations in breast milk is exceedingly complex and involves all of the above-mentioned physical properties, the most important factor governing transfer to milk being the concentration of unbound agent(s) in the plasma (Anderson, 1977). The variability of protein concentrations in plasma and milk, the differences in pH and ionization of the chemical and the changes in lipid content during lactation (low in early colostrum and high at later stages of lactation) as well as daily variations (peak fat concentrations at midmorning) are all factors that must be included in any consideration of exposure of the nursing newborn. One example, recently reviewed by Kanto (1982), serves to demonstrate the complexity of this field for the benzodiazepines.

Only in the past decade has genuine concern been raised about the exposure of the developing fetus and nursing neonatal individual to the myriad of chemicals ingested by the mother. While the overt mutagenic and teratogenic potentials of many agents have been studied extensively, the more subtle covert effects on tissue function have been largely ignored. Given the situation that human fetal tissues are sufficiently developed that they can respond to xenobiotic agents acquired transplacentally via passive diffusion and that acquisition may continue into the postnatal lactational period if maternal exposure is continuous, how then can the potential hazards from such agents be assessed using suitable animal models? The fetuses of most rodent species are unresponsive to transplacentally acquired agents, necessitating the use of expensive primate models for such studies. As was shown above, the tissues of the perinatal guinea pig are morphologically, physiologically and biochemically more mature than those of other rodents. In addition, a well-defined trimester pregnancy and a placental structure similar to that of the human are added features of the model.

1. Hepatotoxicity

Research in my own laboratory has centered on the effects of drugs and environmental contaminants on inducible hepatic functions in attempts to answer the following questions:

(a) What influence does an agent administered orally to the pregnant dam have on the ontogenesis of enzymes in the fetal and in the newborn guinea pig?

(b) Are there significant differences between enzyme-inducing chemicals based on high or low lipid solubility associated with protein binding, sequestration and persistence in vivo and ease of biotransformation?

(c) What are the effects of agents used acutely at parturition on the early postnatal development of tissue function(s)?

In such studies, we have employed a systematic three-pronged approach (i) to quantitate tissue residues of the agent and selected biochemical parameters as indices of function and (ii) to examine qualitatively the ultrastructure of target tissue(s). In this manner, we have been able both to see and measure when the perinatal liver responded to known levels of xenobiotic and to correlate observed biochemical changes with morphological alterations.

In one such study, phenytoin, a rather tenaciously protein-bound and slowly biotransformed anticonvulsant agent, was administered orally (25 mg/kg body weight) for 3 consecutive days to pregnant or lactating guinea pigs at different pre- and postnatal periods, the dams, fetuses and pups being killed 24 hours after the third dose. Selected hepatic microsomal monooxygenase activities in the fetuses and pups were measured and comparisons were made with hepatic residues of phenytoin and

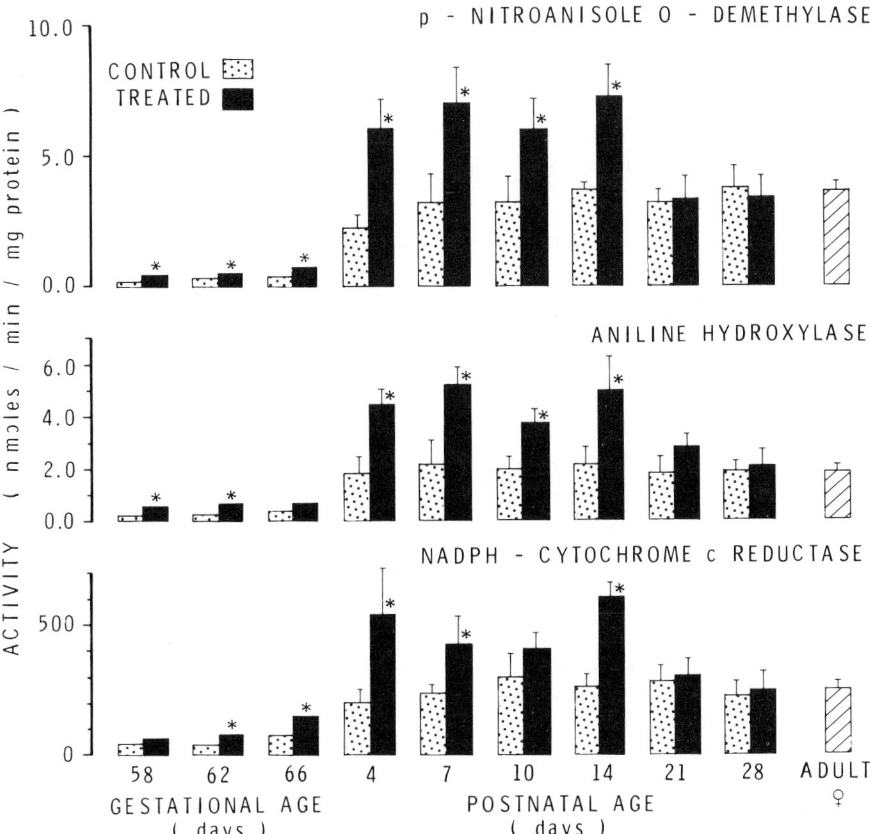

Figure 6. The influence of maternally administered phenytoin on the ontogenesis of guinea pig hepatic microsomal *p*-nitroanisole *O*-demethylase, aniline hydroxylase and NADPH-cytochrome *c* reductase at various pre- and postnatal stages of development. Values are expressed as the amount of product formed per minute per mg of microsomal protein and represent the mean $\pm$ S.D. for five to eight individual samples. Asterisks indicate statistically significant differences from control values at $P < 0.05$. From Lui et al. (1980), with permission.

electron micrographs of the developing perinatal livers (Lui and Ecobichon, 1979; Lui et al., 1980). The enzymatic results for the perinatal monooxygenases are shown in Figure 6. The influence of the transplacental or milk transfer of phenytoin on hepatic function is evident. While the activities in the 58-, 62- and 66-day-old fetuses were very low, they were significantly elevated following the transplacental acquisition of phenytoin, even though the agent had little visible effect on hepatic morphology. Postnatally, the 4-, 7-, 10- and 14-day-old pups, nursed by dams receiving oral phenytoin, demonstrated markedly increased activities concomitant with marked increases in hepatocellular SER. The hepatic monooxygenase systems of 21- and 28-day-old guinea pig pups did not respond to the xenobiotic, due, probably, to the fact that the pups had been weaned by this age. When one considers the results

TABLE 3

THE DIPHENYLHYDANTOIN (DPH) RESIDUE LEVELS IN THE SERUM AND LIVER OF DAMS AND PERINATAL INDIVIDUALS FOLLOWING ADMINISTRATION OF DPH

Age (days)		DPH residue levels					
		Perinate			Dam		
Gestational	Postnatal or postpartum	*n*	Serum (μg/ml)	Liver (μg/g)	*n*	Serum (μg/ml)	Liver (μg/g)
58		5	10.96±2.32	41.00± 5.70	5	12.72±1.89	39.43±3.17
62		5	15.00±1.86	33.60±10.50	6	11.80±3.40	41.60±7.68
66		5	18.91±3.20	23.10± 3.10	4	16.26±2.32	25.50±2.93
	4	9	1.42±1.00	4.20± 1.50	3	1.65±0.03	13.50±0.87
	7	7	1.30±0.92	5.82± 2.22	4	1.12±0.34	13.90±3.04
	10	7	1.63±0.29	5.44± 1.30	3	2.10±0.29	15.90±1.10
	14	5	2.07±0.91	6.80± 0.90	3	1.01±0.10	10.50±2.83
	21	8	−	+ +	3	1.08±0.25	12.50±2.30
	28	6	−	+ +	3	1.01±0.21	14.40±0.85
Nonpregnant, adult female					3	1.88±0.88	19.50±1.76

Values represent mean ±S.D. of tissue residues in the numbers of animals shown. DPH was administered orally at 25 mg DPH/kg/day for 3 consecutive days to the dam. −, Below limit of detection, 0.5 μg/ml; + +, below limit of detection, 2.5 μg/g.

in terms of tissue phenytoin residues, as is shown in Table 3, high and comparable levels of drug were measured in the serum and liver of the dams and fetuses, suggesting equilibrium between the two circulations. The excessively high tissue levels in the pregnant dams in comparison to levels found in similarly treated nonpregnant animals suggested that pregnancy resulted in a lowered rate of biotransformation and clearance. In the postnatal period, the serum and hepatic phenytoin residues of 4-, 7-, 10- and 14-day-old pups were approximately 10 and 20%, respectively, of the residues measured in fetal tissues. Neonatal and maternal serum contained similar concentrations of drug but neonatal liver contained only 30–40% of the concentration measured in maternal liver. Phenytoin residues of 21- and 28-day-old pups were below the limits of detection. The elevated enzyme activities at 14 days of age are puzzling since the dam should have weaned the pups by this age, but, in other studies, we have demonstrated that intestinal absorption of phenytoin is slow, peak plasma levels being acquired only after 12 hours, with a subsequent β-phase half-life of 6.5 hours (Lui and Ecobichon, 1979). The slow elimination of residues is reflected in the persistent serum and hepatic levels in the pups (Table 3).

In contrast to the above study, recent experiments with another anticonvulsant agent, sodium phenobarbital, revealed quite different results. The treatment regimen, 25 mg/kg body weight administered orally to pregnant or lactating dams for 3 consecutive days with analysis of the various parameters in dams, fetuses and pups 24 hours following the terminal dose, was identical to that used for the phenytoin study. This agent, with a more rapid absorption, attainment of peak levels in 4 hours and a longer β-phase half-life of 14.9 hours, exerted little effect on perinatal hepatic microsomal monooxygenases or on hepatic morphology. Only at 62 days of gestation and at 4 days after birth were significant increases in activities observed following acquisition of the drug. There was marked transplacental acquisition of drug residues by the developing fetuses but postnatal acquisition via the milk was not high enough, except in the first 4 days following birth, to influence the enzyme activities. One can see that residues in the serum and liver in dams and in fetuses were comparable, signifying the absence of an effective placental barrier to the drug. The excessively high tissue levels in treated pregnant animals compared to those measured in treated nonpregnant female guinea pigs suggest a markedly reduced rate of biotransformation and/or elimination.

Recent published studies of the influence of d,l-methadone hydrochloride on hepatic drug-metabolizing functions in perinatal guinea pigs using a similar protocol as that used for phenytoin and sodium phenobarbital revealed an interesting problem associated with this drug (Pak and Ecobichon, 1982). This agent, bound to plasma proteins to an extent of 90–95%, has a β-phase half-life of 13.5 hours. Figure 7 shows the distribution of drug residues in plasma, brain, liver and kidney of nonpregnant treated adult guinea pigs and in treated pregnant or lactating dams and their fetuses and pups at 12 hours following the terminal dose. Compared to the residues in nonpregnant animals, plasma methadone was very high in the pregnant dams, though levels dropped sharply in the postnatal period. A similar pattern of distribution was observed in maternal brain, liver and kidney, the residues being much higher than in tissues of nonpregnant treated adults. The most startling result was the markedly elevated levels detected in fetal brain. An examination of the tissue/plasma ratio for methadone revealed that distribution in the pup was different from that in the mother, the brain/plasma ratio for fetuses at 60–65 days of gestation being 4–5-fold higher than in the pregnant dams. To ascertain why this should occur, protein-binding studies were conducted in vitro using an equilibrium dialysis technique, the results presented in Figure 8 showing that, while the protein concentration in blood plasma changed from 35.8 ± 2.7 mg/ml at 50–55 days of gestation to 46.5 ± 2.4 mg/ml at 10 days of age, the amount of methadone bound went from 52 to 93% over the same time period. From these results, it is apparent that much of the transplacentally acquired methadone would not be bound to fetal plasma proteins and would be available for uptake into tissues, particularly the brain. These experimental results illustrate some of the vagaries of protein binding and the necessity of quantitating the bound/free ratio of chemical as an integral part of fetal-neonatal studies in guinea pigs as well as other species.

2. *Nephrotoxicity*

Few toxicological studies have been conducted using the kidney of the perinatal guinea pig. Micturition occurs in utero, with bladders containing urine being

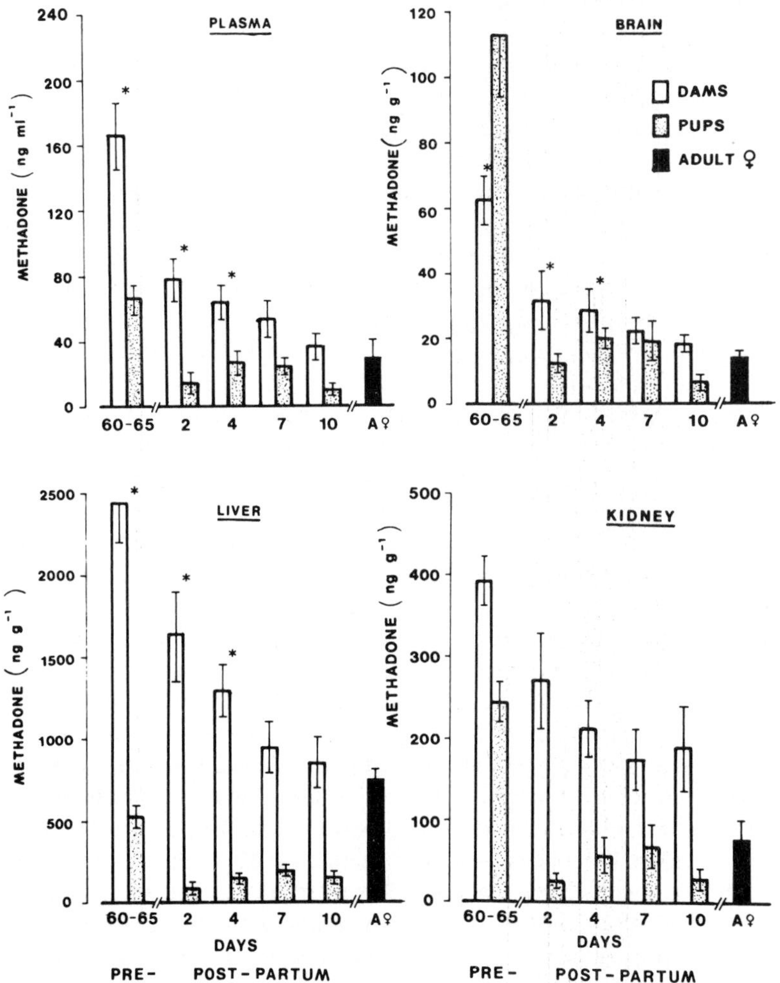

Figure 7. Methadone residues in the plasma, brains, livers and kidneys of nonpregnant females (black bars) and of pregnant and nursing guinea pigs (open bars) and their fetuses and pups (stippled bars). At selected pre- and postnatal intervals, the dams received oral doses of d,l-methadone hydrochloride (25 mg/kg body weight every 12 hours) for 2 consecutive days and the dams, fetuses and pups were killed 12 hours after the final dose. The results presented are mean ($\pm$S.E.) tissue concentrations of the number of experiments shown at the top of each bar. Asterisks signify residue levels in the dams which were significantly different from similarly treated non-pregnant guinea pigs ($P<0.05$). From Pak and Ecobichon (1982), with permission.

observed at 50–55 days of gestation as well as coloration of the amniotic fluid, an indication of excretion. Measurable renal microsomal and cytosolic CE can be found as early as 30 days of gestation, and by 40–50 days of gestation the activity is of the order of 40% of that measured in the adult kidney (Chow and Ecobichon, 1975).

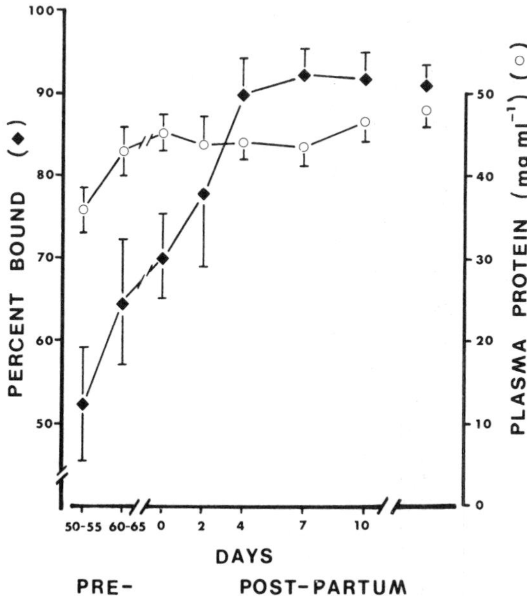

Figure 8. The total protein content of perinatal guinea pig blood plasma (○) and the extent of plasma protein binding of d,l-methadone HCl (◆) in guinea pigs of different pre- and postnatal ages as measured by an equilibrium dialysis method. Each point and bar represents the mean ($\pm$S.D.) value of a minimum of five determinations from individual samples. From Pak and Ecobichon (1982), with permission.

Wachstein and Bradshaw (1965), in an extensive histochemical study of the postnatal development of renal enzymes in the rat, rabbit and guinea pig, found that different rates of appearance occurred. In contrast to observations made for the rat and rabbit, adult activities were detectable in most parts of the neonatal guinea pig kidney, with the intensity of the stain being comparable to that detected in the adult kidney.

A brief search of the literature revealed that only one study had used the perinatal guinea pig in the assessment of covert developmental toxicity from heavy metals such as lead, cadmium, cobalt, mecury, etc. Pregnant guinea pigs were injected with 1.0 μg/kg of radioactively labelled methylmercury at 22, 40, 47, 59 and 66 days of gestation and fetal tissues were examined for radioactivity 24 hours after dosing (Kelman et al., 1980). In general, the amount of mercury absorbed by the whole fetus increased during gestation in parallel with increasing tissue mass, while mercury found in the placentas remained relatively constant. The liver, kidney, blood and brain contained the highest mercury concentrations early in gestation (day 40) and levels decreased as term approached. No morphological or functional studies were undertaken. The administration of methylmercury to adult guinea pigs for 71 consecutive days resulted in the accumulation of the highest levels of the agent in the renal tissue in a dose-related manner (Iverson et al., 1974).

In contrast, methylmercury (4.0 mg Hg/kg) administered to pregnant rats on day 8 of pregnancy was not overtly toxic to the dam but did cause a variety of subtle renal lesions in the neonatal pups (Chang and Sprecher, 1976a, b). Degenerative changes were most prominent in the proximal tubular epithelial cells. Hyperplastic changes in the distal convoluted tubules occurred when the pregnant rats received doses of methylmercury as low as 1.0 mg Hg/kg (Chang and Sprecher, 1976b). The morphological changes were reported to persist into adulthood in these animals. In a recently published study in which renal function was measured, Smith et al. (1983) demonstrated that doses of methylmercury (4.0–6.0 mg Hg/kg) administered on day 8 of gestation had very little influence on the ability of renal slices to accumulate organic ions and to generate glucose. Only high doses (3 $\times$ 4.0 mg Hg/kg) administered on days 8, 10 and 12 of gestation exerted a slight effect on sodium and water elimination when the pups were 42 days of age, giving rise to the conclusion that postnatal renal physiological sequelae to prenatal administration of methylmercury may be less than predicted from histological studies (Smith et al., 1983).

With the size of the guinea pig pup from 45 days of gestation onward and the ample supply of renal tissue compared to that of the rat pup, the effects of heavy metal exposure could be assessed in the fetuses of this animal as well as in the neonate, using tissue slices and the in vitro study of *p*-aminohippuric acid, glucose and ion uptake. I would encourage investigators to try experiments in this animal model since, as was shown by Kelman et al. (1980), the fetal guinea pig appears to take up such ions optimally at mid-gestation, a period of rapid organogenesis and maturation.

3. *Neurotoxicity*

As part of the continuing study of the aftermath of the tragic methylmercury poisoning in Iraq in 1971 from mercurial-treated seed grain (Amin-Zaki et al., 1974; Skerfving and Copplestone, 1976), Marsh et al. (1981) reported that the most severely affected children had been exposed in utero to the methylmercury during the second trimester. Neuropathological evidence of impaired neuronal migration in brains that had been exposed in the 3rd and 4th months of pregnancy was presented by Choi et el. (1978). Both the Iraq and Minamata (Japan) disasters revealed that the fetal and neonatal neurological systems were far more vulnerable to the effects of methylmercury than were those of their mothers or older children. Studies using animal models as divergent as mice and swine have shown that the early periods of gestation (e.g., organogenesis) represent a critical time of toxicity to the nervous system, with doses not toxic to the mother causing overt and covert toxicity in the fetal and neonatal animal (Spyker and Smithberg, 1972; Kelman et al., 1982).

The guinea pig has been shown to be sensitive to methylmercury intoxification, the LD_{50} values being 5.5 mg Hg/kg intraperitoneally and 16.5 mg Hg/kg orally (Iverson et al., 1973). Moderate concentrations of methylmercury were found in various regions of the central nervous system, the levels being approximately 10% of those measured in the kidney and comparable to the levels found in the blood (Iverson et al., 1974). While I am unaware of any studies of the neurotoxic effects of methylmercury using the perinatal guinea pig, this would make an ideal model. The greatest rate of brain growth velocity, expressed as a percentage of adult weight, occurs between 41 and 51 days of gestation (Dobbing and Sands, 1971). Kelman et al. (1980) demonstrated that the maximal uptake of radioactively labelled methylmercury by fetal guinea pig brain occurred at or before 40 days of gestation.

Limited numbers of studies have used the fetal guinea pig to investigate the effects of drugs on the central nervous system. Geddes et al. (1972) demonstrated that following the inhalation of halothane-^{82}Br by pregnant guinea pigs similar concentrations were found in maternal and fetal brains, while the fetal liver contained twice the level found in the maternal liver, these results suggesting that the fetal liver played an important role in the fetal distribution of the anesthetic. That this may not always be true was shown by Pak and Ecobichon (1982), who found that d,l-methadone readily penetrated the brain of fetal guinea pigs, achieving concentrations 2-fold higher than in the maternal brain and causing a reduced viability of newborn pups with obvious difficulty in maintaining spontaneous respiration. Thalidomide, administered at 46–55 days of gestation to pregnant guinea pigs, produced electrical silence in the cortical region (Bergstrom et al., 1963). When administered at 55–62 days of gestation, there were silent intervals interspersed among periods of slow wave activity, whereas in near-term fetuses the electrical responses were not affected. These results suggested that the concentrations of thalidomide gaining access to the fetal guinea pig brain may vary, depending upon the stage of development.

A pertinent question for study concerns the possible effects of cigarette smoke on the functions of the developing fetus. The effects on the human neonate have been investigated extensively and need not be reviewed here. One interesting paper on the effects of marihuana smoke on the maternal and fetal heart rates and electroencephalograms (EEG) was published using the maternal-fetal guinea pig (Singer et al., 1973). Pregnant dams, near term, were anesthetized with diethyl ether, laparotomized and stainless steel needles attached to a metal syringe were pushed through the maternal myometrium and fetal skull into the brain to a depth of 1–2 mm in the central regions, analogous to a biparietal location. Within 3 or 4 hours of closure of the abdomen, the alert dam was placed in the smoking chamber and the externalized leads were connected to a polygraph for recording. The marihuana cigarette consisted of 500 mg of material with a content of 1.4% Δ^9-tetrahydrocannabinol (THC). The results showed that during the exposure to the smoke the maternal EEG remained unchanged, but subsequently changed to a pattern of low-frequency and high-amplitude activity. The fetal EEG changed to a slow-frequency, high-voltage activity pattern during the smoking period and, subsequent to the exposure, the EEG gradually changed to a lower voltage and higher frequency activity. While blood studies of Δ^9-THC levels were not carried out, it would appear that, once again, the fetus was more susceptible to the transplacentally acquired agent than was the dam.

4. *Teratology*

The guinea pig is not the favored animal for teratological experiments because of the difficulty in breeding them, the long gestational period and the limited number of young per litter, the latter factor probably being the most significant drawback. According to Hoar (1976), the guinea pig occupies a position intermediate between rats and mice and the primates and man. The normal organogenesis of the guinea pig fetus has been described in detail by several investigators in the late 1920s and 1930s and relevant papers are referred to by Hoar (1976) in a recent review. Normally, the guinea pig has a relatively low incidence of congenital malformations, a positive feature of the species.

Malformations can be readily induced in fetal guinea pigs. Thalidomide, administered in a three-generation study, caused significant numbers of deformities of the outer ear, cleft palate and shortened limbs (Arbab-Zadeh, 1965). If thalidomide was injected intraperitoneally from 3 days before and for 15 days after mating, the young showed aplasia and bone atrophy of the forelimbs, reminiscent of the malformations seen in humans. Equivocal results have been obtained for other chemicals. The anticholinesterase insecticide, carbaryl, was teratogenic in the guinea pig at doses of the order of 300 mg/kg when administered repeatedly from day 11 to day 20 of gestation or when given in single doses on days during this same time interval (Robens, 1969). Most of the observed defects were skeletal and involved the cervical vertebrae, though the absence of kidneys and genitalia was noted in two fetuses and fused thoracic vertebrae and ribs were seen. Weil et al. (1973) were unable to reproduce malformations in the guinea pig to confirm the earlier results. The azo dye, trypan blue, long used as a positive control chemical in teratological studies, caused fetal malformations when administered on a single day during the period of day 6 to day 13 of gestation (Hoar and Salem, 1961).

As can be seen from the above studies, a major difficulty in the use of the guinea pig is in knowing that the animal is pregnant when treatment must start. The agent(s) must be given in the time interval of days 6–20 following mating, the first trimester and the period of maximum embryonic growth (Fig. 2). Extensive use of this species in studies designed to identify congenital malformations would require a carefully controlled breeding regimen and considerable expertise among the personnel.

5. *Toxicokinetics*

One of the main drawbacks of the guinea pig as an experimental animal is the complete absence of any exposed and handy vessels from which one can obtain suitable blood samples to monitor drug levels. Cardiac puncture can be used with some success, but only at widely spaced intervals or by using larger groups and collecting blood from subgroups at alternate time intervals (Lui and Ecobichon, 1979; Pak and Ecobichon, 1981). This becomes an even greater problem when one wishes to work with pregnant animals and to sample both maternal and fetal circulations.

The best technique that I have seen is that developed by Schenker and his colleagues to study the fetal disposition and elimination of BSP and glucuronide conjugate (Schenker et al., 1964, 1965). The animals used were all within an estimated 2 weeks of delivery so that one had large fetuses and large blood vessels for use.

Anesthesia was induced by the intraperitoneal injection of 6.0 mg of pentobarbital and was maintained by intermittent inhalation of diethyl ether. The pregnant guinea pig was submerged to the neck in an isotonic saline bath at 37°C and strapped in a semirecumbent position permitting unrestricted respiration. The uterus was extruded from the submerged pelvis through an abdominal mid-line incision. The uterus was then opened along its relatively avascular margin and the fetuses were delivered into the bath. The amnion was stripped from the fetus and umbilical vessels (it could be left in place on one or more fetuses if sampling of amniotic fluid was desired to ascertain urinary excretion of drug or metabolite), and the submerged fetus was secured loosely to the wall of the bath with silk ties.

In this preparation, the umbilical and the uterine vessels are visible, the viability of the fetus can easily be monitored by palpating the fetal heart, small blood samples can be readily obtained from either circulatory system and the agent(s) can be administered to the dam orally, intravenously or by inhalation. The system, with care, can remain viable for 2–3 hours, sufficient time for the conduction of most drug distribution and kinetic experiments.

VI. CONCLUSIONS

Many studies over the past three decades have emphasized the ability of xenobiotic agents to stimulate the synthesis of tissue enzymes in the early postnatal young of many species. The hepatic tissue, in particular, has been shown to be very susceptible to such effects. Short et al. (1976) derived a scheme, shown in Figure 9 in modified form, in which three distinct development profiles for enzymes emerge with only minor species differences. One could expand this concept to cover any biochemical or

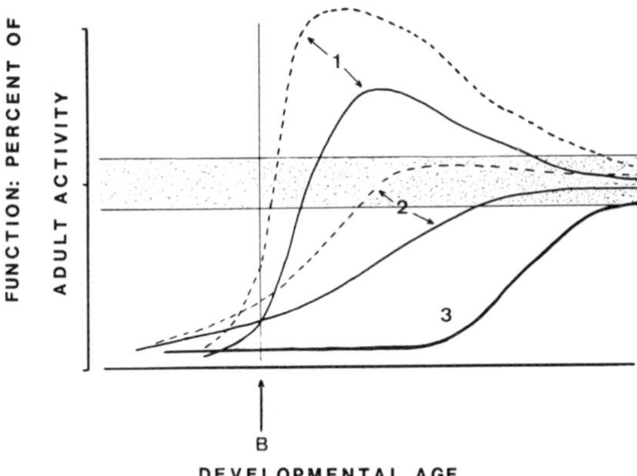

Figure 9. Developmental profiles for tissue functions of perinatal animals. The solid lines represent normal early postnatal (1), intermediate (2) and late postnatal (3) development. The dotted lines represent enhanced development due to exposure to certain xenobiotic agents. The hatched area represents the range of functionality measured in adult animals. Adapted from Short et al. (1976).

physiological function of a tissue. Foreign agents appearing in the 'environment' of the fetus or nursing neonatal individual may alter the pattern of functional ontogenesis significantly, as is shown by the dotted lines for type 1 and type 2 profiles, the functional maturity appearing earlier and at higher levels than under normal developmental conditions. In contrast, few studies have demonstrated that the agents acquired by the perinatal animal cause the opposite effects to those shown in Figure 9, i.e., a retardation of the rate of development and levels of functional maturity achieved. This would appear to be an area of fruitful research yet to be explored systematically. Indeed, given the fact that we know the mechanisms by which some of these xenobiotic agents exert their biological effects in adult animals, these same chemicals might be invaluable tools in elucidating the factors controlling the ontogenesis of function(s).

The precocious perinatal guinea pig, despite its many faults, may provide an excellent animal model, lying between the rodents with their latent and slow development and the primates with their advanced development at mid-gestation. It is hoped that this chapter will convince the reader of the versatility and usefulness of this species in the field of perinatal toxicology.

VII. ACKNOWLEDGMENTS

The financial assistance of the Medical Research Council of Canada in the form of an operating grant (MA-3611) supporting the author's studies of the perinatal guinea pig is gratefully acknowledged.

VIII. REFERENCES

Amin-Zaki, L., Elhassani, S., Majeed, M.A., Clarkson, T.W., Doherty, R.A. and Greenwood, M. (1974) Pediatrics 54, 587–595.

Amoroso, E.C. (1961) Br. Med. Bull. 17, 81–90.

Anderson, P.O. (1977) Drug Intel. Clin. Pharmacol. 1, 208–223.

Arbab-Zadeh, V.A. (1965) Med. Klin. (Munich) 60, 1733–1736.

Bartels, H., Yassin, D.E. and Reinhardt, W. (1967) Resp. Physiol. 2, 149–162.

Bedford, C.A., Challis, J.R.G., Harrison, F.A. and Heap, R.B. (1972) J. Reprod. Fert. Suppl. 16, 1–23.

Bell, J.U., Hansell, M.M. and Ecobichon, D.J. (1975) Can. J. Physiol. Pharmacol. 53, 1147–1157.

Bell, J.U., Hansell, M.M. and Ecobichon, D.J. (1976) Toxicol. Appl. Pharmacol. 35, 165–177.

Bergström, R.M., Bergström, L., Putkonen, D. and Sainio, K. (1963) Med. Exp. 11, 119–127.

Blandau, R.J. (1949) Anat. Rec. 103, 19–48.

Blandau, R.J. (1961) in Sex and Internal Secretions (Young, W.C., ed.), pp. 797–882, Williams and Wilkins, Baltimore, MD.

Blandau, R.J. and Young, W.C. (1939) Am. J. Anat. 64, 303–330.

Boling, J.L., Blandau, R.J., Wilson, J.G. and Young, W.C. (1939) Proc. Soc. Exp. Biol. Med. 42, 128–132.

Bruce, H.M. and Parkes, A.S. (1948) J. Hyg. 46, 434–437.

Castle, W.E. and Wright, S. (1916) Publ. Carnegie Inst., No. 241, 1–129.

Challis, J.R.G., Heap, R.B. and Illingworth, D.V. (1971) J. Endocrinol. 51, 333–345.

Chang, L.W. and Sprecher, J.A. (1976a) Environm. Res. 11, 392–406.

Chang, L.W. and Sprecher, J.A. (1976b) Environm. Res. 12, 218–223.
Choi, B.H., Lapham, L.W., Amin-Zaki, L. and Saleem, T. (1978) J. Neuropath. Exp. Neurol. 37, 719–733.
Chow, A.Y.K. and Ecobichon, D.J. (1975) Biol. Neonate 25, 23–30
Dancis, J. (1964) Fed. Proc. 23, 781–784.
Dancis, J., Money, W.L., Springer, D. and Levitz, M. (1968) Am. J. Obstet. Gynecol. 101, 820–829.
Deanesly, R. (1960) J. Reprod. Fert. 1, 242–248.
Dobbing, J. (1968a) in Malnutrition, Learning and Behaviour (Scrimshaw, N.S. and Gordon, J.E., eds.), pp. 181–202, M.I.T. Press, Boston, MA.
Dobbing, J. (1968b) in Applied Neurochemistry (Davison, A.N. and Dobbing, J., eds.), pp. 287–316, Blackwell, Oxford.
Dobbing, J. and Sands, J. (1970) Brain Res. 17, 115–123.
Dobbing, J. and Sands, J. (1971) Biol. Neonate 19, 363–378.
Dobbing, J. and Sands, J. (1973) Arch. Dis. Child. 48, 757–767.
Donovan, B.T. and Lockhart, A.N. (1972) J. Reprod. Fert. 30, 207–211.
Draper, R.L. (1920) Anat. Rec. 18, 369–392.
Dunkin, G.W., Hartley, P., Lewis-Faning, E. and Russell, W.T. (1930) J. Hyg. 30, 311–330.
Ecobichon, D.J., Dykeman, R.W. and Hansell, M.M. (1978) Can. J. Biochem. 56, 738–745.
Einer-Jensen, N., Edvinsson, L., Falck, B., Owman, C., Sjoberg, N. O. and Walles, B. (1975) Acta Physiol. Scand. 93, 97–103.
Emrys-Roberts, E. (1909) J. Anat. Physiol. 44, 192–202.
Enders, A.C. (1965) Am. J. Anat. 116, 29–68.
Faulkner, A. and Jones, C.T. (1979) Biochem. J. 178, 89–95.
Ford, D.H. and Young, W.C. (1953) Anat. Rec. 115, 495–503.
Fuchs, F. (1952) Acta Physiol. Scand. 28, 162–171.
Garris, D.R. (1980) IRCS Med. Sci. 8, 793–794.
Garris, D.R. and Whitehead, D.S. (1981) Am. J. Physiol. 241, 142–145.
Garris, D.R., Blankenship, L.T. and Whitehead, D.S. (1983) Gynecol. Obstet. Invest. 15, 33–40.
Geddes, I.C., Brand, L., Finster, M. and Mark, L. (1972) Br. J. Anaesth. 44, 542–547.
Goldstein, J., Schenker, S. and Combes, B. (1965) Am. J. Physiol. 208, 573–577.
Goy, R.W., Hoar, R.M. and Young, W.C. (1957) Anat. Rec. 128, 747–757.
Haines, G. (1931) J. Agr. Res. 42, 123–164.
Harned, M.A. and Casida, L.E. (1972) J. Mammal. 53, 223–225.
Heap, R.B. and Deanesly, R. (1966) J. Endocrinol. 34, 417–423.
Hendrickx, A.G. and Houston, M.L. (1970) in Reproduction and Breeding Techniques for Laboratory Animals (Hafez, E.S.E., ed.), pp. 157–176, Lea and Febiger, Philadelphia, PA.
Herschfeld, M.S. and Nemeth, A.M. (1968) J. Lipid Res. 9, 460–468.
Hesselberg, C. and Loeb, L. (1937) Anat. Rec. 68, 103–112.
Hisaw, F.L., Zarrow, M.K., Money, W.L., Talmage, R.V.N. and Abramowitz, A.A. (1944) Endocrinology, 34, 122–134.
Hoar, R.M. (1976) in The Biology of the Guinea Pig (Wagner, J.E. and Manning, P.J., eds.), pp. 269–280, Academic Press, New York.
Hoar, R.M. and Salem, A.J. (1961) Anat. Rec. 141, 173–182.
Hückinghaus, F. (1961) Z. Säugetierk 26, 108–111.
Hunter, R.H.F., Hunt, D.M. and Chang, M.C. (1969) Anat. Rec. 165, 411–430.
Ishii, O. (1920) Biol. Bull. 38, 237–250.
Iverson, F., Downie, R.H., Paul, C. and Trenholm, H.L. (1973) Toxicol. Appl. Pharmacol. 24, 545–554.
Iverson, F., Downie, R.H., Trenholm, H.L. and Paul, C. (1974) Toxicol. Appl. Pharmacol. 27, 60–69.
James, M.O., Foureman, G.L., Law, F.C. and Bend, J.R. (1977) Drug Metab. Dispos. 5, 19–28.
Jones, C.T. and Ashton, I.K. (1976) Arch. Biochem. Biophys. 174, 506–522.
Kanto, J.H. (1982) Drugs 23, 354–380.
Kelman, B.J., Steinmetz, S.E., Walter, B.K. and Sasser, L.B. (1980) Teratology 21, 161–165.
Kelman, B.J., Walter, B.K. and Sasser, L.B. (1982) J. Toxicol. Environ. Hlth. 10, 191–200.

King, B.F. and Enders, A.C. (1971) Am. J. Anat. 130, 409–430.
Kuenzig, W., Kamm, J.J., Boublik, M., Jenkins, F. and Burns, J.J. (1974) J. Pharmacol. Exp. Ther. 191, 32–44.
Lane-Petter, W. and Porter, G. (1963) in Animals for Research. Principles of Breeding and Management (Lane-Petter, W., ed.), pp. 287–321, Academic Press, New York.
Linzell, J.L. (1971) Res. Reprod. 3, 2–3.
Linzell, J.L. (1972) Dairy Sci. Abst. 34, 351–360.
London, W.T., Money, W.L. and Rawson, R.W. (1963) Endocrinology 73, 205–209.
Lucier, G., Sonawane, B.R. and McDaniel, O.S. (1977) Drug Metab. Dispos. 5, 279–288.
Lui, E.M.K. and Ecobichon, D.J. (1979) Can. J. Physiol. Pharmacol. 57, 517–523.
Lui, E.M.K., Hansell, M.M. and Ecobichon, D.J. (1980) Toxicol. Appl. Pharmacol. 55, 55–66.
Marcus, G.J. (1974) J. Endocrinol. 63, 89–97.
Marsh, D.O., Myers, G.J., Clarkson, T.W., Amin-Zaki, L., Tikriti, S. and Majeed, M.A. (1981) Clin. Toxicol. 18, 1311–1318.
McKeown, T. and MacMahon, B. (1956) J. Endocrinol. 13, 195–200.
Mepham, T.B. and Beck, N.F.G. (1973) Comp. Biochem. Physiol. A. 45, 273–281.
Miller, R.K. and Berndt, W.O. (1975) Life Sci. 16, 7–30.
Mirkin, B.L. (1974) Clin. Pharmacol. Therap. 14, 643–647.
Muñoz, L. (1970) Canca, Talleres Editoriales del Departamento Popayan.
Neims, A., Warner, M., Loughnan, P.M. and Aranda, J.V. (1976) Annu. Rev. Pharmacol. Toxicol. 16, 427–445.
Nelson, W.L., Kaye, A., Moore, M., Williams, H.H. and Herrington, B. (1951) J. Nutr. 44, 585–594.
Pak, R.C.K. and Ecobichon, D.J. (1981) Drug. Metab. Dispos. 9, 170–171.
Pak, R.C.K. and Ecobichon, D.J. (1982) Biochem. Pharmacol. 31, 2941–2947.
Porter, D.G. (1971a) J. Reprod. Fert. 26, 251–253.
Porter, D.G. (1971b) J. Reprod. Fert. 27, 219–226.
Porter, D.G. (1972) Biol. Reprod. 7, 458–464.
Raghunathan, R. and Arinze, I.J. (1977) Int. J. Biochem. 8, 737–743.
Reed, M. and Hounslow, W.F. (1971) J. Endocrinol. 49, 203–211.
Robens, J.F. (1969) Toxicol. Appl. Pharmacol. 15, 152–163.
Roberts, C.M. and Perry, J.S. (1974) in Biology of Hystricomorph Rodents (Rowlands, I.W. and Weir, B.J., eds.), pp. 333–360, Academic Press, London.
Robinson, B.H. (1976) Biol. Neonate 29, 48–55.
Rowlands, I.W. (1949) J. Hyg. 47, 281–287.
Schenker, S., Dawber, N.H. and Schmid, R. (1964) J. Clin. Invest. 43, 32–39.
Schenker, S., Goldstein, J. and Combes, B. (1965) Am. J. Physiol. 208, 563–572.
Schmidt, M. (1929) Kunst und Kultur von Peru, Propyläen Verlag, Berlin.
Short, C.R., Kinden, D.A. and Stith, R. (1976) Drug. Metab. Rev. 5, 1–42.
Singer, P.R., Scibetta, J.J. and Rosen, M.G. (1973) Am. J. Obs. Gyn. 117, 331–340.
Sisk, D.B. (1976) in Biology of the Guinea Pig (Wagner, J.E. and Manning, P.J., eds.), pp. 63–98, Academic Press, New York.
Skerfving, S.B. and Copplestone, J.F. (1976) Bull. W.H.O. 54, 101–112.
Smith, J.H., McCormack, K.M., Brazelton, W.E. and Hook, J.B. (1983) Environ. Res. 30, 63–71.
Sonawane, B.R. (1982) Ped. Pharmacol. 2, 223–229.
Spector, S. (1956) in Handbook of Biological Data (Spector, S., ed.), p. 50, W.B. Saunders, Co., Philadelphia, PA.
Spyker, J. and Smithberg, M. (1972) Teratology 5, 181–187.
Stockard, C.R. and Papanicolaou, G.N. (1917) Am. J. Anat. 22, 225–283.
Stockard, C.R. and Papanicolaou, G.N. (1919) Biol. Bull. 37, 222–245.
Wachstein, M. and Bradshaw, M. (1965) J. Histochem. Cytochem. 13, 44–56.
Wagner, J.E. (1976) in Biology of the Guinea Pig (Wagner, J.E. and Manning, P.J., eds.), pp. 1–4, Academic Press, New York.

Weil, C.S., Woodside, M.D., Bernard, J.B., Condra, N.I., King, J.M. and Carpenter, C.P. (1973) Toxicol. Appl. Pharmacol. 26, 621–638.
Weir, B.J. (1974) in Biology of Hystricomorph Rodents (Rowlands, I. W. and Weir, B.J., eds.), pp. 437–446, Academic Press, London.
Wender, M. and Waligora, Z. (1961) J. Neurochem. 7, 259–263.
Wender, M. and Waligora, Z. (1964) J. Neurochem, 11, 243–246.
Whelan, G., Hoch, J., Schenker, S. and Combes, B. (1970) J. Lab. Clin. Med. 70, 775–789.
Wilson, J.T., Brown, R.D., Cherek, D.R., Dailey, J.W., Hilman, B., Jobe, P.C., Manno, B.R., Manno, J.E., Redetzki, H.M. and Stewart, J. J. (1980) Clin. Pharmacokin. 5, 1–66.
Wong, C.T. and Morgan, E.H. (1973) Q. J. Exp. Physiol. Cog. Med. Sci. 58, 47–58.
Wright, S. (1960) J. Cell. Comp. Physiol. 56, 123–151.
Young, W.C., Dempsey, E.W. and Myers, H.I. (1935) J. Comp. Physiol. Psychol. 19, 313–335.
Young, W.C., Dempsey, E.W., Hagquist, C.W. and Boling, J.L. (1939) J. Comp. Physiol. Psychol. 27, 49–68.
Zarrow, M.X. (1947) Proc. Soc. Exp. Biol. Med. 66, 488–491.

S. Kacew and M.J. Reasor (eds), *Toxicology and the Newborn*
© 1984 Elsevier Science Publishers B.V.

Chapter 3

Effects of Cationic Amphiphilic Drugs on the Developing Animal

MARK J. REASOR[a], SAM KACEW[b] and DEBRA L. THOMA-LAURIE[c]

[a]*Department of Pharmacology and Toxicology, West Virginia University Medical Center, Morgantown, WV 26506, U.S.A.*, [b]*Department of Pharmacology, School of Medicine, University of Ottawa, Ottawa, Ontario, K1H 8M5, Canada and* [c]*Syntex, Inc., Palo Alto, CA 94304, U.S.A.*

CONTENTS

I. INTRODUCTION

The repeated administration of a number of cationic amphiphilic drugs to animals, and in certain cases also humans, leads to the appearance of abnormal inclusions in many of the tissues of the body (Lüllmann-Rauch, 1979). This phenomenon has been studied extensively in the adult, while, in contrast, relatively little has been reported concerning the development of the disorder in the fetus or newborn. The purpose of this chapter is to examine this response to cationic amphiphilic drugs following in utero exposure or administration to the newborn. Comparisons of the sensitivities of these age groups and the adult will be presented where studied. In order to introduce the reader to this area, the initial discussion will present information obtained following drug administration to the adult.

II. MORPHOLOGIC CHARACTERISTICS

When examined with the electron microscope, the drug-induced inclusions appear either lamellated, reticular or crystalloid in nature (Lüllmann-Rauch, 1979). Their prevalence is a function of the drug used and the tissue studied; they are often found in the same cell and may occur in the same inclusion. In general, the lamellar inclusions are the most common and consist of membranous material arranged in a concentric pattern. The lamellated material may display a simple periodicity of 40–50 angstroms or a more complex arrangement and may be unicentric or multicentric in configuration.

Because phospholipids assume a lamellar configuration in an aqueous environment (Stoeckenius, 1962), it was initially assumed that the inclusions were rich in phospholipids, and subsequently this was confirmed biochemically (Matsuzawa and Hostetler, 1980a). Accordingly, increases in whole-tissue phospholipid levels are demonstrable (Yamamoto et al., 1971; Seiler and Wassermann, 1975; Kacew, 1982).

Ultrastructural evidence indicates that the aberrant inclusions arise from lysosomes. The structures contain acid phosphatase activity and concentrate material phagocytized by the cell (Vijeyaratnam and Corrin, 1972; Lüllmann-Rauch, 1979; Matsuzawa and Hostetler, 1980a). In addition, electron microscopic studies have shown inclusions transforming from the electron-dense lysosomal matrix to the lamellar configuration (Reasor, 1981). Following their administration to rats and examination of the liver, chloroquine and diethylaminoethoxyhexestrol (two cationic amphiphilic drugs) have been shown to concentrate only in the lysosomes, which also was the only subcellular fraction where an elevation in phospholipid content occurred (Matsuzawa and Hostetler, 1980a, b). Evidence is, therefore, compelling that this drug-induced disorder is lysosomal in origin.

III. MECHANISMS OF INDUCTION OF PHOSPHOLIPIDOSIS

A list of drugs shown to induce a phospholipidosis in adult animals or humans is presented in Table 1. While belonging to a wide range of therapeutic classes, these

TABLE 1

CATIONIC AMPHIPHILIC DRUGS CAUSING PHOSPHOLIPIDOSIS IN ANIMALS AND HUMANS

Class/drug	Representative references	Class/drug	Representative references
Anorectic		Tranquilizer	
Chlorphentermine	1–3	AC-3579	27, 28
Cloforex	4		
Fenfluramine	5	Interferon inducer	
		S3458-0	29
Antidepressant		Tilorone	29
1-Chloramitriptyline	6		
1-Chloro-10,11-dehydroamitriptyline	6	Cholesterol biosynthesis inhibitor	
Imipramine	6	AY-9944	14, 15
Iprindole	7, 8	Boxidine	11
Maprotiline	9	Haloperidol	11
Zimelidine	10	Triparanol	11
Chlorimipramine	52	20,25-diazacholesterol	15
Antihistaminic		Antimalarial, antiinflammatory	
Chlorcyclizine	11–13	Chloroquine	16, 17
Cyclizine	11	Mepacrine	18, 19
Norchlorcyclizine	11		
Homochlorcyclizine	11	Antianginal	
Hydroxyzine	11	Amiodarone	10, 20
Meclizine	11	Perhexiline	21
Coronary vasodilator		Antiestrogenic	
4, 4′-Diethylaminoethoxy-hexestrol	17, 24	Tamoxifen	22
		Serotonin uptake inhibitor	
Antithrombotic		Fluoxetine	23
RMI 10.393	25		
		Secretolytic	
Neuroleptic		Bromhexine	50
Clozapine	26	Ambroxol	50
Schistosomicidal		Antibiotic	
IA-3	26	Gentamicin	51

References: 1, Franken et al. (1970); 2, Kacew and Narbaitz (1977); 3, Reasor et al. (1979); 4, Magnusson and Magnusson (1972); 5, Lüllmann-Rauch and Reil (1974a); 6, Lüllmann-Rauch and Scheid (1975); 7, Vijeyaratnam and Corrin (1974); 8, McNulty and Reasor (1981b); 9, Stäubli et al. (1978); 10, Bockhardt et al. (1978); 11, Hruban et al. (1972); 12, Reasor et al. (1982);13, Kacew (1982); 14, Hill and Greselin (1967); 15, Dietert and Scallen (1969); 16, Nelson and Fitzhugh (1948); 17, Matsuzawa and Hostetler (1980a); 18, Staiger (1974); 19, Gidion and Wassermann (1978); 20, Marchlinski et al. (1982); 21, Lhermitte et al. (1976); 22, Lüllmann and Lüllmann-Rauch (1981); 23, Wold et al. (1976); 24, Yamamoto et al. (1971); 25, Karabelnik et al. (1974); 26, Haussenpflug (1976); 27, Ghys et al. (1975); 28, Laurent et al. (1975); 29, Thelmo and Levine (1978); 30, Lüllmann-Rauch and Stoermer (1982); 31, Shikata et al. (1972); 32, Fedorka (1967); 33, Lüllmann-Rauch (1975a); 34, Sakuragawa et al. (1977); 35, Lüllmann-Rauch (1974); 36, Pühlhorn and Theil (1976); 37, Hendry et al. (1969); 38, Drenckhahn (1977); 39, Kacew and Narbaitz (1981a, b); 40, Drenckhahn and Lüllmann-Rauch (1977); 41, Seiler and Wassermann (1975); 42, De la Iglesia et al. (1974); 43, Gloster et al. (1976); 44, Reasor (1981); 45, Hruban et al. (1965); 46, Elleder et al. (1977); 47, Klinghardt (1974); 48, Drenckhahn and Lüllmann-Rauch (1976); 49, Fischer and Nelson (1974); 50, Von Wichert et al. (1977); 51, Kosek et al. (1974); 52, Sgaragli et al. (1983).

drugs have a similar chemical characteristic; they are cationic and amphiphilic in nature. Physicochemically, the molecule contains both a hydrophobic portion and a cationic hydrophilic region. The hydrophobic component of the molecule consists of a ring system which is usually aromatic but may contain both aromatic and aliphatic moieties. The ring system is often substituted with a halogen atom, making the molecule even more amphiphilic. The hydrophilic property resides in a nitrogen group which is highly charged at physiological pH (Lüllmann and Wehling, 1979).

The induction of a phospholipidosis in tissues appears to occur as a result of an inhibition of catabolism of phospholipids arising either intra- or extracellularly. Cationic amphiphilic drugs have been shown in vitro to inhibit the activities of lysosomal phospholipases (Matsuzawa and Hostetler, 1980c; Hostetler and Matsuzawa, 1981), but it is not clear as to whether this occurs as a result of drug interaction with the enzymes or with the phospholipids (the latter resulting in the formation of an indigestible complex). Under in vitro conditions, certain of these drugs do interact with phospholipids (Lüllmann and Wehling, 1979; Seydel and Wassermann, 1976); however, the extent of inhibition of hydrolysis of phospholipids by phospholipase A does not appear to correlate with the affinity of the drugs for the lipids (Lüllmann and Wehling, 1979; Pappu and Hostetler, 1984).

There is no indication that the storage of phospholipids is due to a deficiency of lysosomal enzymes, as occurs with the inborn lysosomal storage diseases; however, in one study, Sakuragawa et al., (1977) reported a reduction in sphingomyelinase activity in the livers of rats treated with AY-9944. It was suggested by these authors that the reduction in activity was due to impaired enzyme synthesis.

Additional factors may be involved in the accumulation of phospholipids within the cell. As cationic amphiphilic drugs accumulate within the lysosome, the molecule becomes protonated (Lüllmann et al., 1978). As this occurs, the level of protons may diminish sufficiently to raise the pH within the organelle, as demonstrated in macrophages (Okuma and Poole, 1978) and fibroblasts (Hollemans et al., 1981). If the pH is elevated enough to impair acid phospholipase catabolic activity, phospholipids could accumulate. An increase or redirection in synthesis may also contribute to the elevated tissue content of phospholipids (Brindley et al., 1975).

1. Potency

The ability of cationic amphiphilic drugs to produce tissue phospholipidosis is dependent on certain pharmacokinetic factors as well as on physicochemical characteristics of the molecules. It has been established that the amphiphilic nature of the drug plays a role in the degree of phospholipidosis seen (Lüllmann et al., 1975; Lüllmann-Rauch, 1979). Of possibly greater importance are factors such as absorption, retention, metabolism and/or excretion of the compounds administered. The potency of certain amphiphilic drugs to induce phospholipidosis in various tissues has been compared by numerous investigators (for review, see Lüllmann-Rauch, 1979).

TABLE 2

TISSUES IN WHICH PHOSPHOLIPIDOSIS HAS BEEN INDUCED BY CATIONIC AMPHIPHILIC DRUGS

Tissue	Representative references	Tissue	Representative references
Adenohypophysis	30	Liver	9, 41, 42
Adrenals	5, 15, 31	Lung	16, 43, 44
Blood cells	31, 33	Lymphatics	5, 22, 31
Bone marrow	31	Neurohypophysis	22
Central nervous system	22, 34, 35	Pancreas	31, 45
Cornea	36	Peripheral nervous system	46, 47
Corpus luteum	5	Retina	22, 34
Heart	31, 37	Skeletal muscle	48
Inner ear	38	Spleen	5, 31, 34
Kidney	29, 31, 39	Testis	11, 15
Lens	34, 40	Vascular endothelium	49

For references, see Table 1.

2. *Additional factors*

Amphiphilic drug-induced phospholipidosis is a generalized phenomenon occurring in a variety of mammalian species and tissues. A list of tissues in which this drug-induced disorder has been observed is presented in Table 2. The fact that a phospholipidosis is induced in virtually all tissues in which cells are engaged in phagocytic activity and in which there is active lipid metabolism may account for the widespread appearance of this disorder in the organism. However, this phenomenon is not universal and certain exceptions, which still remain unexplained, have been reported. For example, rat liver, a major site of lipid metabolism, appears relatively unresponsive to the phospholipidotic effect of chlorphentermine (Lüllmann-Rauch and Reil, 1973). In contrast, chlorphentermine induces a phospholipidosis in other rat tissues, including lung, kidney, adrenal, testes, etc. (Lüllmann et al., 1975). Why the liver of rat responds in a distinctly different manner is not known, as chlorphentermine does produce hepatic phospholipidosis in mouse, rabbit and guinea pig (Lüllmann-Rauch and Reil, 1973; Lüllmann-Rauch and Stoermer, 1982).

The extent and degree of drug-induced phospholipidosis is species-dependent. Although this disorder has been reported to occur in rat, mouse, guinea pig, rabbit, dog and pig, and in both sexes where studied, differences in morphologic responsiveness exist. In the case of pulmonary tissue, a phospholipidosis is readily induced with chlorpentermine in the lungs of rats, but only weakly, if at all, in rabbit (Lüllmann-Rauch and Reil, 1974b; Reasor and Walker, 1979). Mice and guinea pigs are intermediate between these two species in their pulmonary sensitivity to this disorder. Among species, the response observed in the lung is qualitatively different than that seen in the adrenals. Rabbits show a pronounced induction of phospholipidosis in the adrenal cortex while in the mouse this tissue is affected much less severely.

Although it has not received much attention, another factor which may play a role in the development of a drug-induced phospholipidosis is the sex of the organism. The tricyclic antidepressant imipramine was reported to induce a phospholipidosis in lungs of adult rats of either sex (Lüllmann-Rauch and Scheid, 1975). However, the extent or degree of differences in phospholipidosis between sexes was not indicated. In a recent study, Ginsburg et al. (1982) demonstrated that the uptake and retention of imipramine and desmethylimipramine in lung was several-fold higher in females compared to males. It is conceivable that phospholipidosis is dependent on tissue drug concentrations, and thus the degree of morphologic change may differ qualitatively and quantitatively in females and males.

3. *Functional consequences*

Although the phospholipidosis occurs in many tissues of the adult, the effects on organ or cellular function have not been studied extensively. Chlorphentermine-induced phospholipidosis in rat lung results in an impairment in clearance of inhaled particles from this tissue (Ferin, 1982). When the function of macrophages isolated from drug-treated rats was studied divergent effects were noted, depending on the length of treatment. The administration of chlorphentermine for 2–3 days leads to an impairment of phagocytosis by macrophages in vitro (Lehnert and Ferin, 1983). In contrast, treatment of rats for 4 weeks with either chlorphentermine or iprindole results in an activation of the cells, as seen by an enhanced respiratory burst activity and increased phagocytic and bactericidal function (McNulty and Reasor, 1981a, b).

The induction of phospholipidosis in rat kidney by chlorphentermine is associated with an impairment in renal function (Lüllmann et al., 1981). Affected rats had decreased abilities to concentrate and dilute the urine. In addition, a rise in plasma urea level occurred.

IV. EXPOSURE OF THE FETUS TO CATIONIC AMPHIPHILIC DRUGS

1. *Induction of phospholipidosis*

The administration of either chlorphentermine, chlorcyclizine or chloroquine to pregnant animals or AY-9944 directly into the fetus leads to the development of a phospholipidosis in many tissues of the offspring whether the affected animal is examined pre- or postpartum. Table 3 lists studies where this phenomenon has been reported.

Several points are apparent from these studies. Under a variety of treatment schedules, a phospholipidosis can be induced in the fetuses of three animal species. Relatively short treatment periods are effective since only 2 days after intra-fetal injection of AY-9944 lamellar inclusions appeared in the lungs of fetal rabbits

(Kikkawa and Motoyama, 1973). In addition, administration of chlorphentermine to pregnant rats during only the last 5 days of gestation resulted in a pronounced phospholipidosis in lungs of offspring when the animals were examined during the first day after birth (Thoma-Laurie et al., 1982, 1983). Lamellar inclusions were observed in many pulmonary cell types, and the newborn lungs contained about 35% more phospholipid (on a dry weight basis) than did lungs from newborns whose mothers had received vehicle while pregnant. Of the individual phospholipid classes examined, the relative proportions of each remained about the same, with only disaturated phosphatidylcholine showing a significant increase over controls.

As in the adult, many tissues are affected by prepartum exposure to cationic amphiphilic drugs (Table 3). The degree of induction of the disorder is probably a function of the retention of the drug by the tissue and the level of phospholipid metabolism occurring at that time in development.

Where comparisons have been made, maternal prepartum drug treatment leads to a more severe phospholipidosis in the tissues of the dam than in the offspring (Lüllmann-Rauch and Stoermer, 1982; Thoma-Laurie et al., 1983). This difference is probably due to several factors, including differences in phospholipid metabolism in mature versus fetal tissues. Also, a lower drug concentration may be present in fetal tissues than in maternal tissues because of initial maternal uptake or elimination of some of the drug prior to it reaching the placenta (Thoma-Laurie et al., 1983).

TABLE 3

INDUCTION OF PHOSPHOLIPIDOSIS BY IN UTERO EXPOSURE TO CATIONIC AMPHIPHILIC DRUGS

Drug	Species	Tissue affected	Reference
Chlorphentermine	Rat	Lungs, heart	Lüllmann-Rauch (1973)
	Rat	Brain, viscera	Adachi et al. (1976)
	Rat	Lungs	Thoma-Laurie (1982), Thoma-Laurie et al. (1982, 1983)
	Rat and guinea pig	Lungs, liver, kidney, spleen, adenohypophysis, adrenal glands, spinal cord, neurohypophysis, hypothalmus	Lüllmann-Rauch and Stoermer (1982)
Chlorcyclizine	Rat	Lungs, liver, kidney spleen, adenohypophysis, adrenal glands, spinal cord neurohypophysis, hypothalmus	Lüllmann-Rauch and Stoermer (1982)
Chloroquine	Rat	Adenohypophysis, adrenal glands, spinal cord, hypothalmus	Lüllmann-Rauch and Stoermer (1982)
AY-9944	Rabbit	Lungs	Kikkawa and Motoyama (1973)

2. *Toxicological manifestations*

The prepartum maternal administration of chlorphentermine or AY-9944 results in toxicity to the offspring. In the case of AY-9944, a decrease in fetal body weight of rabbits was noted (Kikkawa and Motoyama, 1973), while treatment with chlorphentermine resulted in lower body weights of newborn rats when compared to the offspring of vehicle-treated rats (Thoma-Laurie et al., 1982). Within 24–48 hours of birth most of the neonates exposed to chlorphentermine had died (Adachi et al., 1976; Thoma-Laurie et al., 1982). In contrast, treatment of newborn rats with chlorphentermine resulted in no overt signs of toxicity to the animals (Kacew and Narbaitz, 1977; Kacew, 1982).

Thoma-Laurie et al. (1982) examined the mortality response to prepartum chlorphentermine in an attempt to understand the mechanisms by which death occurred. Cross-fostering studies indicated that abnormal maternal behavior was not involved in the neonatal mortality. Approximately 1 hour after birth, litters from chlorphentermine-treated dams were placed with control dams, and vice versa. Even when placed with control dams, the same incidence of mortality still occurred in the litters exposed to chlorphentermine. Control litters showed no mortality when placed with chlorphentermine-treated dams. Additionally, the drug-induced mortality was not due to starvation from lack of neonatal feeding.

The possibility of a direct effect of chlorphentermine on the fetus was examined (Thoma-Laurie, 1982). Prior to death, neonates were observed gasping for breath, indicating that an impairment in pulmonary function may have contributed to the mortality. Since biochemical changes occurred in the lungs as a result of chlorphentermine treatment, pulmonary maturation may have been affected such that, following birth, the neonates failed to maintain adequate respiration. By certain biochemical criteria, the lungs of affected neonates were mature; their glycogen levels were the same as controls and the content of disaturated phosphatidylcholine, the major surface-active lipid in the lungs, in fact was elevated over that present in control neonates. In contrast, the level of surface-active material was lower in the amniotic fluid of drug-treated mothers when measured 1 day prior to term, indicating that there may be an impairment in the secretion of this essential material.

Glucocorticoids are believed to be important in the maturation of the lung in vivo, which allows the newborn to survive outside the womb (Liggins and Howie, 1972; Murphy, 1973). When dexamethasone was administered to pregnant rats concurrently with chlorphentermine, neonatal mortality was reduced but not prevented totally (Thoma-Laurie, 1982). Following dexamethasone treatment, the level of surface-active material was increased in the amniotic fluid of chlorphentermine-treated females; however, not to the level found in controls. These results indicated that diminished prepartum release of surface-active material into the alveolar spaces of the lung may have resulted in compromised pulmonary gas exchange and thus contributed to the neonatal mortality of rats exposed in utero to chlorphentermine. In addition to biochemical changes in the lungs of affected neonates, regions of the lungs appeared atelectic at 12 hours postpartum. This lack of inflation is consistent with an impairment in maturation of the lungs as a result of exposure to chlorphentermine.

Kikkawa and Motoyama (1973) reported a similar apparent discrepancy (a retardation in lung development in light of elevated surfactant in the lung) following the injection of AY-9944 directly into the fetus. The drug was administered to fetal rabbits on gestational day 24 and the fetuses examined on day 26 (full term being 30 days). Morphologically, maturation of the lungs appeared to cease completely during the time of drug treatment. However, there was an increased accumulation of lamellar bodies in type II cells, indicating elevated surfactant levels within the cell. Concurrently, a striking increase in the amount of membranous material was present in the alveolar spaces; no biochemical measurements were made, however, to assess the levels of surface-active lipids in the lungs of the AY-9944-treated fetuses.

In addition to alterations in the morphological appearance of the neonatal rat lung following in utero exposure to chlorphentermine, Thoma-Laurie (1982) reported the presence of pathological change. In some, but not all, animals damage was present in the arterioles of the lungs. At the light microscopic level, this had the appearance of a vacuolization of the endothelial cells. When examined by electron microscopy the endothelial cells were partially detached from the basement membrane, resulting in spaces between the two structures. The cells protruded noticeably into the arteriolar lumen. Whether these changes in the arterioles contributed to the neonatal death is unknown.

The relationship between the development of the pulmonary phospholipidosis and the neonatal mortality is unclear. The observation that the prepartum administration of phentermine, a cationic amphiphilic drug structurally and pharmacologically related to chlorphentermine, to rats does not induce a pulmonary phospholipidosis nor cause neonatal mortality (Thoma-Laurie et al., 1982) indicates that this association needs further investigation.

V. ADMINISTRATION OF CATIONIC AMPHIPHILIC DRUGS TO NEWBORNS

l. Induction of phospholipidosis

In addition to observing phospholipidosis in newborns following in utero exposure to cationic amphiphilic drugs, this disorder can be induced by direct administration of the drugs to newborns. Table 4 lists the compounds and tissues in which this phenomenon has been reported. While Adachi et al. (1976) found the presence of foam cells in livers of newborn rats administered chlorphentermine for 12 weeks, no apparent ultrastructural alterations were observed in hepatic tissue in animals given this drug for 3 weeks (Kacew and Narbaitz, unpublished data). In contrast to liver, Kacew et al. (1978, 1981a) demonstrated the presence of a foam cell reaction in lung and kidney after a 1-week treatment. As in the case of adults, data suggest that newborn rat liver appears less susceptible to the morphologic action of chlorphentermine than are lung and kidney. In addition to differences in susceptibility of organs

TABLE 4

MORPHOLOGIC AND METABOLIC ALTERATIONS, IN NEWBORNS, INDUCED BY CATIONIC AMPHIPHILIC DRUGS

Drug	Species	Tissue affected	Reference
Chlorphentermine	Rat	CNS, liver	Adachi et al. (1976)
		Lung	Kacew et al. (1979)
		Kidney	Kacew and Narbaitz (1981a)
		Liver	Kacew and Calderwood (1980)
	Mouse	Peripheral nerve, spinal cord	Anzil et al. (1977)
Chlorcyclizine	Rat	Lung	Kacew (1982)
AY-9944	Mouse	Peripheral nerve	Rawlins and Uzman (1970)
	Rat	Peripheral nerve	Suzuki and DePaul (1972)
		Lung	Kikkawa and Suzuki (1977)
		Liver	Sakuragawa et al. (1977)
Triparanol	Rat	Nervous system	Schutta and Neville (1968)

within one species to drug-induced phospholipidosis, there is variation between amphiphilic drugs in their ability to induce morphologic responses. In a comparative study between chlorphentermine and chlorcyclizine, Kacew (1982) reported that both drugs produced an accumulation of hypertrophic macrophages in the lungs. However, the degree of phospholipidosis as based on a foam cell quantitation was far greater with chlorphentermine. It is of interest that Lüllmann-Rauch and Stoermer (1982) demonstrated that the susceptibility of adult rat lung to ultrastructural changes produced by chlorcyclizine was quantitatively less than that observed with chlorphentermine.

2. *Morphologic comparison to adults*

Extensive studies have demonstrated that administration of chlorphentermine results in an accumulation of masses of foam cells in pulmonary alveoli and kidneys of adult rats (Lüllmann et al., 1975; Lüllmann-Rauch, 1975b). In order to compare the ultrastructural changes observed in mature rodents with those in newborns, 1-day-old rat pups were administered orally chlorphentermine (20 or 60 mg/kg/day) for 1 week. No or few hypertrophic macrophages were apparent in lungs and kidneys, respectively, of newborns receiving the lower dose of this amphiphilic agent (Kacew, 1984). In contrast to neonates, numerous macrophages were present in lungs from all adult rats treated for 1 week with 20 mg/kg chlorphentermine. Karabelnik et al. (1974) also reported that treatment with 20 mg/kg/day chlorphentermine for 8 days produced a massive foam cell reaction in lungs of mature rats. Data thus suggest that developing rats may be less susceptible to the cytological effects of chlorphentermine. Regardless of age, the chlorphentermine-induced foam cell reaction was dependent on dose. It is of interest that differences in the morphologic responsiveness of newborns compared to adults has also been reported in animals exposed to ozone (Ospital et al., 1977), oxygen (Bonikos et al., 1976), nitrogen dioxide (Freeman et al., 1974) and thiourea (Dieke and Richter, 1945).

Kacew and Narbaitz (1981a) found that treatment of newborns with either 20 or 60 mg/kg/day phentermine, doses which do not induce a phospholipidosis in adults, for 7 days produced no apparent alteration in lung morphology, a response opposite to that noted in chlorphentermine-treated pups. Daily administration of both doses of phentermine significantly reduced the incorporation of thymidine into newborn lung DNA, a metabolic pattern of response found to differ from that reported for chlorphentermine. Thus, these data show that morphologic and metabolic changes produced in newborn lung are also dependent on the chemical structure of the amphiphilic agent. In studies with the amphiphilic agent chlorcyclizine, comparative responses between newborn and adult yielded results that differed from those observed with chlorphentermine. Recently, Kacew (1982) demonstrated that a 1-week daily treatment of 60 mg/kg chlorcyclizine produced an accumulation of hypertrophic macrophages in newborn lung. In contrast, the same treatment failed to produce an apparent change in adult lung morphology. However, extension of this treatment regimen to 2 weeks resulted in the development of a foam cell reaction in adult lung. The observation that the development of foam cells was greater in newborns compared to adults indicated that newborns seemed more susceptible to this morphologic action of chlorcyclizine. Irrespective of age, the chlorcyclizine-induced accumulation of pulmonary hypertrophic macrophages was both dose- and time-dependent.

3. *Biochemical studies*

The chlorphentermine- or chlorcyclizine-induced accumulation of foam cells was associated with phospholipid accumulation in lung. In newborn lung, both drugs were equally effective in producing a rise in pulmonary total phospholipid (TPL) and phosphatidylcholine (PC) levels after 1 week. Extension of chlorcyclizine administration to 14 days also increased TPL and PC without a change in other individual phospholipid classes examined. However, in the case of chlorphentermine not only were TPL and PC increased but there was also a rise in the levels of sphingomyelin (S), phosphatidylserine (PS) plus phosphatidylinositol (PI) as well as phosphatidylethanolamine (PE) plus phosphatidylglycerol (PG). A similar elevation in all phospholipid classes examined and in TPL occurred in adult rat lung following chlorphentermine treatment (Kacew and Reasor, 1983). Several other investigators also demonstrated that, in addition to TPL and PC, chlorphentermine elevated the levels of S, PS, PI, PE and PG in adult rat lung (Schmien et al., 1974; Karabelnik and Zbinden, 1975; Gloster et al., 1976). As in the case of newborns, chlorcyclizine produced a time-related increase only in TPL and PC levels in adult lung. The finding that chlorcyclizine appeared to elevate only TPL and PC while chlorphentermine increased all individual phospholipid classes examined suggests that the metabolic actions exerted by these compounds on lung may differ. It is of interest that Kacew (1982, 1984) demonstrated that the morphologic responsiveness of lung to these amphiphilic agents also differed.

In newborns, morphological changes in a tissue are not always accompanied by biochemical alterations. While lamellar inclusions were observed in newborn rat brain and liver after 12 weeks of chlorphentermine treatment, no increase in TPL was evident (Adachi et al., 1976). The possibility exists that inclusions occurred only in specific areas of the brain and liver and that use of whole tissue was inappropriate to relate TPL content with morphological change at a specific site.

In mammalian lung glycogen is believed to be a major source of carbohydrate substrate utilized in the synthesis of PC, and glycogen depletion is sequentially followed by increased PC synthesis. Treatment with chlorphentermine was found to increase PC and TPL without a significant change in newborn lung glycogen. Similarly, the chlorphentermine-induced increase in pulmonary TPL in adult rats occurred without a marked change in glycogen. In contrast to chlorphentermine, the chlorcyclizine-stimulated rise in lung PC was accompanied by a fall in glycogen levels. These data, in agreement with the findings of Brehier and Rooney (1981), indicate that glycogen degradation in lung may not simply serve in the role of precursor for the product TPL.

Proliferation of cells is a common, unspecific result of chemical-inflicted injury to the lung, kidneys and liver and has been reported to be associated with increased DNA synthesis and elevation in cyclic AMP levels. Kacew and Narbaitz (1977, 1978) demonstrated that the chlorphentermine-induced rise in cyclic AMP was accompanied by an elevation in thymidine incorporation into adult rat lung DNA. However, in newborn rats treated with chlorphentermine an increase in pulmonary cell number and incorporation of thymidine into DNA was associated with no marked change in cyclic AMP levels (Kacew and Narbaitz, 1981b). In contrast, the chlorphentermine-induced increase in renal lamellar inclusions was associated with enhanced incorporation of thymidine into kidney DNA and elevated cyclic AMP levels (Kacew and Narbaitz, 1981a; Kacew and Calderwood, 1980). At present, the basis for the divergence in responsiveness between tissues is not known. However, the finding that the butylated hydroxytoluene-stimulated increase in mouse lung DNA synthesis was also accompanied by no marked change in cyclic AMP levels (Witschi et al., 1976) supports the view that cyclic AMP may not serve as a necessary trigger for chlorphentermine-induced DNA synthesis in newborn lung. The observation that chlorphentermine stimulated thymidine incorporation into hepatic DNA without an associated morphologic change (Kacew and Calderwood, 1980; Lüllmann-Rauch and Stoermer, 1982) suggests that estimation of DNA synthesis appears to be a more sensitive indicator of drug-induced effects on liver. Further support for the view that cyclic AMP may not play a role as a modulator of DNA synthesis was the finding that chlorphentermine decreased cyclic nucleotide levels in newborn liver (Kacew and Calderwood, 1980).

VI. PHARMACOLOGICAL MANIPULATIONS

1. *Interaction between chlorphentermine and phenobarbital*

The chlorphentermine-induced accumulation of masses of foam cells in pulmonary alveoli and kidney is modified by phenobarbital (Kacew and Narbaitz, 1981a; Kacew et al., 1981a). Daily treatment of newborn rats with 60 mg/kg chlorphentermine for 1 week resulted in a development of foam cells in lung and kidney. However, in rat pups concurrently administered chlorphentermine and phenobarbital for 7 days, the foam cell reaction was reduced or prevented. In addition to reduction and/or prevention of the morphologic effect of chlorphentermine on newborn lung, phenobarbital produced an increase in the activity of pulmonary aminopyrine *N*-demethylase (Kacew et al., 1981a). It was suggested that phenobarbital may have provided protection against chlorphentermine-induced pulmonary phospholipidosis through stimulation of drug-metabolizing enzymes, leading to an enhanced conversion of chlorphentermine to metabolites ineffective in inducing the disorder. It is of interest that phenobarbital also blocked the chlorphentermine-stimulated increase in foam cell accumulation in adult lung and kidney (Svendsen, 1977; Kacew et al., 1981b). The observed effect in lung was associated with stimulation in the drug-metabolizing enzyme aminopyrine *N*-demethylase. In a subsequent study, Kacew and Reasor (1983) demonstrated that phenobarbital also prevented the chlorphentermine-stimulated rise in pulmonary PC and TPL levels in adult rats.

2. *Effect of withdrawal*

In order to examine whether the chlorphentermine-induced accumulation of pulmonary and renal hypertrophic macrophages was reversible, newborn rats were administered 60 mg/kg/day anorectic for 1 week and subsequently maintained without additional treatment for 7 or 14 days. Kacew et al. (1979) demonstrated that a 7-day withdrawal from drug treatment in rat pups previously given chlorphentermine resulted in a marked reduction in the number of hypertrophic macrophages. Complete disappearance of these cells from pulmonary alveoli occurred after a 2-week recovery period, indicating that the chlorphentermine-induced cytological alterations were reversible upon drug withdrawal. In addition to the disappearance of drug-induced morphologic alterations, withdrawal from treatment results in a return of elevated DNA synthesis to approximate control levels in lung. It was observed that the chlorphentermine-stimulated increase in incorporation of thymidine into renal and hepatic DNA of newborns also returns to normal upon drug cessation (Kacew et al., 1978). Similarly, recovery of adult rats for 2 weeks after an initial chlorphentermine treatment resulted in a clearance of pulmonary lipid histiocytes from lung (Woodward, 1981). Recently, Kacew and Reasor (1983) reported that a 7-day recovery from chlorphentermine treatment in adult rats previously injected with drug for 2 weeks resulted in a return to control in the levels of pulmonary PC and TPL. It is of interest that the chlorphentermine-induced phospholipidosis in alveolar macrophages also disappeared by 2 weeks after cessation of drug administration (Reasor and Koshut, 1980). Evidence thus indicates that the chlorphentermine-induced morphologic and metabolic changes in lung, liver and kidney are reversible in both newborn and adult rat. In general, it takes 2 or more weeks for tissues to appear morphologically and metabolically indistinguishable from controls. It has been postulated that following cessation of drug administration, the equilibrium favors movement of drug from tissue (Lüllmann et al., 1978). As the putative drug-lipid complex is eliminated, the phospholipids are free to undergo metabolism, with a subsequent return to normal in tissue phospholipid content.

3. *Effect of hyperoxia*

In view of the fact that neonates are less susceptible to the toxic actions of high concentrations of oxygen on lung (Bonikos et al., 1976) and hyperoxygenation is known to modify drug-induced pulmonary changes (Witschi and Côté, 1977), it was of interest to examine the interaction between chlorphentermine and hyperoxygenation on pulmonary morphology. Exposure to hyperoxia for 3 days or administration of 20 mg/kg/day chlorphentermine for 1 week produced no apparent phospholipidotic changes in newborn lung (Kacew and Narbaitz, 1980; Kacew et al., 1981c). However, in newborns exposed to 95% O_2 for 3 days followed by chlorphentermine for 1 week or in rat pups simultaneously exposed to oxidant gas and drug for 3 days, an accumulation of hypertrophic macrophages occurred. These data thus demonstrated that hyperoxygenation modified the susceptibility of neonatal rat lung to the morphologic action of chlorphentermine. The lack of a morphological response of newborn lung to phentermine was not altered by hyperoxia (Kacew and Narbaitz, 1981b).

VII. CONCLUSIONS

It has been known for some time that the administration of certain cationic amphiphilic drugs to adult animals can result in a phospholipidosis in many tissues. It is now clear that this disorder can be induced in both the fetus and newborn as well. With prepartum treatment, the severity of the phospholipidosis in the offspring is less marked than found in the dam. When examined in newborns, the drug-induced response may be greater or less than in the adult, depending upon the agent studied. Treatment of newborns with cationic amphiphilic drugs for 1 week has no apparent adverse affect on their health. In contrast, in utero drug exposure can result in lethality to neonates within a short time after birth. It is, therefore, apparent that the response to cationic amphiphilic drugs is quantitatively and qualitatively different depending upon the age of the organism.

VIII. REFERENCES

Adachi, M., Tsai, C.Y., Greenbaum, M., Mask, B. and Volk, B.W. (1976) in Current Trend in Sphingolipidoses and Allied Disorders (Volk, B.W. and Schenck, L., eds.), pp. 429–451, Plenum Press, New York.

Anzil, A.P., Herrlinger, H. and Blinzinger, K. (1977) in Neurotoxicology (Roizin, L., Shiraki, H. and Grcevic, N., eds.), pp. 485–496, Raven Press, New York.

Bockhardt, H., Drenckhahn, D. and Lüllmann-Rauch, R. (1978) Verh. Anat. Ges. 72, 417–423.

Bonikos, D.S., Bensch, K.G. and Northway, W.H., Jr. (1976) Am. J. Pathol. 85, 623–650.

Brehier, A. and Rooney, S.A. (1981) Exp. Lung Res. 2, 273–287.

Brindley, D.N., Allan, D. and Mitchell, R.H. (1975) J. Pharm. Pharmacol. 27, 462–464.

De la Iglesia, F.A., Feuer, G., Takada, A. and Matsuda, Y. (1974) Lab. Invest. 30, 539–549.

Dieke, S.H. and Richter, C.P. (1945) J. Pharmacol. Exp. Ther. 83, 195–202.

Dietert, S.C. and Scallen, T.J. (1969) J. Cell Biol. 40, 44–60.

Drenckhahn, D. (1977) Virchows Arch. B. Cell Pathol. 23, 87–92.

Drenckhahn, D. and Lüllmann-Rauch, R. (1976) Virchows Arch. B. 20, 343–364.

Drenckhahn, D. and Lüllmann-Rauch, R. (1977) Exp. Eye Res. 24, 621–632.

Elleder, M., Jirasek, A. and Smid, F. (1977) Virchows Arch. B. 26, 93–96.

Fedorka, M.E. (1967) J. Clin. Invest. 46, 1932–1946.

Ferin, J. (1982) Exp. Lung Res. 4, 1–10.

Fischer, V.W. and Nelson, J.S. (1974) Acta Neuropathol. (Berl.) 29, 65–72.

Franken, G., Lüllmann, H. and Seigfriedt, A. (1970) Arzneim. Forsch. 20, 417.

Freeman, G., Juhos, L.T., Furiosi, N.J., Mussenden, R. and Weiss, T.A. (1974) Am. Rev. Respir. Dis. 110, 754–759.

Ghys, A., Thys, O., Hildebrand, J. and Georges, A. (1975) Toxicol. Appl. Pharmacol. 31, 13–20.

Gidion, U. and Wassermann, O. (1978) Naunyn-Schmiedeberg's Arch. Pharmacol. 302, R4.

Ginsburg, E., Hirokata, Y. and Gram, T.E. (1982) Life Sci. 30, 757–760.

Gloster, J., Heath, D., Hasleton, P. and Harris, P. (1976) Thorax 31, 558–564.

Haussenpflug, J. (1976) Naunyn-Schmiedeberg's Arch. Pharmacol. 293, R57.

Hendry, R.J., Abraham, R. and Grasso, P. (1969) J. Ultrastruct. Res. 29, 485–495.

Hill, P. and Greselin, E. (1967) Toxicol. Appl. Pharmacol. 11, 245–256.

Hollemans, M., Ellferink, R.O., DeGroot, G., Strijland, A. and Tager, J.M. (1981) Biochim. Biophys. Acta 643, 140–151.

Hostetler, K. and Matsuzawa, Y. (1981) Biochem. Pharmacol. 30, 1121–1126.

Hruban, Z., Swift, H. and Slesers, A. (1965) Lab. Invest. 14, 1652–1672.

Hruban, Z., Slesers, A. and Aschenbrenner, I. (1972) Toxicol. Appl. Pharmacol. 26, 72–85.

Kacew, S. (1982) Toxicol. Appl. Pharmacol. 65, 100–108.

Kacew, S. (1984) Fed. Proc., in press.

Kacew, S. and Calderwood, G.A., Jr. (1980) J. Toxicol. Environ. Hlth. 6, 141–154.

Kacew, S. and Narbaitz, R. (1977) Exp. Mol. Pathol. 27, 106–120.

Kacew, S. and Narbaitz, R. (1978) Fed. Proc. 37, 2489–2495.

Kacew, S. and Narbaitz, R. (1980) Experientia 36, 673–674.

Kacew, S. and Narbaitz, R. (1981a) Virchows Arch. Cell Pathol. 36, 59–63.

Kacew, S. and Narbaitz, R. (1981b) Drug Chem. Toxicol. 4, 123–132.

Kacew, S. and Reasor, M.J. (1983) Biochem. Pharmacol. 32, 2683–2688.

Kacew, S., Dubas, T.C. and Stevenson, A.J. (1978) Toxicology 10, 77–90.

Kacew, S., Narbaitz, R. and Dubas, T.C. (1979) Toxicol. Appl. Pharmacol. 47, 185–191.

Kacew, S., Parulekar, M.R., Narbaitz, R., Ruddick, J.A. and Villeneuve, D.C. (1981a) J. Toxicol. Environ. Hlth. 8, 873–884.

Kacew, S., Narbaitz, R., Ruddick, J.A. and Villeneuve, D.C. (1981b) Exp. Mol. Pathol. 35, 98–107.

Kacew, S., Calderwood, G.A., Jr. and Parulekar, M.R. (198lc) Biochem. Pharmacol. 30, 341–347.

Karabelnik, D. and Zbinden, G. (1975) Hoppe-Seyler's Z. Physiol. Chem. 356, 1151–1160.

Karabelnik, D., Zbinden, G. and Baumgartner, E. (1974) Toxicol. Appl. Pharmacol. 27, 395–407.
Kikkawa, Y. and Motoyama, E. (1973) Lab. Invest. 28, 48–54.
Kikkawa, Y. and Suzuki, K. (1972) Lab. Invest. 26, 441–447.
Klinghardt, G.W. (1974) Acta Neuropathol. (Berl.) 28, 117–141.
Kosek, J.C., Mazze, R.I. and Cousins, M.J. (1974) Lab. Invest. 30, 48–57.
Laurent, G., Hildebrand, J. and Thys, O. (1975) Lab. Invest. 32, 580–584.
Lehnert, B.L. and Ferin, J. (1983) J. Reticuloendothel. Soc. 33, 293–303.
Lhermitte, F., Fardeau, M., Chedru, F. and Mallecourt, J. (1976) Br. Med. J. II, 1265.
Liggins, G.C. and Howie, R.N. (1972) Pediatrics 50, 515–525.
Lüllmann, H. and Wehling, M. (1979) Biochem. Pharmacol. 28, 3409–3415
Lüllmann, H. and Lüllmann-Rauch (1981) Toxicol. Appl. Pharmacol. 61, 138–146.
Lüllmann, H. Lüllmann-Rauch, R. and Mosinger, E.U. (1981) Arzneim. Forsch. 31, 795–799.
Lüllmann, H., Lüllmann-Rauch, R. and Wassermann, O. (1975) CRC Crit. Rev. Toxicol. 4, 185–218.
Lüllmann, H., Lüllmann-Rauch, R. and Wassermann, O. (1978) Biochem. Pharmacol. 27, 1103–1108.
Lüllmann-Rauch, R. (1973) Virchows Arch. Abt. B. Zellpathol. 12, 295–302.
Lüllmann-Rauch, R. (1974) Acta Neuropathol. (Berl.) 29, 237–249.
Lüllmann-Rauch, R. (1975a) Toxicol. Appl. Pharmacol. 32, 32–39.
Lüllmann-Rauch, R. (1975b) Virchows Arch. B. Cell Pathol. 18, 51–60.
Lüllmann-Rauch, R. (1979) in Lysosomes in Biology and Pathology (Dingle, J.T., Jacques, P.J. and Shaw, I.H., eds.), Vol 6, pp. 49–130, North-Holland Publishing Co., Amsterdam.
Lüllmann-Rauch, R. and Reil, G.H. (1973) Virchows Arch. Abt. B. Zellpathol. 13, 307–320.
Lüllmann-Rauch, R. and Reil, G.H. (1974a) Naunyn-Schmiedeberg's Arch. Pharmacol. 285, 175–184.
Lüllmann-Rauch, R. and Reil, G.H. (1974b) Toxicol. Appl. Pharmacol. 30, 408–421.
Lüllmann-Rauch, R. and Scheid, D. (1975) Virchows Arch. B. Cell Pathol. 19, 255–268.
Lüllmann-Rauch, R. and Stoermer, B. (1982) Virchows Arch. Cell Pathol. 39, 59–73.
Magnusson, G. and Magnusson, O. (1972) Beitr. Path. Bd. 146, 79–88.
Marchlinski, F.E., Gansler, T.S., Waxman, H.L. and Josephson, M.E. (1982) Ann. Intern. Med. 97, 839–845.
Matsuzawa, Y. and Hostetler, K.Y. (1980a) J. Lipid Res. 21, 202–214.
Matsuzawa, Y. and Hostetler, K.Y. (1980b) Biochem. Biophys. Acta. 620, 592–602.
Matsuzawa, Y. and Hostetler, K. (1980c) J. Biol. Chem. 255, 5190–5194.
McNulty, M.J. and Reasor, M.J. (1981a) J. Reticuloendothel. Soc. 30, 534–549.
McNulty, M.J. and Reasor, M.J. (1981b) Exp. Lung Res. 2, 57–69.
Murphy, B.E.P. (1973) J. Obstet. Gynecol. 115, 521–530.
Nelson, A.A. and Fitzhugh, O.O. (1948) Arch. Pathol. 45, 454–462.
Okuma, S. and Poole, B. (1978) Proc. Natl. Acad. Sci. U.S.A. 75, 3327–3331.
Ospital, J.J., Hacker, A.D., Elsayed, N., Mustafa, M.G. and Lee, S. D. (1977) Am. Rev. Resp. Dis. 115, 5235.
Pappu, A. and Hostetler, K.Y. (1984) Biochem. Pharmacol. 33, 1639–1644.
Pühlhorn, G. and Thiel, H.J. (1976) Albrecht von Graefes Arch. Klin. Exp. Opthalmol. 201, 89–98.
Rawlins, F.A. and Uzman, B.G. (1970) Lab. Invest. 23, 184–189.
Reasor, M.J. (1981) Toxicology 20, 1–33.
Reasor, M.J. and Koshut, R.A. (1980) Toxicol. Appl. Pharmacol. 55, 334–341.
Reasor, M.J. and Walker, E.R. (1979) Gen. Pharmacol. 10, 83–88.
Reasor, M.J., Koshut, R.A. and Castranova, V. (1979) Exp. Molec. Pathol. 31, 297–307.
Reasor, M.J., Heyneman, C.A. and Walker, E.R. (1982) Res. Commun. Chem. Pathol. Pharmacol. 38, 235–245.
Sakuragawa, N., Sakuragawa, M., Kuwabara, T., Pentchev, P.G., Barranger, J.A. and Brady, R.O. (1977) Science 196, 317–319.
Schmien, R., Seiler, K.U. and Wassermann, O. (1974) Naunyn-Schmiedeberg's Arch. Pharmacol. 283, 331–334.
Schutta, H.S. and Neville, H.G. (1968) Lab. Invest. 19, 487–493.

Seiler, K.U. and Wassermann, O. (1975) Naunyn-Schmiedeberg's Arch. Pharmacol. 288, 261–268.
Seydel, J.K. and Wassermann, O. (1976) Biochem. Pharmacol. 25, 2357–2364.
Sgaragli, G.P., Corte, L.D. and Gremigni, D. (1983) Pharmacol. Res. Commun. 15, 231–246.
Shikata, T., Kanetaka, T., Endo, Y. and Nagashima, K. (1972) Acta Pathol. Jpn. 22, 517–531.
Staiger, G.R. (1974) Experientia 30, 385–386.
Stäubli, W., Schweizer, W. and Suter, J. (1978) Exp. Mol. Pathol. 28, 177–195.
Stoeckenius, W. (1962) J. Cell. Biol. 12, 221–229.
Suzuki, K. and DePaul, L.D. (1972) Lab. Invest. 26, 534–539.
Svendsen, O. (1977) Toxicol. Appl. Pharmacol. 40, 171–173.
Thelmo, W.L. and Levine, S. (1978) Am. J. Pathol. 91, 355–358.
Thoma-Laurie, D.L. (1982) Ph.D. Dissertation, Postnatal Toxicity in Rats Exposed Prenatally to Chlorphentermine, West Virginia University, Morgantown, WV.
Thoma-Laurie, D.L., Walker, E.R. and Reasor, M.J. (1982) Toxicology 24, 85–94.
Thoma-Laurie, D.L., Walker, E.R. and Reasor, M.J. (1983) Exp. Mol. Pathol. 38, 310–321.
Vijeyaratnam, G.S. and Corrin B. (1972) J. Pathol. 108, 105–113.
Von Wichert, P., Bavendamm, U., Von Teichmann, M., Müller, G., Thalheim, E., Wilke, A. and Weigers, U. (1977) Naunyn-Schmiedeberg's Arch. Pharmacol. 297, 269– 273.
Witschi, H. and Côté, M.G. (1977) Chem. Biol. Interact. 19, 279–289.
Witschi, H., Kacew, S., Tsang, B.K. and Williamson, D. (1976) Chem. Biol. Interact. 12, 29–40.
Wold, J.S., Joost, R.R., Griffing, W.J., Marroquine, P. and Harris, P.N. (1976) Toxicol. Appl. Pharmacol. 37, 118.
Woodward, S.C. (1981) J. Toxicol. Environ. Hlth. 7, 569–583.
Yamamoto, A., Adachi, S., Ishikawa, K., Yokomura, T., Kitani, T., Nasu, T., Imoto, T. and Nishikawa, M. (1971) J. Biochem. (Tokyo) 70, 775–784.

S. Kacew and M.J. Reasor (eds), *Toxicology and the Newborn*
© 1984 Elsevier Science Publishers B.V.

Chapter 4

Alcohol and the Newborn Infant

PETER A. FRIED

Department of Psychology, Carleton University, Ottawa, Ontario, K1S 5B6, Canada

CONTENTS

I. HISTORICAL PERSPECTIVE

As alcohol is produced endogenously in the gut, it can be said to be as old as mankind. Although alcohol's history as a beverage may not go back quite as far, there is evidence that it has its beginnings very early in civilization. 23 centuries before the dynasty of King Tutankhamen there was a brewery in Egypt. The writings of the ancient Chinese and Indian cultures of 2000 B.C. include discussions of alcohol. Considering the length of time that alcohol has been associated with human societies it is, at first blush, somewhat surprising that the interaction of alcohol and pregnancy has been recently 'discovered' by researchers in the past decade. 'Rediscovered' might be a better term.

In the Old Testament, Judges 13:7, there is the warning: "Behold, thou shalt conceive and bear a son; and now drink no wine or strong drink". The recipient of this admonition was the mother of Samson. In ancient Greece, where social gatherings were termed symposia (meaning 'drinking together'), Plato proposed that the laws of Carthage include the prohibition of wine "at night .... to any person of either sex contemplating the procreation of children" (translation by Taylor, 1971). Aristotle continued this line of thought by declaring that "foolish, drunken or harebrain women for the most part bring forth children like unto themselves, *morosos et languidos*" (cited in Rosett, 1980). In Roman mythology, Vulcan, the deformed god of fire and metal working was said to be the product of a conception while under the influence of alcohol.

Possibly the most outstanding historical case of public and political awareness of alcohol's ramifications upon offspring occurred during Britain's gin epidemic of the 18th century. In the first half of that century the British parliament passed legislation that encouraged the growing and the distillation of grain. Licences to distill were essentially done away with, the need to serve a 7-year apprenticeship was discontinued and distillers and retailers of gin were exempted from having to house soldiers, which other innkeepers and stablekeepers had to do (George, 1925). The government of the time expected that the trade of distilling would substantially increase the demand for grain and would thereby provide considerable revenue both to the land owners (who were greatly overrepresented in parliament) and to the British treasury, due to the export to other countries of the gin produced. However, due to abundant supply of gin, it became extremely cheap and the poor of Britain (particularly in London) became the principal consumers. The quantity drunk was staggering. In 1685 approximately half a million gallons were drunk. 30 years later that figure had quadrupled and by 1750 it had reached an amazing 11 million gallons. On a per capita basis it is estimated that the London population downed over ten and a half gallons of gin per year (Coffey, 1966). In the largest parish in London one house in five was licenced to sell gin. Possibly the first coin-operated vending machine came into existence during this period. Passers-by were urged to place money into the mouth of a metal cat that was on a window sill, whisper "Puss, give me 2d worth of gin", and down a pipe would come a shot of gin (Coffey, 1966).

As mentioned earlier, the reasons for the rise in consumption were acts of parliament motivated by the landed gentry's desire for increased revenue. The reasons for the subsequent decline were also attributable to acts of parliament — this time in the form of taxes. From the high of 11 million gallons in the middle of the century, the consumption dropped to 2 million by 1785 and to about a million gallons by 1790. Taxes were imposed because of public pressure that built up with the recognition of the tremendous social consequences that resulted from the flood of gin. Much of the poverty and criminality of the age was associated with the virtually unlimited sale of gin (Coffey, 1966). In addition, one of the major consequences that contemporary writers attributed to the distilled product was the decline in London's population. Only one child in four who was born in London between 1730 and 1749 reached the age of five (George, 1925). A historian writing in 1751 stated: "The diminution of births set out from the time that the consumption of these liquors by the common people became enormous .... As this consumption hath been continually increasing since that time, the amount of the births hath been continually diminishing .... Can it be necessary to add to this shocking loss .... the sickly loss .... the sickly state of such infants as are born, who with difficulty pass through the first stages of life and live very few of them to years of manhood?" (cited by George, 1925).

It is noteworthy that the denunciation of gin drinking and the role it played among those ".... Unhappy mothers (who) habituate themselves .... (whose) children are born weak and sickly ...." (quoted in George, 1925, p. 34) did not extend to all alcohol-containing beverages. For example, in 1751 William Hogarth produced a print entitled 'Gin Lane' which depicted many of the horrific consequences (particularly those associated with the care of children) related to gin. However, as part of the same series of moral lessons Hogarth also printed 'Beer Street' in which the consumption of that British staple, beer, was associated with happiness and productivity.

William Sullivan, a physician to a Liverpool prison, published a study in 1899 that may have been the first empirical study on maternal alcoholism (Sullivan, 1899). He examined 600 offspring of 120 jailed drunkards. In contrast to non-alcoholic female relatives, the alcoholic women had a stillbirth and infant mortality rate that was 56% higher than the comparison group. Paternal drinking habits did not appear to affect mortality rates but the risk increased with successive pregnancies as the women's alcoholism progressed. If the woman was forced to abstain from alcohol during pregnancy — as might happen if she were imprisoned — the cycle of adverse outcome was reported often to be broken.

During the first half of this century, relatively little work was reported on the influence of alcohol on the fetus. It was assumed that if alcohol did have a measurable effect in infants and children it did so via sociological and environmental routes rather than some direct mechanism. Factors such as maternal malnutrition during pregnancy and poor postnatal maternal care were thought to be what led to the physical, behavioural and mental abnormalities seen in the offspring of alcoholics.

II. THE FETAL ALCOHOL SYNDROME

Not until 1973 did the pendulum swing back once more to the recognition of the importance of direct intrauterine exposure to alcohol. In that year, Jones et al. (1973) published a pivotal work that described eight unrelated children, all born to chronic alcoholic mothers, who had a similar pattern of physical abnormalities and growth reduction. A somewhat ironic note (from an historical perspective) was a summary statement by the authors that "This seems to be the first reported association between maternal drinking and aberrant morphogenesis in the offspring". Just a few months later, Jones and Smith (1973) published further cases and also brought to the attention of researchers some of the historical reports pertaining to this issue. It was in this publication that the term 'Fetal Alcohol Syndrome' (FAS) was coined to describe the cluster of anomalies that were a distinct outcome arising from in utero exposure to maternal alcoholism. During the next 8 years, over 800 clinical and research studies were published (Abel, 1981) dealing with prenatal exposure to alcohol. It was recognised as well that in the 1960s there had been a report from France (Lemoine et al., 1968) describing the offspring of alcoholics. In that French report the description of the infants was very similar to those discussed in the later, Jones et al. (1973), American study.

There are three main features that comprise the FAS: (a) prenatal and/or postnatal growth retardation (especially microcephaly (small head circumference)), (b) distinctive abnormal facies, including short palpebral fissures (eye slits), epicanthic folds, short, upturned nose, indistinctive philtrum (the parallel ridges lying between the nose and mouth), thin upper lip and underdeveloped midface and (c) central nervous system involvement that might be manifested as retarded mental and motor development, hyperactivity or tremulousness. Further, children who have been identified as demonstrating the FAS frequently have other congenital physical malformations, including limb abnormalities (unusual palmar creases and joint anomalies), cardiac defects and genito-urinary anomalies. Detailed descriptions (Table 1) of the principal features of the FAS can be found in Clarren and Smith (1978) and Streissguth et al. (1980).

As reported by Rosett et al. (1981), it has been recommended that the diagnosis of FAS only be made when a patient has signs in each of the three main areas as described above. Neugut (1981) has noted that an important and problematic aspect of the FAS is that, except for the facial features (which are not the easiest to assess objectively), the principal features of the syndrome are far from unique in their association with alcohol. This certainly adds to the difficulty in establishing a causal relationship between maternal alcohol consumption and the features observed in the offspring.

The general consensus among researchers with respect to the frequency of occurrence of FAS in the general population is in the range of one or two per thousand but, as pointed out by Abel (1981), the estimates are very often based on the identification of very few cases and the prevalence rate must be considered tentative at this time. Among women who have been identified in clinical reports as

TABLE 1

CLINICAL FEATURES OF THE FETAL ALCOHOL SYNDROME

Feature	Symptoms
Growth deficiency	
Prenatal	Length and weight
Postnatal	Diminished adipose tissue
Head	Reduced circumference of skull
Abnormal facial characteristics	
Eyes	Short eye slits, vertical fold of skin on either side of nose
Nose	Short, upturned. Indistinct ridges between nose and mouth
Mouth	Thin upper lip, smallness of jaws
Face	General underdevelopment of mid-face
Central nervous system involvement	
Intellectual	Mild-to-moderate retardation
Neurologic	Poor motor co-ordination, flaccid motor tone
Behavioural	Irritability during infancy, hyperactivity in childhood

alcoholics (Olegard et al., 1979) or who have been identified as severe alcoholics in a sample derived from a large data base (Jones et al., 1974), the incidence of offspring showing the FAS is approximately 30%, although this figure varies considerably from one study to the next, influenced, it appears, by the interaction with socio-economic factors and the severity of the alcoholism. In other studies, frequently prospective in nature, in which the alcohol consumption or the evidence of alcoholism may not be as striking (e.g., Ouellette et al., 1977; Sokol et al., 1980), although the degree of drinking is still clearly a case of alcohol abuse, the estimate of the full FAS is approximately 3%.

Several reports (Jones et al., 1974; Kaminski et al., 1978; Sokol et al., 1980) have confirmed Sullivan's (1899) observations that maternal alcohol abuse is related to a history of pregnancy loss and/or increased neonatal and infant mortality. Among the offspring it has become evident in recent years that the child with the full FAS represents the extreme end of the spectrum of the consequences of maternal alcohol abuse. Based on information gathered from viable offspring there is accumulating data to show that even if a child does not meet the criteria of the FAS there are still a multitude of ways in which the mother's alcoholism can manifest itself. Not only does this include children who demonstrate only some aspects of the FAS — mental deficiencies in the absence of physical anomalies, for example (Jones et al., 1974; Streissguth et al., 1979) — but also a variety of effects that are not required for the diagnosis of FAS. Included among these is the report by Clarren et al. (1978) describing four cases of brain malformations related to maternal alcohol consumption. One baby was stillborn and the remaining three survived from 68 hours to 10 weeks. In each of the cases the maternal drinking habits were quite different. One woman was described as a chronic alcoholic, and her infant was diagnosed as having the FAS. A second woman drank several times a week, consuming as much as a gallon of wine at a time. Her infant displayed the facial features of the FAS. The remaining two women drank only occasionally, but both reported 'binge' drinking (five or more drinks at one sitting). One of the offspring born to these women demonstrated partial features of the FAS, whereas the other showed none. Among the four infants the neuropathological findings appear to be more severe in the babies of the two women who drank heavily. The malformations in the brain of the offspring of alcoholic women have also been reported by Majewski (1981).

A number of functional disturbances have been reported in infants who do not meet the criteria for the diagnosis of the FAS. Rosett and his co-workers (Ouellette et al., 1977; Rosett et al., 1979; Rosett and Weiner, 1980; Rosett, 1980) reported that women who drank heavily, averaging 5.8 ounces of absolute alcohol per day, were significantly more likely to have infants that were jittery, hypotonic and have a poor suck compared to women who drank moderately or rarely. The offspring of these heavily drinking women also were characterized as having significantly more congenital malformations and growth retardation but, although demonstrating components of the FAS, no one child (out of 42) showed the complete syndrome. Infants born to the heavy drinkers also showed a disturbance in their sleep/wake regulation. Their total sleep was less and their quiet sleep episodes were interrupted more frequently. Researchers have reported behavioural and learning deficiencies in the offspring of alcoholic mothers, even in the absence of marked morphological signs of FAS (Streissguth et al., 1978) or in the absence of impaired intelligence (Shaywitz et al., 1980). A number of authors (Streissguth et al., 1978, 1980; Majewski, 1981) have reported a correlation between the extent of FAS consistent anomalies and the degree of intellectual impairment. However, other investigators have not found this association (Golden et al., 1982).

While considering maternal alcohol abuse to produce a continuum of effects, some authors have attempted to estimate the risk of fetal alcohol effects (FAE) as distinct from the full-blown FAS. Sokol et al. (1980), in a prospective cohort study based on over 12,000 pregnancies, reported that among 204 women identified as alcohol abusers the risk for adverse perinatal outcome was 50% — 20 times as frequent as that for the complete FAS among the babies of those 204 women. Rosett et al. (1977), using a high risk population, found the percentage of FAE infants born to heavy drinkers (as defined above) was double that found among the babies born to light or moderate drinkers.

The issue of whether the symptoms in the offspring of alcohol-abusing mothers are permanent or not has been the subject of a number of investigations. Only one report has indicated that with increasing age the characteristic facies associated with the FAS may attenuate (Majewski, 1981), while both that study and Golden et al. (1982) report that microcephaly persists and actually becomes proportionally more pronounced with increasing age.

Particular attention has been placed upon the permanence of mental deficiences in those offspring exposed to large amounts of alcohol in utero. Although mental impairment cannot be used as a criterion for the diagnosis of either FAS or FAE at birth, a large number of studies have emphasized the mental deficiencies found in children or young adults who have been labelled as having the FAS on the basis of the criteria mentioned earlier. Streissguth and her co-workers (Jones et al., 1973, 1974; Streissguth, 1976; Streissguth et al., 1978) consistently found the average mental scores, although varying considerably, to fall within the range of mild-to-moderate retardation. These results cannot be attributed to poor postnatal environments, as impaired intelligence was also found in those cases in which the patients were reared in foster homes. Many of the subjects in these studies were identified as having the FAS only after being referred to professionals because of intellectual or developmental retardation, and thus their status in infancy is not known.

Golden et al. (1982) reported a prospective study involving 12 infants who were identified at birth as having possible FAE. At approximately 1 year of age these babies were contrasted to other infants who were matched in terms of gestational age, sex and race. The infants in the experimental group showed delayed mental and motor development (falling in the borderline range), a greater number of physical abnormalities and growth retardation. As pointed out by the authors, these results must be interpreted cautiously, not only because of the small sample size but also because details with respect to the mother's drinking habits were not available. Further, whereas 11 of the 12 mothers who abused alcohol also smoked, only one of the control mothers did so. Consistent with these findings was a second prospective study conducted by Darby et al. (1981). In a preliminary report the authors describe eight children ranging in age from 14 to 80 months who were given age-relevant developmental and intelligence tests. Four of these children had been identified at birth as having the FAS while the remaining four had been so identified between 5 and 8 months. At the time of the follow-up testing, six of the eight children were in foster homes. The average score on the tests was 76.

In Germany, Majewski (1981) tested 18 children ranging from 3.5 to 9 years of age who displayed varying degrees of FAE. It is not apparent from his report when these subjects were initially diagnosed as suffering from the consequences of in utero alcohol exposure. There were five children who had very marked symptoms of maternal alcohol abuse. These symptoms included pronounced growth retardation, pronounced facial anomalies and severe visceral malformations. In this group of FAS children the average intelligence score was 66. In four cases in which the alcohol symptoms were more moderate the average score was 79 and in the nine cases in which the FAE were relatively mild the intelligence score averaged 91. In this latter group there was a considerable range of performance.

Together, these data suggest that the long-term prognosis for normal mental development in those children showing marked effects of antenatal alcohol exposure is not very promising. It must be recognized, however, that those instances in which the newborn or the very young infant is labelled as an FAS baby presumably represent the most severe cases. In instances in which the FAE are milder a more optimistic forecast for their future appears possible in situations in which intervention programs coupled with a stable environment are instituted.

The wide range of effects seen in the offspring of alcohol-abusing women emphasizes the complex multitude of mechanisms that come into play when the fetus is exposed in utero to this substance. Unlike a drug such as thalidomide, which produced its tragic results only when taken at particular stages of pregnancy (Stern, 1982), the number of systems that are affected when large amounts of alcohol are ingested indicates that ethanol abuse imposes a risk upon the fetus throughout gestation as the development and growth of various systems proceed. Recently, Rosett and Weiner (1982) discussed this aspect of the FAS.

As the FAS includes so many diverse aspects of fetal development, it is not unexpected that the full syndrome is only seen in the offspring of women who have abused alcohol thoughout their pregnancy. Majewski (1981) has argued that more important than the amount of alcohol consumed by the alcoholic is the chronicity of her alcoholism. When other things are equal, the longer the woman has been an alcoholic the greater are the physiological consequences of the alcohol abuse. Majewski based this conclusion on his finding that among children born to the same alcohol-abusing mother the younger siblings were more affected than the older siblings. This, incidentally, is consistent with Sullivan's (1899) report of increasing risk among alcoholic women with successive pregnancies. In addition to the chronicity and the volume of alcohol drunk, other variables that enter into the equation for predicting the occurrence of the FAS are genetic influences and concomitant risk factors, such as low socio-economic status, poor nutrition and the use of other soft drugs (Rosett, 1980). There is also evidence (Clarren et al., 1978) that the pattern of drinking, particularly binge drinking, may be a very important variable in contributing to FAE. It has been postulated that a high blood alcohol level at particular stages of fetal development may be the underlying etiology in circumstances in which offspring manifest only parts of the FAS (Rosett, 1980). Binge drinking early in pregnancy may affect organ development (including the nervous system), while binge drinking later in pregnancy may affect the growth and integration of systems (again including the nervous system) (Fried, 1983). The pathogenetic mechanisms that might be involved in the etiology of the FAS and FAE have been reviewed in detail by Henderson et al. (1981).

If alcohol abuse can affect the fetus at all stages of development, attempts to get women to reduce their heavy alcohol consumption even after they have become pregnant would be of considerable benefit. Details of such programs have been presented elsewhere (Little et al., 1980; Little and Streissguth, 1981; Rosett et al., 1977, 1981) and the evidence for their success in reducing the degree of FAE are quite striking (Rosett et al., 1977).

Research from two centres indicated that beer may have a comparatively greater effect than either wine or liquor for some of the FAS characteristics. In a large cohort study based on 9,236 pregnancies from 13 French institutions in the 1960s Kaminski et al. (1978) reported that the proportion of small-for-date infants and the stillbirth rate were significantly greater among heavy beer drinkers as compared to women who did not drink beer. The results were interpreted cautiously, as cider was included with beer in the categorization of the women and, in a country where wine is the type of alcohol consumed by the vast majority of drinkers, the women who consume beer heavily (to the exclusion of wine) may have differed on other important, unspecified parameters. Sokol and his co-workers (Bottoms et al., 1982; Kuzma and Sokol, 1982) have also found suggestive data indicating that beer drinking may contribute to a special degree to lowered birth weight. Beer contains thiocyanate, which has been implicated as a contributing factor in diminished fetal growth found among cigarette smoking women (Meberg et al., 1979), and it has been proposed that it may serve as a possible link between beer and small-for-date infants. Interestingly, in a recent study that found an association between spontaneous abortion and maternal drinking (Kline et al., 1980), beer was not found to differ from either wine or liquor in its contribution to the risk for this form of fetal loss.

III. NON-ALCOHOLIC LEVELS OF DRINKING

Although there is little question that large amounts of alcohol consumed during pregnancy impose a risk for the fetus there is much less certainty with respect to the issue of more moderate drinking, including what is often termed 'social drinking'. Quite frequently, the amount of alcohol consumed by non-alcoholic women is categorized in such a fashion that it is very difficult to ascertain at what drinking levels effects in the offspring have actually been observed.

There have been two reports that have linked moderate drinking during pregnancy with an increased risk of spontaneous abortion. Kline at al. (1980) found that women who were interviewed after being admitted to hospital because of spontaneous abortion reported drinking two times a week or more, twice as often as control subjects. Although matched for a number of variables, the two groups of subjects may have differed in a number of important respects (e.g., recall of alcohol consumption might have been more vivid among those women who lost their baby). Further, although the authors concluded that there is a "strong association between spontaneous abortion and drinking as seldom as twice a week", it should be noted that there was no differentiation between those women drinking from twice a week up to those women drinking six times per week. In a prospective study Harlap and Shiono (1980) analyzed data collected from questionnaires that had been filled in by 32,019 women early in pregnancy. Among those women who reported drinking between one and two drinks (approximately 0.7–1.5 ounces of absolute alcohol) per day during pregnancy the risk for a spontaneous abortion was about twice as great as the risk for women who were categorized as drinking 2–6 times per week. Because of the manner in which the data were collected, it is not possible to determine if there was any greater risk among those women who drank almost every day and those who drank twice a week or less.

The relationship between FAE and non-alcoholic levels of maternal drinking has been addressed in numerous studies, with not only varying results but also varying interpretations of a given set of results. In a widely cited study, Hanson et al. (1978) reported that if maternal ingestion during pregnancy is in the range of 1–2 ounces of absolute alcohol per day the risk of FAE approaches 10% while drinking 2 or more ounces per day puts the risk level at almost 20%. Dealing with the latter risk level first: it was derived from the finding that of 16 women who consumed 2 or more ounces per day three gave birth to babies that showed FAE. However, the three infants that showed such effects were all born to women who had actually drunk 5 or more ounces on a daily basis. Thus, by including them among the 16 women in the drinking category of 2 or more ounces it is very easy to misinterpret the statement of a 20% risk associated with drinking 2 or more ounces. The risk level of 10% among those who drank 1–2 ounces per day also can be somewhat misleading. Among the women who drank virtually no alcohol there was a 3% incidence of FAE (as described earlier many of the FAE are not unique to alcohol effects). Thus, the difference in risk levels between very light drinkers and those who drank between 1 and 2 ounces per day is not as striking as it might appear initially (Thompson, 1979). Adding additional caution to the interpretation of the results of Hanson et al. (1978) are the failure of both Tennes and Blackard (1980) and Hingson et al. (1982) to find FAE in the offspring of non-alcoholic drinkers, with the quantities consumed, particularly in the latter study, being relatively similar to those in the Hanson et al. (1978) work.

The effect of non-alcoholic levels of drinking upon intrauterine growth is also an area of inconsistent results. Kaminski et al. (1981) reported a small but significant decrease in birthweight (60 g) among women who drank 1.6 ounces or more of absolute alcohol per day (how much more was not specified) in two prospective studies but not in a retrospective investigation carried out by the same investigator. While Little (1977), using a regression analysis, found that drinking an ounce of absolute alcohol per day late in pregnancy was associated with a 160 g deficit in birthweight, Tennes and Blackard (1980) and Hingson et al. (1982), using similar statistical approaches, failed to find a significant association.

Neonatal behavioural effects in the offspring of non-alcoholic women have been examined by Streissguth and her associates at Seattle, WA, and have recently been summarized (Streissguth et al., 1980, 1981). Briefly, the results were interpreted as indicating that maternal alcohol use at non-alcoholic levels (defined in various ways but approximately 1 ounce or more of absolute alcohol per day or 0.75 ounce or more per day coupled with occasional binge drinking) was associated with lower Apgar scores, poorer habituation and lower arousal, increased tremulousness and decreased body activity measured during naturalistic observation periods, and decreased sucking pressure. The same group of researchers (Streissguth et al., 1980) reported a significantly lower mental and motor development in 8-month-old infants whose mothers had drank at least 2 ounces of absolute alcohol per day during pregnancy. However, in this study the data suggest that the alcohol effects are primarily due to the children born to women who, in fact, drank more than twice that amount. The longer-term behavioural development of the infants of non-alcoholic women has also been reported upon by the Seattle group of researchers (Landesman-Dwyer et al., 1981). Included in a sample of 128 middle-class women and their 4-year-old children were 67 women who averaged more than 2 ounces of alcohol per day.

The children of this subsample, while being observed at home, tended to be less attentive, less compliant with parental commands and more fidgety than were the children of light and non-drinkers. These behavioural differences were small and their clinical significance remains to be determined.

IV. THE OTTAWA PRENATAL STUDY

The neonatal effects associated with non-alcoholic levels of drinking are also being studied in an ongoing prospective investigation in Ottawa, Canada, that is primarily directed at determining the effects of marihuana use during pregnancy. The procedures being followed in this research have been described in detail elsewhere (Fried et al., 1980). Since 1979 mothers-to-be have been informed of a study concerning prenatal lifestyle habits by their obstetricians or notices in reception rooms of prenatal clinics in three of the largest hospitals in Ottawa. Upon volunteering to participate (typically by returning a prepaid postcard that is attached to the information pamphlet), each subject is interviewed once during each of the trimesters remaining in her pregnancy. Approximately 80% of the 600 participants to date have been interviewed at least twice prior to giving birth. During each of the interviews, usually conducted in the homes of the mother-to-be, information that is collected includes socio-demographic data, the mother's health both prior to the pregnancy and currently, father's health history, obstetrical history of previous pregnancies, a 24-hour dietary recall (including caffeine), which is then broken down into units of nutrients and contrasted to recommended allowances for specific weight and trimester categories, and past and present drug use, with emphasis upon alcohol, cigarette and marihuana usage. Drug histories are gathered for both the year before pregnancy and each trimester of pregnancy. Alcohol information is collected with respect to types of alcoholic beverages, quantity consumed and the pattern of drinking. The offspring are examined at birth, 9 and 30 days postnatally and approximately every 6 months thereafter, with age-relevant mental and motor tests.

When assessing variables such as nutrition and drug habits there is the overriding problem of both validity and reliability. A number of points must be made. Despite the obvious shortcomings of self-reporting, there are no practical alternative methods for gathering the type of information needed for this type of study. What is possible, however, is to incorporate a number of procedures that will increase the probability of obtaining an accurate report. A feeling of confidence in the interviewer is vital. In the Ottawa prenatal study the same interviewer 'followed' a given subject throughout her pregnancy and the interview sessions were always conducted so as to maximize privacy and the feeling of confidentiality. Further, by repeating the questionnaire (once during each trimester) a test-retest reliability was possible. The multiple interview procedure also had the advantage of shortening the period of time for the woman to have to recollect her drug use during pregnancy. Biochemical techniques are being employed to assess the use by the women of cannabinoids, amphetamines and opiates (Fried, 1984).

Although the major thrust of the Ottawa prenatal study is to examine the neurological and behavioural consequences of marihuana use during pregnancy, two substudies pertaining to drinking at non-alcoholic levels and neonatal development are pertinent to the topic of this chapter. Staisey and Fried (1983) reported the relationship between moderate alcohol consumption during pregnancy and the infant's development up to 30 days of age. 59 mother-infant pairs were included in this study. The mean absolute alcohol level in the year before pregnancy was 0.5 ounce per day, with the maximum being 2.5 ounces. During pregnancy the average dropped to 0.2 ounce per day, with the maximum being 2.1 ounces. No relationship was found between maternal alcohol consumption, either pre-pregnancy or during pregnancy, with respect to birth weight when cigarette use (which was correlated with alcohol) was statistically controlled through partial correlation techniques. The Prechtl Neurological (Prechtl and Beintema, 1964) examination was administered at each infant's home by two trained examiners when the infant was 9 and 30 days of age. The items tested during the neurological inventory were classified into six main categories: (1) physical characteristics, (2) motor activity, (3) tone, (4) startles, (5) reflexes and (6) eye characteristics.

At 9 days of age, scores which measured changes in infant muscle tone were found to be related negatively to maternal alcohol consumption during pregnancy when other risk factors were controlled. The type of tests that demonstrated this relationship included a weaker strength of overall movement, a lesser amount of muscle tonus during movement, a diminished knee jerk reflex, a slowed, prolonged glabella reflex and an exaggerated extension of the legs when supine. An increased number of spontaneous startles was also observed to be related to the use of alcohol during pregnancy. No relationship was found between alcohol consumption during pregnancy and the physical characteristics, general motor activity or eye characteristics. At 30 days of age most of the negative relationship between the mother's drinking and the measures of muscle tone had attenuated.

Hypotonia or weakened muscles has been listed frequently as a consequence of alcohol abuse (Lemoine et al., 1968; Ouellette and Rosett, 1976), and neonatologists have emphasized the importance of muscle tone as a predictor of later development (Parmalee and Michaelis, 1971). The data described by Staisey and Fried (1983) suggest a lesser but possibly parallel finding in moderate drinkers when other risk factors are controlled. The absence of marked effects at 30 days of age may be due to a sufficient or even compensatory maturation. As an alternative explanation it is possible that at 30 days the neurological test has a decreased discriminatory sensitivity, as ceiling effects were noted on many items.

An additional alcohol-related finding that arose out of the Ottawa prenatal study was based on an examination of the relationship between maternal alcohol consumption and the developmental status of the offspring at 13 months (Gusella and Fried, 1984). The subjects were 84 children who were a consecutively selected subsample of offspring born to women who had volunteered to participate in the overall study. The child was tested at home using the Bayley Scales of Infant Development (Bayley, 1969), including the Infant Behaviour Record. In addition to the global indices of mental and motor performance, three clusters of dependent variables were derived to examine the maturity of spoken language, verbal comprehension and fine motor skills.

Prior to pregnancy one subject reported consuming an average of 2.5 ounces of absolute alcohol per day, while all the other women reported drinking less than 2.0 ounces daily. The average pre-pregnancy consumption per day was 0.5 ounce. During pregnancy all but one woman consumed an average of less than 1.5 ounces per day and the average daily amount drunk was 0.21 ounce. Reported binge drinking during pregnancy was too infrequent to consider as a separate variable in the analysis, with only 6% of the women reporting such a pattern. For these women, the binge drinking was a very atypical mode of drinking behaviour.

Social drinking during pregnancy was found to be related to a significant decrease in the scores on the overall mental component of the test. The mental scale consists of many items which sample the child's ability to comprehend instructions, vocalize words or sounds, imitate actions and solve problems. When language-related items were extracted, both verbal comprehension and spoken language scores were found to decrease with an increase in maternal alcohol consumption. This relationship persisted when controlling for postnatal demographic factors and did not appear attributable to temperamental differences (which might inhibit language production) as alcohol use was not related to scores on the Infant Behaviour Record.

An examination of the data suggests that the critical level of alcohol consumption for the effects noted is approximately 0.6 ounce (one drink) per day. This is somewhat lower than the risk level found by Streissguth et al. (1980) when those researchers tested 8-month-old babies using the same developmental tests. This may very well reflect the increased range of skills that can be examined when the child is older. It must be emphasized that although there was a significant relationship between non-alcoholic levels of drinking and some of the developmental scores the range of performance at the low end was, with one exception, within 1.5 S.D. of the norms established for that age group. Thus, the association between prenatal drinking at social levels is not one that has obvious clinical implications. At this state of knowledge it is perhaps more accurate to characterize the effects as ones that may be contributing to factors that impede a child from attaining a level of performance that he or she might otherwise achieve.

V. CONCLUSIONS

Although there can be no quarrel with the 1981 Surgeon General's Advisory on Alcohol and Pregnancy (1981) that "a woman who consumes alcohol at amounts consistent with diagnosis of alcoholism risks bearing a child with a specific cluster of severe physical and mental defects", knowledge about the other end of the drinking spectrum is much less definitive. Evidence is mounting that non-alcoholic levels of drinking can produce a number of effects in offspring — many of which appear to be mild forms of those observed among the babies of blatant alcohol abusers. From this, however, it does not automatically follow that there is a threshold below which alcohol consumption is 'safe'. Like all socially used drugs with the potential to be abused during pregnancy, alcohol will interact with other exogenous and endogenous risk factors. Certainly, the 'safe' approach is for professionals to advise patients who are pregnant or who are planning to become pregnant to refrain from any drinking whatsoever. However, as emphasized recently by Rosett and Weiner (1982), there is no objective, scientific evidence that drinking less than a drink a day during pregnancy has any measurable effects upon the developing fetus. This is not to say that such effects do not exist. Rather, it means that to imply that research has shown such levels to be harmful is both misleading and an exaggeration — the consequences of which can have important repercussions. If the credibility of one aspect of prenatal alcohol research is called into question it will become extremely difficult to maintain the credibility of findings pertaining to the consequences of heavier drinking or possible future findings related to lesser amounts of alcohol consumption.

VI. ACKNOWLEDGEMENTS

The research described in this chapter carried out by the author and his associates was funded by grants from the National Research Council of Canada and the Department of Health and Welfare, Canada.

VII. REFERENCES

Abel, E.A. (1981) Psychol. Bull. 90, 564–581.

Bayley, N. (1969) Manual for the Bayley Scales of Infant Development, Psychological Corporation, New York.

Bottoms, S.F., Judge, N.E., Kuhnert, P.M. and Sokol, R. (1982) Alcoholism: Clin. Exp. Res. 6, 391–395.

Clarren, S.K. and Smith, D.W. (1978) N. Engl. J. Med. 298, 1063–1067.

Clarren, S.K., Alvord, E.C. Jr., Sumi, S.M., Streissguth, A.P. and Smith, D.W. (1978) J. Pediatr. 92, 64–67.

Coffey, T.G. (1966) Q. J. Stud. Alcohol 27, 669–692.

Darby, B.L., Streissguth, A.P. and Smith, D.W. (1981) Neurobehav. Toxicol. Teratol. 3, 157–159.

Fried, P.A. (1983) Pregnancy and Life Style Habits, General, Toronto.

Fried, P.A. (1984) in Neurobehavioral Teratology (Yanai, J., ed.), pp. 275–285, Elsevier, Amsterdam.

Fried, P.A., Watkinson, B., Grant, A.G. and Knights, R.M. (1980) Drug Alcohol Depend. 6, 323–343.

George, M.D. (1925) London Life in the Eighteenth Century, Kegan Paul, London.

Golden, N.L., Sokol, R.J., Kuhnert, B.R. and Bottoms, S. (1982) Pediatrics 70, 931–934.

Gusella, J. and Fried, P.A. (1984), Neurobehav. Toxicol. Teratol. 6, 13–17.

Hanson, J.W., Streissguth, A.P. and Smith, D.W. (1978) J. Pediat. 92, 457–460.

Harlap, S. and Shiono, P.H. (1980) Lancet 2, 173–176.

Henderson, G.I., Patwardha, R.V., Hoyumpa, A.M. Jr. and Schenker, S. (1981) Neurobehav. Toxicol. Teratol. 3, 73–80.

Hingson, R., Alpert, J.J., Day, N., Dooling, E., Kayne, H., Morelock, S., Oppenheimer, E. and Zuckerman, B. (1982) Pediatrics 70, 539–546.

Jones, K.L. and Smith, D.W. (1973) Lancet 2, 999–1001.

Jones, K.L., Smith, D.W., Ulleland, C.N. and Streissguth, A.P. (1973) Lancet 1, 1267–1271.
Jones, K.L., Smith, D.W., Streissguth, A.P. and Myrianthopoulos, N. C. (1974) Lancet 1, 1074–1076.
Kaminski, M., Rumeau, C. and Schwartz, D. (1978) Alcoholism: Clin. Exp. Res. 2, 155–163.
Kaminski, M., Franc, M., Lebouvier, M., Du Mazaubrun, C. and Rumeau-Rouquette, C. (1981) Neurobehav. Toxicol. Teratol. 3, 173–181.
Kline, J., Shrout, P., Stein, Z., Susser, M. and Warburton, D. (1980) Lancet 2, 176–180.
Kuzma, J.W. and Sokol, R.J. (1982) Alcoholism: Clin. Exp. Res. 6, 396–402.
Landesman-Dwyer, S., Ragozin, A.S. and Little, R.E. (1981) Neurobehav. Toxicol. Teratol. 3, 187–193.
Lemoine, P., Harousseau, H., Borteyru, J.P. and Menuet, J.C. (1968) Ouest Med. 25, 476–482.
Little, R.E. (1977) Am. J. Publ. Hlth. 67, 1154–1156.
Little, R.E. and Streissguth, A.P. (1980) Can. Med. Assoc. J. 125, 159–164.
Little, R.E., Streissguth, A.P. and Guzinski, G.M. (1980) Alcoholism: Clin. Exp. Res. 4, 185–189.
Majewski, F. (1981) Neurobehav. Toxicol. Teratol. 3, 129–144.
Meberg, A., Sande, H., Foss, O.P. and Stenwig, J.T. (1979) Acta Paediatr. Scand. 68, 547–552.
Neugut, R. (1981) Early Human Dev. 5, 411–429.
Olegard, R., Sable, K.G., Aronsson, M., Sandin, B., Johansson, P. R., Carlsson, C., Kyllerman, M., Iverson, K. and Hrbek, A. (1979) Acta Paediatr. Scand. Suppl. 275, 112–121.
Ouellette, E.M. and Rosett, H.L., (1976) Ann. N. Y. Acad. Sci. 273, 123–129.
Ouellette. E.M., Rosett, H.L., Rosman, N.P. and Weiner, L. (1977) N. Engl. J. Med. 295, 528–530.
Parmalee, A.H. and Michaelis, R. (1971) in Exceptional Infants: Studies in Abnormalities (Hellmuth, J., ed.), Vol. 2, pp. 3–21, Bruner/Mazel, New York.
Prechtl, H. and Beintema, D. (1964) The Neurological Examination of the Full-term Newborn Infant, Lippincott, Philadelphia.
Rosett, H.L. (1980) in Alcohol and Drug Problems in Women (Kalant, O.J., ed.), Vol. 5, pp. 595–652, Plenum Press, New York.
Rosett, H.L. and Weiner, L. (1980) Neurobehav. Toxicol. 2, 267–270.
Rosett, H.L. and Weiner, L. (1982) Pediatrics 69, 813–816.
Rosett, H.L., Ouellette, E., Weiner, L. and Owens, E. (1977) in Currents in Alcoholism (Sexias, F.A., ed.), Vol. 2, pp. 419–430, Grune and Stratton, New York.
Rosett, H.L., Snyder, P., Sandor, L.W., Lee, A., Cook, P., Weiner, L. and Gould, J. (1979) Dev. Med. Child Neurol. 21, 464–473.
Rosett, H.L., Weiner, L. and Edelin, K.C. (1981) Obstet. Gynecol. 57, 1–7.
Shaywitz, S.E., Cohen, D.J. and Shaywitz, B.A. (1980) J. Pediat. 96, 978–982.
Sokol, R.J., Miller, S.I. and Reed, G. (1980) Alcoholism: Clin. Exp. Res. 4, 135–145.
Staisey, N.L. and Fried, P.A. (1983) J. Stud. Alcohol 44 (2).
Stern, L. (1982) Dev. Pharmacol. Ther. 4, 10–18.
Streissguth, A.P. (1976) Ann. N.Y. Acad. Sci. 273, 140–145.
Streissguth, A.P., Herman, C.S. and Smith, D.W. (1978) Alcoholism: Clin. Exp. Res. 2, 165–170.
Streissguth, A.P., Little, R.E., Herman, C. and Woodell, S. (1979) Alcoholism: Clin. Exp. Res. 3, 197.
Streissguth, A.P., Barr, H.M., Martin, D.C. and Herman, C.S. (1980a) Alcoholism: Clin. Exp. Res. 4, 152–164.
Streissguth, A.P., Landesman-Dwyer, S., Martin J.C. and Smith, D.W. (1980b) Science 209, 353–361.
Streissguth, A.P., Martin, D.C., Martin, J.C. and Barr, H.M. (1981) Neurobehav. Toxicol. Teratol. 3, 223–233.
Sullivan, W.C. (1899) J. Ment. Sci. 45, 489–503.
Surgeon General's Advisory on Alcohol and Pregnancy (1981) FDA Drug Bull. 11, 9–16.
Taylor, A.E. (translator) (1971) Laws, 2:674b in Plato: The Collected Dialogues (Hamilton, E. and Cairns, H., eds.), 6th ed., p. 1270, Princeton University Press, Princeton.
Tennes, K. and Blackard, C. (1980) Am. J. Obstet. Gynecol. 138, 774–780.
Thompson, R.J. (1979) J. Pediat. Psychol. 4, 265–276.

S. Kacew and M.J. Reasor (eds), *Toxicology and the Newborn*
© 1984 Elsevier Science Publishers B.V.

Chapter 5

Maternal Drug Abuse and Subsequent Effects on the Newborn

NADIA Z. MIKHAEL[a] and HAROLD W. PEEL[b]

[a]*Associate Professor of Pathology, University of Ottawa, and Head, Pharmacopathology Unit, Ottawa General Hospital, Ottawa, Ontario, K1H 8M5, and* [b]*Chief Scientist — Toxicology, Central Forensic Laboratory, Royal Canadian Mounted Police, Ottawa, Ontario, K1A 0R2, Canada*

CONTENTS

I. INTRODUCTION

For centuries men and women have been seeking not only the analgesic but also the euphoric effects of drugs of abuse. In the last century, Sir William Osler described this situation so well when he said "The desire to take medicine is, perhaps, the greatest feature which distinguishes man from animals" (Cushing, 1925).

During the last decade, increasing numbers of pregnant drug-dependent women have been admitted to medical facilities; some only to deliver their infants and others to receive ongoing prenatal care. In general, the pregnant addict has a low standard of self care and, prior to this decade, nearly three-quarters of these women never saw a physician during their pregnancies.

Despite the increased intake of drugs of abuse by women in many countries the exact magnitude of drug dependency in pregnant women has been difficult to determine. Unfortunately, in the past, these women did not wish to risk confrontations with legal authorities, and therefore did not seek medical care. Therefore, as identified in the United Nations Bulletin on Narcotics, addiction in pregnancy has become an important health problem due to the increased incidence of morbidity and mortality in the mother and infant (Finnegan, 1979).

Leaving aside her exposure to household and industrial chemicals, a woman on the average consumes nine drugs during pregnancy (Harbison, 1980). Owing to the combined intake of drugs and the interaction of other environmental factors, it is often difficult to establish the causal-effect relation of congenital malformations and other reproductive hazards in man. In an attempt to appraise adverse reactions to drugs used in hospital practice, Campbell et al. (1981) recommended avoidance of all drugs as a useful precaution for the pregnant woman. It is now believed that 2–3% of congenital malformations in man are related to drugs and environmental chemicals (Wilson, 1973) and drug-induced liver injury in neonates has been documented (Mikhael et al., 1979).

Since it is beyond the scope of this chapter to include all drugs with potential for abuse, a focus will be made only on the drugs more commonly prone to abuse, their pertinent pharmacological features and teratogenic effects.

II. TRANSPLACENTAL TRANSFER

In the adult human, metabolic and functional parameters undergo considerable change in the gravid female, and therefore drug disposition is modified. Unfortunately, minimal information exists in this regard despite the high intake of drugs throughout gestation. Very little is known about the absorption of drugs, although the absorption of certain nutrients seems to be enhanced during pregnancy. Studies of drug-metabolizing capacity in pregnant rats have shown that a decreased metabolism exists for oxidative and reductive pathways, whereas sulphation is increased. The mechanism behind these changes during pregnancy is not fully understood, though it may be related to the known hormonal changes (Finnegan, 1979).

Many of the rate-limiting processes which operate to modulate the transplacental passage of pharmacologic agents are poorly understood and probably some have not been identified. Relevant characteristics of the placenta and the drug passing through it include: lipid solubility, degree of drug ionization, molecular weight, placental blood flow, placental metabolism of drugs, protein binding of drugs, and ageing of the placenta (Mirkin, 1973).

The mechanisms involved in the transfer of both exogenous and endogenous substances across the placenta include simple diffusion, facilitated diffusion, active transport and special processes. The effect of fetal circulation on drug transfer must also be considered. If circulation is impaired, secondary to maternal heart failure, erythroblastosis fetalis or maternal drug intoxication, it will significantly decrease drug transfer rates between the maternal and fetal compartments. Placental circulation may be affected by drugs, and in turn produce changes both in drug transfer and transport of oxygen and nutrients to the fetus.

III. CANNABIS

Probably the most widely available and extensively used illicit drugs of abuse in the world are the cannabis derivatives, such as marijuana, hashish and liquid hashish. Originally cultivated as a source of hemp, modern society has diverted the cannabis plant to be the most widely used illegal drug. *Cannabis sativa* grows wild or is cultivated in most tropic or temperate regions of the world. It was once used in the form of tinctures to treat assorted medical problems, such as headaches, insomnia, hallucinations and certain pains, but was removed from use after 1937. Cannabis and its derivatives are now regulated in some manner as a controlled substance in most developed countries.

Cannabis contains over sixty cannabinoid compounds and some 400 other compounds. The most pharmacologically active cannabinoid, which is extracted from the plant in a resin, is 1-Δ^9-tetrahydrocannabinol (THC). Marijuana, which consists of a mixture of mainly leaves with stems and some flowering resinous tops of the plant, can contain 2–4% THC, depending upon source. Within the last decade, selective breeding and 'good gardening' practices have produced plants which contain much higher concentrations of THC. The highly potent variety called 'sinsemilla' is produced by elaborate agricultural techniques, including breeding, plucking the leaves to make a bushier plant, and weeding out the less potent or less resinous male plant, so that the resin-producing female plant proliferates. 'Sinsemilla' can have a THC content as high as 10% (Hawks, 1982).

Whereas the crude cannabis product is marijuana (also known as bhang, kif or dagga), other products are prepared from the plant. Since the psychoactive cannabinoids occur in the resin, modifications are made to prepare more potent products, such as ganga (which is a mixture of the flowering tops), hashish (which is the resinous exudate itself) or hashish oil (which is a concentrated form of resin). Marijuana, hashish and hash oil are commonly used in smoking preparations in North America and Europe and in oral preparations in India.

The variation in these cannabis products accounts for the wide psychoactive potency exhibited with each product. Thus, persons whose experience has been primarily with the low-potency marijuana preparations may have a different view of cannabis effects than other persons, who use the more potent products of hashish and hash oil. The pharmacological classification for cannabis is difficult to assign, unless the dose level is specified, and can range from stimulant, sedative, analgesic to psychomimetic (Harris, 1979).

In 1982 a survey in the United States found that marijuana was the most commonly used of all the non-legal psychoactive drugs, with the age group 18–25 years consistently showing the highest rate of current use (Relman, 1982). The report further states that by 1979 more than 50 million individuals in the United States had tried marijuana at least once. In 1981, it was estimated that approximately 3 million Canadians, one-third of whom were teenagers, had used cannabis products within the last year, and recent observations point towards a shift to the more potent products of hashish and hash oil (Fahlman, 1982).

The effects of marijuana when smoked are usually felt within a few minutes, reach their peak in 10–30 minutes and linger on for a few hours. The dose, the environment and the expectation of the user greatly determine the effects experienced. Low doses may produce a sense of well-being or euphoria, with feelings of relaxation. Doses of 2.5 and 5 mg produce effects on mood, memory, motor coordination and cognitive ability (Hollister, 1974). With much stronger doses, the effects are increased dramatically and can cause distortion, hallucinations, loss of personal identity, resulting in a psychotic situation (Hembree et al., 1979). Tolerance does occur where frequent and high doses of cannabis are given (Hembree et al., 1979).

Tissue distribution studies in animals indicate that ^{14}C-labelled THC is transferred across the placenta and accumulates in fetal tissues and amniotic fluid (Harbison and Mantilla-Plata, 1972), reaching highest concentrations in fetal brain (Kennedy and Waddell, 1972). THC or its metabolites are covalently bound to maternal and fetal tissues, and such covalent binding of reactive metabolites may produce adverse effects in the developing embryo or fetus (Evans and Harbison, 1977). THC and its metabolites are secreted into the milk and substantial amounts of radioactivity were found in the liver, brain, stomach, spleen, heart and lung of suckling pups after the subcutaneous administration of ^{14}C-labelled THC to lactating rats (Jakubovic et al., 1973).

Marijuana smoke, extracts from cannabis resin and the plants as well as pure THC have been tested for embryotoxic and teratogenic actions in laboratory mammals by several investigators. Interspecies differences have been observed in the teratogenic activity of the resin of cannabis. High incidences of resorptions and stunting of fetuses, without apparent malformations, occurred in mice (Persaud and Ellington, 1967). On the other hand, injections of cannabis extract to pregnant rats produced not only marked increase in fetal resorption and stunting, but also a wide variety of congenital malformations, such as phocomelia, amelia, syndactyly, encephalocele, and eventration of abdominal viscera (Persaud and Ellington, 1968). Extracts from marijuana plant injected into hamsters and rabbits during the period of major organogenesis were markedly embryocidal in rabbits, but produced multiple malformations in hamsters (Geber and Schramm, 1969). Pace et al. (1971), however, were unable to duplicate the marijuana extract teratogenicity in hamsters. These workers also reported that treatment of gravid rats and rabbits with marijuana extract produced erratic results.

Rosenkrantz et al. (1978) exposed rats and mice to marijuana smoke during gestation, with THC doses equivalent to those consumed by heavy chronic marijuana users. No adverse effects were noted on the pregnancy rate, maternal weight gain, litter size and weight and sex ratio for both species. On the other hand, marijuana smoke produced embryotoxic effects, but did not cause any soft tissue anomalies or skeletal abnormalities in either species. The presence of carbon monoxide in the marijuana smoke may have been a contributory factor in producing embryotoxicity because of diminished oxygen supply to the fetus (Rosenkrantz, 1979).

No congenital anomalies were observed in the offspring of rhesus monkeys given THC before and during pregnancy, although the incidence of resorptions, abortions, fetal death, stillbirth and neonatal deaths were higher in treated dams than in the controls (Sassenrath et al., 1979).

In summary, the overwhelming majority of animal studies including primates indicate that marijuana smoke, crude marijuana extract and pure THC are embryotoxic/fetotoxic but not teratogenic. However, the isolated reports on cannabis-related congenital defects in mice (Harbison et al., 1977), rabbits (Fournier et al., 1976), hamsters (Geber and Schramm, 1969) and rats (Persaud and Ellington, 1968) deserve serious consideration and warn against using cannabis during pregnancy. Some of the discrepancies may be attributed to variations in dose, route of administration and species; however, the most important factor is probably variability of cannabinoid content in marijuana (Fleischman et al., 1980).

In human studies, Fried (1982) studied 420 subjects, including several infants born to marijuana users, and concluded that a shorter gestation period and a reduced maternal weight gain were associated with heavy marijuana use. However, no association between marijuana and birth weight, birth abnormalities or difficulties at birth were observed. The relationship reported previously by the same investigator (Fried, 1980) between marijuana and aspects of neonatal behaviour, such as increased tremors and startles and altered visual responsiveness, remained a consistent finding in the 60–80-hour-old babies. However, based on a 'limited' number of babies, these effects were less striking at 9 days, whereas by 30 days they no longer distinguished the offspring of the heavy marijuana users. Further, at 1 year of age, no motor, mental or general behavioural attributes appeared to characterize the offspring of the marijuana users.

Thus, the preliminary human results (Fried, 1982) suggest that the measurable correlates in newborns of regular marijuana use during pregnancy diminish with age. Whether this is because the neurological abnormalities present at birth are overcome or compensated for with maturity, or whether the tests used at the later ages have a decreased discriminatory sensitivity to subtle differences that may exist, can only be answered by increasing the sample size and further follow-up of these infants.

IV. DEPRESSANT DRUGS

A wide variety of drugs are included in the group of depressant drugs: barbiturates, non-barbiturate hypnotics and sedatives, as well as major and minor tranquillizers. The pattern of use and the effects of these drugs are similar. The abuse of depressants includes the episodic intoxication in younger persons who gain their supply from the family medicine chest to the chronic user whose sources can be from neglectful physicians, illegal prescriptions, thefts or illicit manufacture. These substances include problems of subtle development of addiction and cross-tolerance with other depressants. The extent of the non-medical use of the 'downers' (slang term for depressants) is not accurately known, but is believed to exceed greatly that of the narcotics. The non-barbiturate depressant drugs comprise a very wide range of compounds, including benzodiazepines, methaqualone, bromides, chloral hydrate, meprobamate, glutethimide and antihistamines.

1. Barbiturates

Barbiturates are usually taken orally, with the effects occurring in about 20 minutes. The injection of a barbiturate causes a warm 'rush', which is considered different than the explosive (flash) effect achieved by a methamphetamine or cocaine injection. Although the barbiturates vary in potency, latency and duration of effects, there is general overlap in their characteristic properties. Normal medical applications are for the sedative-hypnotic or anticonvulsant effects using a dose of 100–200 mg. These low doses usually cause general relaxation or drowsiness, with a heightened sense of well-being. In some persons, a low dose may cause short-term excitement, which can lead to aggressive actions or loss of inhibitions. As the dose is increased, stronger sedative effects occur, with less control of emotions, until a drunk-like or stuporous effect results. Finally, at higher doses of 10–20 times above therapeutic, fatal situations occur from respiratory arrest and cardiovascular collapse. All these effects are potentiated by concomitant use of alcohol and other drugs.

Transport of barbiturates occurs at least as early as the 4th month of gestation (Pomerance and Yaffe, 1973), and cord serum levels achieve, on average, 95% of the concentration in the maternal serum (Sobel, 1960). All barbiturates cross the placenta very rapidly after maternal administration. They reach the fetus in significant concentration within 2 minutes after intravenous injection (Flowers, 1957) and within 30 minutes after maternal intramuscular injections (Ploman and Persson, 1957). Fetal exposure to barbiturates may cause central nervous system depression in the newborn in varying degrees, but correlation between the depth of this depression and the cord-blood barbiturate level is poor (Adamsons and Joelsson, 1966).

A barbiturate withdrawal syndrome has been described in the neonate (Bleyer and Marshall, 1973; Desmond et al., 1972; Hill and Stern, 1979). Infants born to mothers receiving barbiturates throughout pregnancy or throughout the 3rd trimester may show symptoms similar to those seen in infants of heroin-addicted mothers, though the former show up later than the latter, appearing by 10 days to 2 weeks of age (Hill and Stern, 1979). Withdrawal symptoms include irritability, high-pitched crying, tremulousness, etc. Symptoms were observed in infants of mothers receiving as little as 60 mg/day of barbiturates during the last weeks of pregnancy (Hill and Stern, 1979).

2. *Non-barbiturate depressants*

(a) Benzodiazepines

The benzodiazepine-type drugs are among the most widely used medicaments in the Western world, with their application as anticonvulsants, anxiolytics and muscle relaxants. Since they are regularly prescribed for treatment of anxiety, tension or insomnia, the increased occurrence of their misuse has become an issue of concern (Balter et al., 1974). As their actions are similar to other classes of drugs, they are often inappropriately termed 'minor tranquillizers'.

Fetal and neonatal effects resulting from administration of tranquillizers and antidepressants have not been studied adequately (Pomerance and Yaffe, 1973). Benzodiazepine derivatives, such as chlordiazepoxide and diazepam, cross the human placenta and appear in cord blood in concentrations similar to those in the mother. Some studies do report that there is no depression in infants born to mothers on benzodiazepines (Decanq et al., 1965; Cavanagh and Condo, 1964), whereas others report lower-than-average Apgar scores, i.e., evaluation of newborn's physical well-being based on numerical values assigned to heart rate, respiratory effort, muscle-tone, skin colour and reflex irritability (Lean et al., 1968; Owen et al., 1972). The causative factor remains unknown.

Hill and Stern (1979) report an increase in the incidence of central nervous system abnormalities in infants exposed to chlordiazepoxide. This correlation was present only if exposure occurred in the first 42 days of pregnancy. Athinarayanan et al. (1976) described late onset irritability and tremors in twins born to a mother receiving 30 mg of chlordiazepoxide per day. Infants born to mothers taking mood elevators demonstrate an exaggerated colic-like syndrome, lasting for 9 months (Hill and Stern, 1979). Cree et al. (1973) described an increased incidence of operative deliveries, resuscitation, hypothermia, apnea and hypotonia, with hypotonia lasting for 9–12 months. Safra and Oakley (1975) reported a 4-fold greater incidence of cleft lip and palate in infants of mothers who had received diazepam in the first trimester of their pregnancy. Two separate reports described early onset of withdrawal symptoms, consisting of tremors, hypertonia and hyperreflexia in infants of mothers receiving 10–15 mg of diazepam daily during the last 2–4 months of pregnancy (Rementeria and Bhatt, 1977; Mazzi, 1977).

V. STIMULANTS

1. *Cocaine*

Cocaine is derived from coca paste extracted from the leaves of the bush *Erythroxylon coca.* A crude mixture of coca paste results when coca leaves are steeped with kerosene to extract the raw drug, followed by alternate washes with sulphuric acid, alkali, and then kerosene. Further processing of the paste with hydrochloric acid can yield a relatively pure, white, flakey (or powdered) product of cocaine hydrochloride. Before being distributed illicitly, the cocaine product is usually diluted from two to eight times with such compounds as sugar (lactose, mannitol or inositol), local anaesthetics (procaine, lidocaine, tetracaine or benzocaine), or sometimes with other substances such as flour or talc.

Although cocaine has had considerable use as a local anaesthetic, most medical applications of the drug are now limited to eye disorders and in certain types of surgery. Since 1975, there has been a very significant increase in the illegal use of cocaine and its production from the source countries in South America. It is now reported to be the second most popular illicit drug (after marijuana) in Canada (MacLennen, 1982). Although an earlier study by Finkle and McClosky (1977) reported few cocaine deaths relative to the population, a later report by Caffery (1982) described a quadruple increase in the United States.

Cocaine is abused in a variety of ways, ranging from chewing the raw coca to inhalation, smoking or injection. Users most commonly consume the drug by 'snorting' or 'inhaling' the powder directly into the nose. A total dose can range from 15 to 125 mg of cocaine. More recently, users have started to inject or smoke cocaine. Smoking cocaine involves a prior process called free-basing, where the cocaine alkaloid is isolated from the street samples and concentrated on the end of a burning cigarette (marijuana or tobacco) and then sprinkled thoughout the cigarette. The manner of use determines the particular effect that is experienced by the user. Smoking is a less efficient procedure of administration than intravenous injection (Perez-Reyes et al., 1982). Cocaine may be also mixed with heroin to enhance the effects of either. Thus, the common pharmacology text may not include the description of adverse effects of heavy cocaine abuse (Byck and Van Dyke, 1977; Seigal, 1977).

The teratogenicity of cocaine was the subject of study by many investigators. [^{3}H]Cocaine was found to be quickly transferred across the mouse placenta, and the largest amounts of radioactivity were concentrated in the fetal liver (Evans and Harbison, 1977). Cocaine hydrochloride is teratogenic in CF-1 mice, as shown by Mahalik et al. (1980). Single subcutaneous injections of 60 mg/kg/day given on gestational days 7–12 were nontoxic to the mother, but produced significantly high incidences of anencephaly, cryptorchidism, hydronephrosis, anophthalmia, lens malformations, delayed ossification of skull or paws, and a wide variety of skeletal defects. As opposed to the saline controls, the resorptions were increased in the treated group, while the mean fetal weight remained unchanged. It was postulated that the cocaine-induced anomalies result from reduction in uterine blood flow and the subsequent decrease in oxygen supply to the fetus (Mahalik et al., 1980). Reports on human studies are few and not well established. Kushnick et al. (1972) described a malformed child with 45X Turner's syndrome and bilaterally absent fifth toes born to a primigravida with a history of nasal usage of both cocaine and heroin prior to and during early pregnancy. The validation of cocaine as the definite causative agent remains unconfirmed.

2. *Amphetamines*

A wide variety of amphetamines and related drugs are manufactured for various conditions, such as obesity, depression, narcolepsy and types of hyperactivity in children. Abuse of amphetamines has occurred with night-shift workers, students and long-distance truck drivers, who use the drugs to alleviate fatigue. Prominent abuse of amphetamines developed to a point in the 1960s where the practice of injecting the drugs, particularly methamphetamine, became a major concern (Le Dain, 1973). A related problem has recently occurred in the 1980s where tablets and capsules are prepared to look like many of the popular abusable amphetamines. These 'look-alike' stimulants, which contain caffeine, ephedrine or phenylpropanolamine and which closely resemble prescription amphetamines, are usually sold by direct mail mainly to adolescents.

In animal studies, following parental administration, dextroamphetamine causes a high incidence of heart, eye and skeletal defects in mice, although it is inactive in both rats and rabbits. When injected intravenously, methamphetamine produces eye, palate and brain abnormalities in mice and rabbits, but is non-teratogenic when given orally to primates. Daily oral administration of amphetamine sulphate (50 mg/kg) to mice thoughout pregnancy causes significantly higher fetal mortality and slightly greater incidences of cleft palate and umbilical herniation than the control group (Yasuda et al., 1965). Amphetamine is non-teratogenic in the rat (Schardein, 1976). Intrauterine exposure of rats to d,l-amphetamine produces neurochemical and behavioural changes in male offspring and long-lasting effects on the sexual behaviour of female progeny but no changes in sex cycle duration and ovulation. These postnatal effects of amphetamine are attributed to the modified catecholamine and 5-hydroxytryptophan turnover rates in the brain (Ramirez et al., 1979).

Human data indicate that there are some teratogenic risks with amphetamines. From a retrospective study of 184 mothers, Nora et al. (1970) found a higher incidence of cardiovascular anomalies in children of dextroamphetamine users than in 108 infants born to matched control mothers. However, in a prospective study, Levin (1971) found five cases of biliary tract atresia in infants exposed prenatally to dextroamphetamine or methamphetamine, but no evidence of congenital heart disease. Methamphetamine was linked with microcephaly and mental retardation with motor dysfunction in offspring of a woman who received this drug along with phenobarbital during the first and second trimesters of pregnancy (McIntyre, 1966). Eriksson et al. (1978) conducted a retrospective survey of 23 amphetamine abusers, six of whom had discontinued their abuse in early pregnancy, while the remaining 17 continued the abuse throughout pregnancy. One infant was still-born, with myelomeningocele, and another live-born child showed extensive telangiectasis. Six of the 22 babies were preterm, and three were small for their gestational age. Two of the full-term infants exhibited extreme lassitude and required tube feeding. Four of the 22 infants were markedly jaundiced (Eriksson et al., 1978).

VI. HALLUCINOGENS

Hallucinogenic substances include those from natural sources, e. g., mescaline from the peyote cactus and psilocybin from certain mushrooms, and from synthetic sources, e.g., lysergic acid diethylamide (LSD) and phencyclidine (PCP). Hallucinogenic drugs distort the perception of the user to objective reality. It may often become difficult for the user, who is hallucinating due to a high dose of the drug, to distinguish between fact and fantasy.

1. LSD

The teratogenic potential of LSD has been evaluated in several animal species, including primates. Most studies have shown non-teratogenesis or inconsistent results. ^{14}C-labelled LSD quickly traverses the placentas of hamsters (Idanpaan-Heikkila and Schoolar, 1969a) and mice (Idanpaan-Heikkila and Schoolar, 1969b), and autoradiographic results suggest that the distribution pattern of radioactivity in the fetus closely resembles that of the mother. Alexander et al. (1967) observed increased incidence of early resorption, stillbirths, and growth retardation, but no malformations in rats when single doses of LSD (5 μg/kg) were injected on the 4th day of pregnancy. Subsequent studies from several laboratories (Warkany and Takacs, 1968; Nosal, 1969; Roux et al., 1970; Uyeno, 1970) have failed to confirm these results and found no effects on litter size or fetal weight of LSD-treated rats. A single intraperitoneal injection of LSD (0.05–1 μg/mouse) into 7-day pregnant mice caused a 10 and 57% incidence of brain and facial malformations, respectively, in treated embryos examined 4 days post-treatment (Auerbach and Rugowski, 1967). On the other hand, Scheufler (1972) reported that daily intraperitoneal administration of 100 μg of LSD on days 1–12 of pregnancy was embryocidal, but not teratogenic in mice. A similar lack of teratogenic actions of LSD was reported in rats, mice and hamsters (Roux et al., 1970), rabbits (Fabro and Sieber, 1968) and rhesus monkeys (Wilson, 1969). The results of a behavioural study detected no significant differences in the locomotion or learning abilities in 20-day-old, 2-, 3- or 4-month-old offspring of rats injected with 2.5, 5 and 10 μg/kg LSD on day 4 of gestation. Further, the brain morphology remained unchanged in the progeny of LSD-treated dams (Uyeno, 1970).

The cytogenetic and teratogenic aspects of LSD in humans have been reviewed (Long, 1972; Sankar, 1975). Conflicting reports have appeared in the medical literature on the occurrence of LSD-related congenital malformations. Severe limb defects and central nervous system anomalies were reported in infants following maternal ingestion of LSD (Zellweger et al., 1967; Eller and Morton, 1970; Assemany et al., 1970; Apple and Bennet, 1974). In all these retrospectively reported cases, mothers confessed to having taken unknown amounts of LSD and, in some cases, both parents had used illicit drugs before and during pregnancy. On the other hand, the results of a prospective study of ten mothers known to have ingested hallucinogenic doses of LSD (once or on several occasions) during pregnancy showed no evidence of teratogenic effects in any of the babies (Aase et al., 1970). From a retrospective study involving 121 pregnancies with parental exposure to both medically administered and illicit LSD, McGlothlin et al. (1970) reported that the incidence of spontaneous abortions, premature births and congenital anomalies fell within the normal range. These authors, however, pointed out that the tendency towards spontaneous abortions among LSD users was higher than normal. The normal incidence of spontaneous abortions in women ranges from 15 to 20% (Warburton and Fraser, 1964). In another survey, 140 pregnant women and their consorts with personal histories of LSD usage (either in both parents or in only one parent) were followed through 148 pregnancies. While LSD ingestion was a common denominator of all the pregnancies, the relationship between LSD exposure and increased reproductive risk could not be established because of the interplay of several other factors, such as combined drug usage, maternal malnutrition and infections during pregnancy (Jacobson and Berlin, 1972). After a comprehensive review of the literature, Long (1972) identified LSD-related limb deformities in five of 161 children born to parents who took the drug before or during pregnancy. More recently, Verschaeve and Hens (1979) attempted to evaluate the genetic danger of LSD, and concluded that this drug does not seem to present a great genetic danger to humans, but that simultaneous use with other drugs is more hazardous. The foregoing suggests that there is no definite evidence regarding the teratogenic action of LSD in animals and man. Nonetheless, caution dictates that the use of this psychedelic agent should be avoided during pregnancy.

2. PCP

PCP (called: peace pill, angel dust) can be taken orally, by smoking or by injection, and is often sold as being LSD. At lower doses (1–5 mg), it produces adverse effects similar to alcohol and barbiturates. Cohen (1977) found that PCP produced disinhibition at low doses of 1–5 mg, toxic reaction psychosis at 5–15 mg, schizophreniform psychosis at doses higher than 15 mg. Chronic users can consume 100–1000 mg per day, and tolerance was reported to occur in these individuals (Peterson and Stillman, 1978).

Cooper et al. (1977) observed that following intramuscular administration prior to delivery PCP readily crosses the placenta of the sow, and the concentration of PCP in the newborn piglet plasma was 10 times greater than in maternal plasma. The plasma half-life of PCP in the piglet was 1–20 hours, compared with 2–4 hours in the sow. The drug was detectable in the piglet plasma for up to 48 hours. Recently, Law (1981) postulated that in the rat PCP is biotransformed to a reactive metabolite which binds irreversibly to liver, lung and kidney proteins. Whether the reactive metabolite of PCP causes cytotoxicity in animals and man remains to be verified.

Recently, Golden et al. (1980) described an infant with facial dysmorphogenesis and dislocated hip, born to a mother with a history of both marijuana and PCP abuse throughout pregnancy. At the age of 2 months, the infant had generalized spasticity, showed roving eye movements and coarse tremors, exacerbated by auditory and tactile stimuli. This appears to be the second report suggesting possible association between PCP abuse during pregnancy and adverse neonatal effects in the human. In an earlier report, Walker and Seig (1973) linked the maternal ingestion of PCP to increased incidence of limb reduction defects and triploidy in the offspring. These reports warrant a continued surveillance on the teratogenic risks of PCP.

VII. NARCOTICS

1. *General considerations*

The narcotic drugs have traditionally included the natural alkaloids of the opium poppy, the semi-synthetic derivatives of these compounds and other synthetic compounds with similar pharmacological properties.

Opium obtained from the dried juice of the unripened pod of the poppy plant — *Papaver somniferum* — is the parent substance for the isolation or synthesis of many narcotic drugs. Morphine, which accounts for 4–20% by weight of opium, is one of the most effective analgesic drugs known. It is also the precursor material for the production of the widely abused drug, diacetylmorphine or heroin, and the commonly used analgesic, codeine.

First used as a pain remedy in 1896, heroin became widely accepted in medical practice until its potential for addiction later became recognized. In its pure form, it is a white powder but can be seen in illicit preparations in a variety of colours. It is rarely sold on the street in pure form because it is diluted or cut to add bulk and profit. Sugar, starch, powdered milk, quinine and metapyrilene are examples of such diluents. Street heroin, called 'junk', 'smack', 'horse' or 'H', varies considerably in concentration and often contains only 2–4% drug. Significant heroin-user populations exist in the United States (450,000), Western Europe (200,000) and Canada (20,000) (Fahlman, 1982). Heroin is usually taken intravenously, termed 'mainlining' or 'shooting up', subcutaneously, termed 'skin popping', or sometimes by 'sniffing' or 'snorting'. Although heroin abuse reached extraordinary proportions in the 1960s and early 1970s in the United States, medical use of heroin in some situations, e.g., painful terminal cases, is becoming strictly regulated in some countries.

There are many synthetic narcotic drugs that have been prepared, primarily with the objective of maximizing their analgesic properties without the accompanying dangers of tolerance and dependence. Meperidine is a commonly used synthetic narcotic that has become an abused drug. Methadone is also a narcotic drug, but because of its less severe withdrawal symptoms it is widely used in detoxification programs for heroin addicts. Finally, pentazocine, which was once considered to be a non-narcotic analgesic, has been shown to be a drug with definite addiction properties (Mungavin, 1969). A more recent development since 1977 in the illicit market has been the abuse of pentazocine in combination with the antihistamine, tripelennamine. The mixture called 'T's and Blues', which refers to the product Talwin® (pentazocine) and to the light blue colour of pyribenzamine tablets (tripelennamine), has become popular with some heroin users in the United States (Poklis and Whyatt, 1980).

2. *Animal studies*

Morphine, codeine, methadone and meperidine have been shown to produce central nervous system defects in hamsters and mice (Schardein, 1976). Animal studies data are hard to interpret because all these drugs depress food intake and respiration, both of which are known to cause congenital defects. Single daily injections of morphine (15–45 mg/kg) to rats on days 5–18 of gestation had no effect on the litter size, but produced a significant reduction in pup birth weight and high pup mortality during the first week of life. However, postnatal behaviour in the offspring remained unaltered (Davis and Lin, 1972). Single subcutaneous injections of heroin (80 mg/kg) to mice on day 9 of pregnancy produced central nervous system malformations, whereas codeine and papaverine were practically devoid of any teratogenic activity in this species (Jurand, 1980).

Treatment of male rats with methadone (10 mg/kg/day for 12 days) prior to mating results in significantly lower birth weight of the progeny, and higher postnatal mortality than the saline control group (Soyka et al., 1978). Similarly, pre-treatment of male rats with methadone or morphine 24 hours before mating with untreated females increases the neonatal mortality of their offspring in a dose-dependent manner (Smith and Joffe, 1975).

3. *Human studies*

Maternal narcotic addiction constitutes a serious problem for the fetus and newborn, with increased risks of intrauterine growth retardation, perinatal mortality and neonatal morbidity (Harper et al., 1977; Fricker and Segal, 1978). The incidence of infant mortality in populations of mothers dependent on heroin and methadone is higher than in similar control groups (Finnegan et al., 1977). Withdrawal symptoms in newborn babies have been described following maternal ingestion of narcotic drugs, morphine, heroin, codeine, methadone and meperidine. Maternal narcotic addiction may also cause fetal addiction, resulting in neonatal narcotic withdrawal syndrome (Ananth, 1976; Ashton, 1977; Finnegan, 1981; Pierog, 1977). The signs and symptoms of withdrawal include restlessness, respiratory difficulty and cyanosis, vomiting, diarrhoea and poor suckling, yawning and stretching, sweating and fever, convulsions and, occasionally, death. The morphine and heroin withdrawal symptoms usually begin during the first 24–48 hours, whereas withdrawal symptoms from methadone may be noted as late as the 4th to 12th day after birth. The severity of symptoms is parallel to the degree of maternal dependence and the time lapse of the mother's last dose. Deprivation of the opiate-dependent mother from the drug prior to delivery can cause fetal withdrawal signs in utero, leading to increased fetal movements and sometimes fetal death (Ananth, 1976; Ashton, 1977; Pierog, 1977). While establishing the etiology of sudden infant death in the babies of addict mothers, it is important to investigate not only the maternal use of narcotics before and during pregnancy, but also the use of these drugs by the father. In a review of the effects of narcotics on pregnancy and the newborn, Finnegan (1981) commented on the significant potential hazard to the fetus and neonate, as they are continuously exposed to an adverse physical and local milieu.

VIII. VOLATILE SOLVENTS

There are a very large number of volatile substances that can be used to achieve a state of intoxication. They are readily vapourized at room temperature and usually easily absorbed by the lungs to cause altered states of consciousness, changes in mood and, often, hallucinations.

Terms such as 'sniffing', 'glue sniffing' or solvent abuse generally encompass the various practices of volatile substance abuse. Included in this general category is the less readily available product of nitrous oxide and ether. The solvents of abuse include those compounds listed in Table 1.

A 1982 report on solvent abuse and health education included various data on the incidence in Britain and the United States (Woodcock, 1982). It was estimated that there were 1–1.25 million current users of volatile substances in the United States, with 6.5–8.5 million persons having tried using solvents at least once. About 9% of the age group of 12–17 years old and about 16% of the 18–25 year olds were reported to have abused solvents at some time in their lives. Reports on the various aspects of volatile solvents abuse, primarily in the United Kingdom, was the topic of a special issue of Human Toxicology in 1982. The extent of the problem is not clearly defined, although there are serious occurrences in Britain (Anderson et al., 1982; Gay et al., 1982).

The methods of abuse of volatile substances are varied, and depend on the product used. Glue products may be squeezed into a polyethylene or paper bag and then the open end of the bag placed over the nose and the mouth, with deep breathing taking place until the euphoric effects occur. This procedure is obviously not limited to glue products and has included the solvents emanating from other products. Other methods of inhalation are described by Watson (1982).

TABLE 1

VOLATILE SUBSTANCES OF ABUSE

Category	Compounds
Hydrocarbons	Toluene, hexanes, butane
Chlorinated hydrocarbons	Methylene chloride, carbon tetrachloride, trichloroethylene
Fluorinated hydrocarbons	Trichlorofluoromethane, difluorodichloromethane
Ketones	Acetone, methylethylketone
Esters	Ethylacetate, isopropylates

TABLE 2

ADVERSE EFFECTS OF DRUGS OF ABUSE RELATED TO THE HUMAN NEWBORN

Drug	Response	Reference
Cannabis	Abnormalities in neurological neonatal behaviour	Fried, 1980
	Shorter gestation period, reduced maternal weight gain	Fried, 1982
Barbiturates	CNS depression in the newborn	Adamsons and Joelsson, 1966
	Barbiturate withdrawal syndrome in the neonate	Bleyer and Marshall, 1973 Desmond et al., 1972; Hill and Stern, 1979
Benzodiazepines	Lower-than-average Apgar scores	Lean et al., 1968; Owen et al., 1972
	Hypothermia, apnea, hypotonia in infants	Cree et al., 1973
	Cleft lip and palate in infants	Safra and Oakley, 1975
	Late onset irritability and tremors in infants	Athinarayanan et al., 1976
	Withdrawal and symptoms	Rementeria and Bhatt, 1977; Mazzi, 1977
	CNS abnormalities in infants and colic-like syndromes	Hill and Stern, 1979
Cocaine	Malformation with 45X Turner's syndrome and bilaterally absent fifth toes	Kushnick et al., 1972
	Microcephaly and mental retardation with motor dysfunction	McIntyre, 1966
Amphetamines	Higher incidence of cardiovascular anomalies in children	Nora et al., 1970
	Biliary tract atresia in infants	Levin, 1971
	Stillbirth with myelomeningocele, telangiectasia, prematurity, small for gestational age, and extreme lassitude	Eriksson et al., 1978
Hallucinogens		
LSD	Severe limb defects and CNS anomalies	Zellweger et al., 1967; Eller and Morton, 1970; Assemany et al., 1970; Apple and Bennet, 1974
	Spontaneous abortions	McGlothlin et al., 1970
	Limb deformities	Long, 1972
PCP	Facial dysmorphogenesis and dislocated hips	Golden et al., 1980
	Limb reduction defects and triploidy	Seigal, 1977
Narcotics	Intrauterine growth retardation, perinatal mortality and neonatal morbidity	Finnegan et al., 1977; Fricker and Segal, 1978
	Neonatal narcotic withdrawal syndrome and withdrawal signs in utero	Ananth, 1976; Ashton, 1977; Pierog, 1977

Most of these volatile compounds have not been investigated fully as they are not used in normal medical procedures. Those that have been studied have usually been considered in lower concentrations pertinent to industrial exposure, rather than acute doses. For some of the compounds, metabolism does occur, although many are excreted chemically unchanged by the lungs. The psychological and physiological effects of these volatile solvents are somewhat similar to that of alcohol in that low doses cause considerable removal of inhibition and euphoria, whereas higher concentrations usually result in general sedation.

To our knowledge the abuse of volatile substances has not been studied in pregnancy, and thus effects on the newborns are not documented. Since the problem has surfaced fairly recently, the biomedical community should be alerted to the potential hazards of these chemicals.

IX. CONCLUSIONS

The epidemic of drug abuse has increased over the past decade, bringing with it numerous complex problems and a significant health dilemma manifested in many countries of the world. One of the major problems has been the abuse of drugs by pregnant women and numerous investigators have reported the extremely high incidence of obstetrical and medical complications among addicts. The morbidity and mortality among newborn infants in these cases far exceeds those found in any other high-risk maternal and infant population. An account of the more common drugs prone to abuse, their pertinent pharmacological features and teratogenic effects have been discussed and their adverse effects in humans are summarized in Table 2.

X. ACKNOWLEDGEMENTS

The authors wish to thank Dr. H.S. Buttar for supplying a literature review and Mrs. Louise Belisle for typing the manuscript.

XI. REFERENCES

Aase, J.M., Laestadius, N. and Smith D.W. (1970) Lancet 2, 100–101.

Adamsons, K., Jr. and Joelsson, I. (1966) Am. J. Obstet. Gynec. 96, 437–460.

Alexander, G.J., Miles, B.E., Gold, G.M. and Alexander, R.B. (1967) Science 157, 459–460.

Ananth, J. (1976) Int. Pharmaco-Psychiat. 11, 246–260.

Anderson, H.R., Dick, B., McNair, R.S., Palmer, J.C. and Ramsay, J. D. (1982) Human Toxicol. 1, 207–223.

Apple, D.J. and Bennet, T.O. (1974) Arch. Opthalmol. 92, 301–303.

Ashton, C.H. (1977) in Textbook of Adverse Drug Reactions (Davies, D.M., ed.), pp. 64–80, Oxford University Press, Oxford.

Assemany, S.R., Neu, R.L. and Gardner, L.I. (1970) Lancet 1, 1290.

Athinarayanan, P., Pierog, S.H. and Nigam, S.K. (1976) Am. J. Obstet. Gynec. 124, 212–213.
Auerbach, R. and Rugowski, J.A. (1967) Science, 157, 1325–1326.
Balter, M.B., Levine, J. and Mankeimer, D.I. (1974) N. Eng. J. Med. 290, 769–774.
Bleyer, W.A. and Marshall, R.E. (1973) J. Am. Med. Assoc. 221, 185–186.
Byck, R. and Van Dyke, C. (1977) in Cocaine 1977 (Petersen, R.C. and Stillman, R.C., eds.), NIDA Research Monograph, No. 13, pp. 97–117. U.S. Government Printing Office, Washington, DC.
Caffery, R.J. (1982) Drug Enforcement 9, 2–5.
Campbell, J.S., Mikhael, N.Z. and Napke, E. (1981) Meth. Achiev. Exp. Pathol. 10, 221–241.
Cavanagh, D. and Condo, C.S. (1964) Current Ther. Res. 6, 122–126.
Cohen, S. (1977) J. Am. Med. Assoc. 238, 515–516.
Cooper, J.E., Cummings, A.J. and Jones, H. (1977) J. Physiol. 267, 17–18.
Cree, J.E., Meyer, J. and Hailey, D.M. (1973) Br. Med. J. 4, 251–255.
Cushing, H. (1925) The Life of Sir William Osler, Vol. 1, Ch. 14.
Davis, W.M. and Lin, C.H. (1972) Res. Commun. Chem. Pathol. Pharmacol. 3, 205–214.
Decanq, H.G., Bosco, J.R. and Townsend, E.H. (1965) J. Pediat. 67, 836–840.
Desmond, M.M., Schwanecke, R.P., Wilson, G.S., Yasunaga, S. and Burgdorff, I. (1972) J. Pediat. 80, 190–197.
Eller, J.L. and Morton, J.M. (1970) N. Engl. J. Med. 283, 395–397.
Eriksson, M., Larsson, G., Windbladh, B. and Zetterstrom, R. (1978) Acta Paediatr. Scand. 67, 95–99.
Evans, M.A. and Harbison, R.D. (1977) in Drug Abuse in Pregnancy and Neonatal Effects (Rementeria, J.L., ed.), pp. 195–208, The C.V. Mosby Company, Saint Louis, MO.
Fabro, S. and Sieber, S.M. (1968) Lancet 1, 639.
Fahlman, R.C. (1982) in Royal Canadian Mounted Police National Drug Intelligences Estimate, 1981, pp. 13, 57, R.C.M.P., Ottawa.
Finkle, B.S. and McClosky, K.L. (1977) in Cocaine 1977 (Petersen, R.C. and Stillman, R.C., eds.), NIDA Research Monograph, No. 13, pp. 153–192, United States Government Printing Office, Washington, DC.
Finnegan, L.P. (1979) Bull. Narcotics 31, 2–58.
Finnegan, L.P. (1981) Ann. N.Y. Acad. Sci. 362, 136–157.
Finnegan, L.P., Reeser, D.S. and Connaughton, J.F. (1977) Drug Alcohol Dep. 2, 131–140.
Fleischman, R.W., Nagui, R.H. and Rosenkranz, H. (1980) J. Environ. Pathol. Toxicol. 4, 471–482.
Flowers, C.E. (1957) Obstet. Gynec. 9, 332–335.
Fournier, E., Rosenberg, E., Hardy, N. and Nahas, G. (1976) in Marijuana: Chemistry, Biochemistry and Cellular Effects, pp. 457–468 (Nahas, G.G., ed.), Springler Verlag, New York.
Fricker, H.S. and Segal, S. (1978) Am. J. Dis. Child. 132, 360–366.
Fried, P.A. (1980) Drug Alcohol Depend. 6, 415–424.
Fried, P.A. (1982) Neurobehav. Tox. Terat. 4, 451–454.
Gay, M., Mellor, R. and Stanley, S. (1982) Human Toxicol. 1, 257–264.
Geber, W.F. and Schramm, L.C. (1969) Toxicol. Appl. Pharmacol. 14, 276–282.
Golden, N.L., Sokol, R.J. and Rubin, I.L. (1980) Pediatrics 65, 18–20.
Harbison, R.D. (1980) in Casarett and Doull's Toxicology: The Basic Science of Poisons, 2nd ed., (Doull, J., Klaassen, C.D. and Amdur, M.O., eds.), pp. 158–175, MacMillan Publishing Co., Inc., New York.
Harbison, R.D. and Mantilla-Plata, B. (1972) J. Pharmacol. Exp. Ther., 180, 446–453.
Harbison, R.D., Mantilla-Plata, B. and Lubin, D.J. (1977) J. Pharmacol. Exp. Ther. 202, 455–465.
Harper, R.G., Solish, G., Feingold, E., Gersten-Woolf, N.B. and Sokal, M.M. (1977) Am. J. Obstet. Gynecol. 129, 417–424.
Harris, L.S. (1979) in Mechanisms of Pain and Analgesic Compounds (Beers, R.F., Jr. and Bassett, E.G., eds.), pp. 467–473, Raven Press, New York.
Hawks, R.L. (ed.) (1982) in Analysis of Cannabinoids, Research Monograph 42, p. 127, National Institute for Drug Abuse, Washington, DC.
Hembree, W.C., Nahas, G.G., Zeindenberg, P. and Huang, H.F.S. (1979) in Marijuana: Biological Effects (Nahas, G.G. and Paton, N.D.M., eds.), pp. 429–439, Pergamon Press, New York.

Hill, R.M. and Stern, L. (1979) Drugs 17, 182–197.
Hollister, L.E. (1974) Clin. Pharmacol. Ther. 15, 18–21.
Idanpaan-Heikkila, J.E. and Schoolar, J.C. (1969a) Lancet 2, 221.
Idanpaan-Heikkila, J.E. and Schoolar, J.C. (1969b) Science 146, 1295–1297.
Jacobson, C.B. and Berlin, C.M. (1972) J. Am. Med. Assoc. 222, 1367–1373.
Jakubovic, A., Hattori, T. and McGeer, P.L. (1973) Eur. J. Pharmacol. 22, 221–223.
Jurand, A. (1980) Develop. Growth Differ. 22, 61–78.
Kennedy, J.S. and Waddell, W.J. (1972) Toxicol. Appl. Pharmacol. 22, 253–258.
Kushnick T., Robinson, M. and Tsao, C. (1972) Am. J. Dis. Child. 124, 772–773.
Law, F.C.P. (1981) Toxicol. Appl. Pharmacol. 57, 263–272.
Lean, T.H., Ratnam, S.S. and Sivasamboo, R. (1968) J. Obstet. Gynecol. Br. Commonwealth 75, 853–855.
LeDain, G. (1973) Final Report of the Commission of Inquiry into the Non-Medical Use of Drugs, pp. 334–338, Information Canada, Ottawa.
Levin, J.N. (1971) J. Pediat. 79, 130–131.
Long, S.Y. (1972) Teratology 6, 75–90.
MacLennen, A. (1982) The Journal 11, No. 7, pp. 7–9, Addiction Research Foundation Press, Toronto.
Mahalik, M.P., Gautierei, R.F. and Mann, D.E. (1980) J. Pharmacol. Sci. 69, 703–706.
Mazzi, E. (1977) Am. J. Obstet. Gynecol. 129, 586–587.
McGlothlin, W.H., Sparkes, R.S. and Arnold, D.O. (1970) J. Am. Med. Assoc. 212, 1483–1487.
McIntyre, M.S. (1966) J. Am. Med. Assoc. 197, 62–63.
Mikhael, N.Z., Campbell, J.S., Napke, E. and McLean, W. (1979) in The Liver and Biliary Systems in Infants and Children (Chandra, K. K., ed.), pp. 229–241, Churchill Livingstone, Edinburgh.
Mirkin, B.L. (1973) Clin. Pharmacol. Ther. 14, 643–647.
Mungavin, J.M. (1969) Lancet 2, 56–57.
Nora, J.J., Vargo, T.A., Nora, A.H., Love, K.E. and McNamara, D.G. (1970) Lancet 1, 1290–1291.
Nosal, G. (1969) Laval Med. 40, 45–55.
Owen, J.R., Irani, S.F. and Blair, A.W. (1972) Arch. Dis. Childhood 47, 107–110.
Pace, H.B., Davis, W.M. and Borgen, L.A. (1971) Ann. N.Y. Acad. Sci. 191, 123–131.
Perez-Reyes, M., DiGuiseppi, S., Ondrusek, G., Jeffcoat, A.R. and Cook, C.E. (1982) Clin. Pharmacol. Therapeutics 32, 459–465.
Persaud, T.V.N. and Ellington, A.C. (1967) Lancet 2, 1306.
Persaud, T.V.N. and Ellington, A.C. (1968) Lancet 2, 406–407.
Petersen, R.C. and Stillman, R.C. (1978) Phencyclidine: A Review, p. 5, National Institute on Drug Abuse, Rockville, MD.
Pierog, S. (1977) in Drug Abuse in Pregnancy and Neonatal Effects (Rementeria, J.L., ed.), pp. 95–102, The C.V. Mosby Company, St. Louis, MO.
Ploman, L. and Persson, B.H. (1957) J. Obstet. Gynecol. Br. Emp. 64, 706–708.
Poklis, A. and Whyatt, P.L. (1980) J. Forensic Sci. 25, 72–78.
Pomerance, J.J. and Yaffe, S.J. (1973) Current Prob. Pediat. 4, 13–17.
Ramirez, O.A., Carrer, H.F. and Nasello, A.G. (1979) Pharmacol. Biochem. Behav. 11, 605–609.
Relman, A.S. (1982) in Marijuana and Health, pp. 34–56, National Academy Press, Washington, DC.
Rementeria, J.C. and Bhatt, K. (1977) J. Pediat. 90, 123–126.
Rosenkrantz, H. (1979) in Marijuana: Biological Effects (Nahas, G.G. and Paton, W.D.M., eds.), pp. 479–499, Pergamon Press, New York.
Rosenkrantz, H., Fleischman, R.W. and Baker, J.R. (1978) Fed. Proc. 37, 737 (Abstract).
Roux, C., Dupuis, R. and Aubry, M. (1970) Science 169, 588–589.
Safra, M.J. and Oakley, G.P. (1975) Lancet 2, 478–480.
Sankar, D.V.S. (1975) in LSD - A Total Study, pp. 470–500, PJD Publications Ltd., Westbury, New York.
Sassenrath, E.N., Chapman, L.F. and Goo, G.P. (1979) in Marijuana: Biological Effects (Nahas, G.G. and Paton, W.D.M., eds.), pp. 501–512, Pergamon Press, New York.
Schardein, J.L. (1976) Drugs As Teratogens, pp. 57–66, 73–75, CRC Press Inc., Cleveland, OH.
Scheufler, V.H. (1972) Biol. Rundsch. 10, 396–399.

Seigal, R.K. (1977) in Cocaine 1977 (Petersen, R.C. and Stillman, R.C., eds.), NIDA Research Monograph, No. 13, pp. 119–136, U.S. Government Printing Office, Washington, DC.
Smith, D.J. and Joffe, J.M. (1975) Nature 253, 202–203.
Sobel, D.E. (1960) Arch. Gen. Psych. 2, 606–611.
Soyka, L.F., Peterson, J.M. and Joffee, J.M. (1978) Pediat. Res. 11, 422 (Abstract).
Uyeno, E.T. (1970) Proc. Western Pharmacol. Soc. 13, 200–203.
Verschaeve, L. and Hens, L. (1979) Acta Psychiat. Belg. 4, 437–458.
Walker, F.A. and Seig, J.A. (1973) Mut. Res. 21, 348–349.
Warburton, D. and Fraser, F.C. (1964) Am. J. Hum. Genet. 16, 1–25.
Warkany, J. and Takacs, E. (1968) Science 159, 731–732.
Watson, J.M. (1982) Human Toxicol. 1, 249–256.
Wilson, J.G. (1969) in Methods for Teratological Studies in Experimental Animals and Man (Nishimura, H. and Miller, J.R., eds.), pp. 16–33, Igaku Shoin Ltd., Tokyo.
Wilson, J.G. (1973) Environment and Birth Defects, pp. 1–10, Academic Press, New York.
Woodcock, J. (1982) Human Toxicol. 1, 331–336.
Yasuda, M., Ariyuki, F. and Nishimura, H. (1965) Okajimas Fol. Anat. Jap. 41, 227–231.
Zellweger, H., McDonald, J.S. and Abbo, G. (1967) Lancet 2, 1066–1068.

S. Kacew and M.J. Reasor (eds), *Toxicology and the Newborn*
© 1984 Elsevier Science Publishers B.V.

Chapter 6

Toxicity of Carbon Monoxide Exposure in Early Development

LAURENCE D. FECHTER

Department of Environmental Health Sciences, The Johns Hopkins University School of Hygiene and Public Health, Baltimore, MD 21205, U.S.A.

CONTENTS

I. INTRODUCTION

There is little question that fetal oxygen deprivation represents a fundamental and well-recognized threat to survival and normal development. While the consequences of acute hypoxia and anoxia are known, the boundary conditions at which oxygen deprivation produces teratogenic effects are undetermined. Given the large range of xenobiotics and pathophysiological conditions which may reduce oxygen-carrying capacity of maternal hemoglobin or decrease uterine perfusion and those agents which may impede oxygen utilization, it is critical to determine fetal susceptibility to oxygen deprivation. This requires a thorough understanding of toxicokinetic factors which might render the fetus particularly susceptible to a chemical asphyxiant, physiologic factors such as maturation of adaptive mechanisms which may protect against toxic effects, and knowledge of critical periods during which hypoxic exposure might disrupt irreparably the development of structural or biochemical processes. Such global goals are based upon more prosaic investigations of the consequences of individual hypoxic agents in development and, eventually, comparisons between specific xenobiotics whose presumed toxicity is mediated through disruption of oxygen delivery and hypoxic hypoxia.

This chapter reviews the literature on toxicity of carbon monoxide exposure during the prenatal and neonatal periods and makes the assumption that hypoxia is a fundamental aspect of carbon monoxide toxicity. The available literature is derived from three different sources: 1, studies of neonatal asphyxiation using carbon monoxide, hypoxic hypoxia, and placental clamping; 2, studies of maternal cigarette smoking or smoke exposure; and 3, chronic prenatal exposures to carbon monoxide, hypoxic hypoxia and dichloromethane. The latter is an organic solvent which is metabolized in vivo to form carbon monoxide.

Clearly, the results of some of these studies may not relate directly to pure carbon monoxide toxicity in development. While these different conditions may well have some unique components, the hypothesis that they also share some fundamental similarities based upon disruption of oxygen delivery is deserving of experimental attention.

II. SOURCES OF CARBON MONOXIDE EXPOSURE

Carbon monoxide (CO) is a ubiquitous pollutant of air, but its presence is highly correlated with human population and industrial development. Mobile sources account for the largest share of CO generated by man, representing in the late 1970s approximately 75% of this total (National Research Council, 1977), but home heating and waste from industrial processes also contribute substantially to community CO levels (Kahn et al., 1974). The relative importance of these sources in elevating CO levels in blood as indexed by population carboxyhemoglobin levels is not, however, related directly to their contribution to total atmospheric carbon monoxide. When considering sources of carboxyhemoglobin (HbCO), the use of tobacco represents the largest source of sustained CO exposure (Wallace et al., 1974; Cole, 1975). Cigarette smoke contains approximately 3–5% (30,000–50,000 ppm) CO. While we might predict an elevation above baseline in the order of 0.5–1.0% in HbCO values due to community air pollution and industrial exposures in a population, cigarette smokers on average show a 5% elevation in HbCO over non-smokers (Stewart et al., 1976; Wallace et al., 1974). Transportation (automobile exhaust), occupational exposures and home heating (including the burning of wood and use of improperly vented stoves) still can represent significant sources of both acute and sustained CO intoxication in specific individuals, although not necessarily in a community-wide survey. Carbon monoxide is also generated endogenously in the degradation of heme proteins and presumably contributes substantially to the background carboxyhemoglobin levels of 0.5–0.75% seen among non-smokers who are unlikely to experience significant environmental CO exposure (Sjostrand, 1949).

A largely unrecognized source of CO exposure is the metabolism of the dihalogenated methanes in vivo. Dichloromethane (DCM), commonly used as a paint remover and as a degreaser, can produce very high HbCO levels (Kubic et al., 1974; Ratney et al., 1974; DiVincenzo and Hamilton, 1975; Stewart and Hake 1976). DCM can cross the placenta in rats, but it is likely that the fetus would be exposed both to CO generated in the maternal liver and to DCM (Anders and Sunram, 1982). Stevens et al. (1980) have shown that other dihalomethanes are converted to CO in the isolated rat hepatocyte preparation and that, at least for DCM, this effect is increased by agents known to induce cytochrome *P*-450 (phenobarbital and 3-methylcholanthrene) and reduced by SKF-525A. While dibromo- and difluoromethane, which are used as chemical intermediaries, may also be metabolized to form CO in vivo, it is not clear from clinical data to what extent they represent a threat to human health.

In evaluating the effects of cigarette smoking on health and, in this review, the consequences of maternal smoking on fetal development, it must be borne in mind that tobacco smoke represents a very complex exposure to many biologically active agents, of which carbon monoxide represents only one component. However, the epidemiologic data with respect to maternal cigarette smoking provide an unusually good resource from which to develop experimental protocols for evaluating CO toxicity in the fetus. This is true due to the unfortunately large population of women who persist in smoking throughout pregnancy. Moreover, similarities between the consequences of maternal smoking on the fetus and those from other hypoxic agents suggest a possible common mechanism of toxicity.

III. BASIS FOR FETAL SUSCEPTIBILITY TO CARBON MONOXIDE

There are both toxicokinetic (dose) and physiologic bases for predicting that the fetus might show a difference to the adult in susceptibility to CO. While CO readily passes across the placenta, Longo and Hill (1977) have shown that the build-up of fetal HbCO lags behind that of maternal HbCO and, similarly, that the washout of CO from the fetal compartment is also slower. This phenomenon is not uncommon in considering the kinetics into and out of the fetal compartment. A practical consequence of this fact, noted by Longo (1977), is that the clinical treatment of the CO-intoxicated pregnant patient with oxygen therapy must take into account the relatively long washout time for fetal CO rather than relying on restoration of low maternal HbCO values as an endpoint.

Fetal CO exposures are likely to exceed adult levels (given a relatively sustained exposure) because of the higher affinity of fetal hemoglobin for CO (Longo and Hill, 1977; Longo, 1977). The extent of the difference in the fetal to maternal 'partition' of CO appears to be species-related, but consistently to render the fetus more susceptible to CO (Longo, 1970). Given these toxicokinetic considerations, it can be predicted that fetal CO exposures will tend to surpass the peak level seen in the adult under all but the briefest exposures. Longo (1970) suggests that the failure in some early studies to find significant elevations of fetal HbCO levels following acute CO intoxications which were lethal to the mother was misinterpreted as resulting from an effective placental barrier to CO rather than from the relatively long time necessary for fetal accumulation of CO.

Several physiologic factors are also likely to increase the likelihood of CO exposure. First, endogenous production of CO is elevated during pregnancy, a finding which reflects the increase in total hemoglobin during pregnancy rather than a true elevation in rate of production (Linderholm and Lundstrom, 1969). Other factors are somewhat more open to conjecture. These include: the relative dissociation of oxygen from fetal vs. maternal hemoglobin in the presence of HbCO (that is, the relative importance of the 'Haldane effect' as a function of p_{O_2} and CO-Hb affinity); maturation of adaptation mechanisms, such as increased cardiac output in response to CO challenge; susceptibility of specific developmental processes, such as cell proliferation, differentiation and migration to CO exposure; and fetal requirements for oxygen. Because there are few data which bear directly on these issues, the greater part of this review will consist of experimental data documenting the consequences of chronic and acute carbon monoxide exposure prenatally and neonatally and demonstrating the susceptibility of the developing organism to this agent. While adaptation responses and protective mechanisms against CO and hypoxia are not considered directly, the toxic consequences of exposure may be viewed as those which result despite such mechanisms.

IV. MECHANISMS OF CARBON MONOXIDE TOXICITY

The most certain mechanism by which CO produces toxicity is by competitive inhibition of oxygen binding to hemoglobin. Given a relative affinity of hemoglobin for CO relative to O_2 of approximately 250, it is clear that even moderate CO exposures will reduce the oxygen-carrying capacity of blood. In addition to reducing directly the oxygen-carrying capacity of blood, there is a second aspect of CO toxicity which is likely to affect the fetus. Carboxyhemoglobin shifts the oxyhemoglobin (HbO_2) saturation curve to the left at a given p_{O_2} by increasing the affinity of the available (unbound) hemoglobin for O_2 (Roughton and Darling, 1944; Longo, 1970). This shift is particularly pronounced at low oxygen tensions such as those maintained in the fetus and means that less oxygen will dissociate from HbO_2 and be delivered to tissue at a given p_{O_2}.

There remains some question as to whether CO might produce some additional toxicity which is not accounted for strictly by its hypoxic effects. Several experiments have shown that extremely high HbCO levels can be tolerated by experimental animals when the CO is administered intraperitoneally (Goldbaum et al., 1976). The explanation given for these findings is that CO is toxic only when dissociated from hemoglobin so that it can bind with intracellular heme proteins. The importance of such a mechanism remains in doubt and its contribution to the toxicity of carbon monoxide is subject to further study.

V. CONSEQUENCES OF PRENATAL CARBON MONOXIDE EXPOSURE

1. *Growth and teratogenesis*

The evidence for a classical teratogenic effect of CO is principally restricted to high-level acute exposures in which the central nervous system appears to be the major, but not exclusive target. Beaudoing et al. (1969) cite lethality and isolated case reports of teratogenesis associated with high-level CO exposure during the first trimester. These include malformation of the hands and legs. They also summarize the more common encephalopathies associated with acute prenatal CO exposure. Of course, these case reports frequently do not provide for clear documentation of dosage and duration of exposure and so it is difficult to predict critical CO exposures likely to yield developmental disorders. Table 1 presents an overview of experimental studies which measured growth, survival and/or teratogenic consequences of carbon monoxide or DCM exposure. Only one such report (Astrup, 1972) has noted (anecdotally) a teratogenic outcome following moderate, chronic exposure. In that study rabbits exposed throughout gestation to 180 ppm CO (HbCO = 16–18%) were reported to have been born with missing limbs. Quantitative data showing dramatic increase in stillbirths and fatalities within 24 hours are presented. Regrettably, while data on the striking increase in fatalities are given (36% in 180 ppm exposed subjects vs. 1% in controls), no frequencies are reported on missing limbs and it is impossible to compare it with a background level in the colony. However, the magnitude of effect seen with this exposure protocol in Astrup's laboratory appears to be somewhat more severe than reported in other species. For example, teratogenesis has not been reported with chronic low-level CO administrations either by casual observation in rats allowed to deliver their offspring (Fechter and Annau, 1977, 1980; Garvey and Longo, 1978) or when systematically investigated in fetal CF-1 mice and New Zealand rabbits (Schwetz et al., 1979). In the latter study, subjects were exposed to 250 ppm CO for either 7 or 24 hours per day (HbCO values approximately 10% in mice and 15% in rabbit). They did report a significant increase in mild skeletal

TABLE 1

EFFECTS OF PRENATAL CARBON MONOXIDE ON GROWTH AND DEVELOPMENT

Exposure	HbCO	Species	Birth weight	Litter size	Survival	Additional comments	References
30 or 90 ppm CO, GD 3–20	4.8 & 8.8%	Rat	–	–	n.d.	Brain edema	Garvey and Longo, 1978
90 or 180 ppm CO	9–18%	Rabbit	↓	–	↓	Some teratogenesis	Astrup, 1972
150 ppm CO	15%	Rat	–	–	–	Reduced growth rate after removal from CO	Fechter and Annau, 1977, 1980
75, 150 and 300 ppm CO	9, 15 & 24%	Rat	↓	–	–		Fechter and Storm, 1984
230 ppm CO, GD 2–PD 21	24%	Rat	↓	–	↓PD4 & 24	Reduced growth rate in CO neonatally	Hoffman and Campbell, 1977
250 ppm CO 7 or 24 hour/day, GD 6–15	10%	Mouse	–	–	↑Resorptions with 7 hours exposure but decreased with 24 hours	Extra lumbar spurs and ribs	Schwetz et al., 1979
250 ppm CO 7 or 24 hour/day, GD 6–18	15%	Rabbit	↑(7 hours only)	–			Schwetz et al., 1979
60, 125, 250 500 ppm CO	n.d.	Rat	↓	n.d	n.d	n.d	Prigge and Hochrainer, 1977
4500 ppm DCM, GD 1–17 or 3 weeks +GD 1–17	n.d.	Rat	↓	–	n.d.	–	Hardin and Manson, 1980
1200 ppm DCM, 7 hours/day, GD 6–15	10%	Rat Mouse	– –	–	– –	– –	Schwetz et al., 1975

GD, gestational day (when not noted exposure occurred throughout pregnancy); PD, postnatal day; n.d., not determined; –, no significant change; ↓, significant decrease reported; ↑, significant increase reported.

variants in the mice (increased number of lumbar ribs and lumbar spurs), which they distinguish from a teratogenic outcome, but failed to replicate Astrup's report of teratogenicity in rabbits. Reduced survival in rats exposed to CO has also been reported in subjects chronically exposed prenatally and neonatally to 230 ppm (HbCO = 24%) (Hoffman and Campbell, 1977), but the relative contribution of prenatal and neonatal exposure is unclear. Finally, neither Hardin and Manson (1980) nor Schwetz et al. (1975) found teratogenic effects of prenatal DCM exposures. Schwetz et al. (1975) used exposure levels yielding HbCO values of approximately 10% in rats and mice. Hardin and Manson (1980) used substantially higher DCM levels (4500 vs. 1250 ppm) and exposed their subjects (rats) for 24 hours per day, but did not report HbCO levels.

While significant effects of CO on litter size, resorptions, sex ratios and survival generally have not been reported, somewhat stronger evidence of depressed birthweights exists. While significant birthweight reductions have not been reported universally, the trends are almost always in the expected direction, and significant depression in birthweight is commonly observed when several CO dosages are included and/or when the number of litters used is relatively large. This is exemplified by a recent study of Fechter and Storm (1984) in which rats exposed throughout gestation to 75, 150 and 300 ppm CO (9, 15 and 25% HbCO) or air were compared for birthweights (see Table 2). Here, using the mean weight from each litter we see a significant overall effect of CO using analysis of variance (ANOVA) and an appropriate dose-effect curve with a trend to birthweight reduction seen even at 75 ppm CO exposure. It should be pointed out that when each individual subject's birthweight is used in statistical analyses that the number of degrees of freedom is greatly inflated, thus making the chances of finding an apparent significant effect greater. Since birthweights of individuals within a litter are almost certainly not 'independent events', it does not seem appropriate to use the individual as the basic unit of analysis. Reduced birthweights were also reported in rabbits (Astrup, 1972), in rats exposed to CO (Penney et al., 1983) and in rats exposed to DCM (Hardin and Manson, 1980).

TABLE 2

PRENATAL CARBON MONOXIDE EXPOSURE (ppm)

	0	75	150	300
Average No. pups	12.6	11.3	11.1	11.6
S.E.	±0.5	±0.7	±1.0	±0.7
Average birthweight (g)	6.49	6.26	6.08	5.45*
S.E	±0.11	±0.17	±0.24	±0.16
Ratio male/female	1.3	1.1	1.1	1.2
S.E.	±0.2	±0.2	±0.2	±0.1

*$P<0.001$.

Several experiments in which HbCO levels of 10% or less were used failed to observe a change in birthweight. This was true in rats exposed to CO (Garvey and Longo, 1978) and in mice exposed to DCM (Schwetz et al., 1975) or CO (Schwetz et al., 1979).

Reduced birthweights have also been observed in offspring of animals born at high altitude (3800 m, Kelley and Pace, 1968) and in hypoxia control groups included in the study of Astrup et al. (1975). Further, Gross et al. (1981) showed reduced birthweights in neonatal rats exposed to 9.1% O_2 for the 9–11 days preceding birth. It is tempting to attribute these similarities to an underlying effect of hypoxia.

The decrease in birthweight observed after CO exposure may complicate the analysis of biological consequences studied later in development. However, reduction in birthweight appears to be a fundamental aspect of CO toxicity, and not a consequence of reduced maternal weight gain during pregnancy (see Fig. 1). Further, as noted below, significant biological effects of CO have been observed in the developing rat after birth, in the absence of significant weight differences at the time of testing.

2. *Central nervous system development*

The central nervous system (CNS) represents, along with the cardiovascular system, the principal target organ for CO toxicity. In the case of the CNS this probably reflects the very high rate of oxygen utilization by this organ system. The data presented below show that acute CO intoxication can kill neurons and that the pattern of cell loss is quite similar to that seen with hypoxic hypoxia and even ischemia.

In neonates, CO asphyxiation can produce changes in cell morphology, behavior and neurochemistry. It is not particularly clear whether these effects are merely

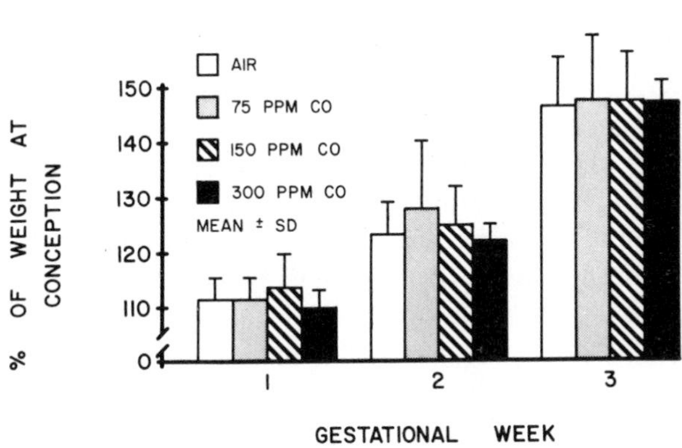

Figure 1. Effects of carbon monoxide exposure on maternal weight gain during each week of gestation in the rat.

correlated or are causally related. The asphyxiation studies do not indicate whether certain developmental processes are more sensitive than others to insult. Evidence that mild, chronic CO exposure during early development may disrupt CNS development is largely indirect, consisting principally of behavioral studies which document altered neuronal function, but which fail to pinpoint the neuroanatomical or biochemical basis for the effects.

The consequences of acute perinatal CO on the brain do not appear to vary greatly from the effects of other asphyxiants or even from ischemia. Ginsberg and Myers (1974a) exposed term-pregnant monkeys to 1000–3000 ppm CO over 1–3 hours, inducing maternal HbCO values above 60%. Fetal delivery was performed as soon as the exposure terminated. In fetuses receiving the 'severe treatment' (fetal arterial p_{O_2} averaging 6–10% for a 1-hour period) moderate-to-marked brain swelling was reported in four out of five subjects. These subjects required mechanical respiration and were killed between 12 and 72 hours after delivery, whenever severe cardiopulmonary distress was noted. They clearly showed abnormal neural signs. Brains of severely exposed neonates showed pathological changes attributable to severe edema, hemorrhage in various brain regions, and softening or necrosis of the basal ganglia, cerebral cortex and, in certain cases, hippocampus and/or cerebellum. The thalamus was affected less severely. Among 'moderate exposure' subjects (fetal arterial p_{O_2} averaging 11–12% for 1 hour), no brain swelling, cortical or subcortical necrosis was reported.

Norton and Culver (1977) asphyxiated 5-day-old rats in 10,000 ppm CO until respiratory failure occurred, resuscitated the subjects, and examined both locomotor activity and development of dendritic spines on caudate neurons. They found enhanced dendritic spine density in CO-exposed subjects present at 2–7 months of age, but not at 6 weeks of age. They correlated this increased spine density with recovery from behavioral hyperactivity which they noted in their juvenile CO-exposed rats (Culver and Norton, 1976). Ginsberg and Myers (1974b, c) exposed anaesthetized juvenile rhesus monkeys to 1000–3000 ppm CO for 75–325 minutes, producing HbCO levels of 62–81%, and studied both the cardio-respiratory responses to this challenge and subsequent neurological function and histopathology. Subsequent neuropathology was correlated with a variety of indices of exposure severity abstracted from the physiologic responses to CO exposure. They reported varying degrees of lesion to cortical white matter which correlated significantly with occurrence of low systolic blood pressure during exposure and with metabolic acidosis. Cortical lesions were bilaterally symmetrical and seen most clearly in the posterior parietal and posterior prefrontal areas. Some animals also showed damage to the anterior commissure, corpus callosum, internal capsule, fornix, globus pallidus and Sommer's sector of the hippocampus.

Such damage is not strikingly different from that reported after ischemia or hypoxic hypoxia (Myers, 1979). It is not particularly clear whether the apparent increased susceptibility of particular cell types to hypoxia is related to rates of cell metabolism, perfusion and proximity to supplying vessels. These theories have been critically reviewed elsewhere (Myers, 1979). The effects of protracted low-to-moderate carbon monoxide exposure or hypoxia on neuronal development is essentially unknown. Fechter and Annau (1977) reported reduced brain protein levels at birth following prenatal exposure to 150 ppm CO, but the permanence of this effect and its significance in terms of brain function are uncertain.

3. Behavioral consequences

Chronic prenatal CO exposure has been shown both to delay maturation of several specific behaviors and to have permanent behavioral consequences. Fechter and Annau (1980) showed that the offspring of rats exposed throughout gestation to 150 ppm CO (15% HbCO) were significantly slower than control subjects in developing negative geotaxic and homing behaviors as neonates. These are commonly used tests for assessing behavioral teratology which rely upon observation of normally occurring behaviors in subjects as they mature. Similarly exposed CO neonates also showed less locomotor activity in an activity monitor than did controls at 14 days of age and were less responsive to pharmacological challenge with the catecholamine precursor 3,4-dihydroxyphenylalanine (L-DOPA) at postnatal ages 1 and 4 days. Thus, while L-DOPA elevated brain dopamine (DA) levels in CO-exposed subjects and consequently increased locomotion, these increases were not as large as those measured among control subjects (Fechter and Annau, 1977). Further interpretation of these data is problematical. While behavioral delays clearly are symptomatic of abnormal development, it is difficult to attribute the disorder to a particular brain region or functional system. Indeed, one might argue for a muscular or neuromuscular explanation for the above data. More recent work by Mactutus and Fechter (1984a) clearly shows that prenatal CO exposure has central nervous system consequences. Juvenile rats which had been exposed to 150 ppm CO or to air were tested for acquisition and retention of a conditioned avoidance task. Subjects were required to respond to a 5-second light and tone stimulus by moving to the opposite side of the test compartment in order to avoid electric shock. 100 trials were given per session. Crossings made between trials were used as a measure of activity and response latency on the first five escape trials as an index of aversiveness of the electric shock. The following day, the test procedure was repeated. The second test day provided an opportunity to measure savings from day 1. The data show a significant deficit in the CO neonates both in original learning and in retention on the second test day. That the data are not a reflection of generalized debilitation is shown by the lack of difference in intertrial crossings or in shock escape latency. Moreover, there were no significant body weight differences found in these subjects.

Mactutus and Fechter (1984b) also found evidence for impaired memory in adult rats which had been exposed prenatally to 150 ppm CO as compared to air subjects. In one such study, adult rats were trained in the conditioned avoidance response task until they were performing at a criterion of 10 successive avoidance responses within the 50 trials which constituted a test session. 1 month after mastering the task, subjects were again tested to measure savings and relearning. The number of trials required to meet criterion was compared between groups (see Fig. 2). As in the case

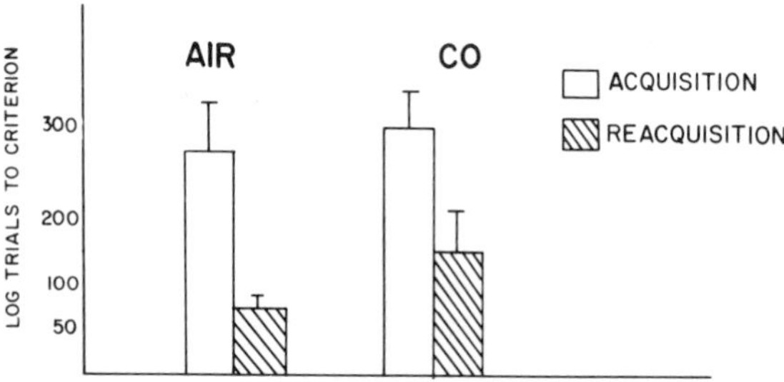

Figure 2. Effects of prenatal CO exposure (150 ppm) on learning and retention of a conditioned avoidance response in adult subjects. The retention test was given 1 month after original learning.

of juvenile rats, cognitive deficits were apparent in the rats exposed prenatally to CO. These data have been replicated in this laboratory in both juvenile and adult rats. They suggest very serious consequences of prenatal CO exposure. Further study to elucidate the generality of this finding to other learning tasks varying, for example, in degree of complexity would be useful. Based upon susceptibility of the cerebral cortex and hippocampal cortex to asphyxiation and the involvement of these structures in learning and memory function, currently we are evaluating the possibility that mild prenatal CO exposure may also damage cells in these brain regions.

4. *Neurotransmitter function*

The synthesis and utilization of a variety of neurotransmitters have been shown to be sensitive to acute hypoxic exposures introduced by carbon monoxide, hypoxic hypoxia and exposure to chemical asphyxiants. Such changes have been demonstrated prior to alteration of cellular energy charge potential or lactate/pyruvate ratio, leading some authors to propose both a vulnerability of the synthesizing enzymes to relatively small decreases in oxygen availability (Davis and Carlsson, 1973a, b; Hedner et al., 1977a, b) and a role of altered neurotransmitter function in the consequences or symptomatology of hypoxia (Brown et al., 1974; Brown and Engel, 1973; Snider et al., 1974). Davis and Carlsson (1973a, b) reported in adult rats that both tyrosine and tryptophan hydroxylase activity measured in vivo were depressed following a 2-hour exposure to 5.6% O_2. They note that these enzymes may not be saturated fully with oxygen under normoxic conditions and suggest a potential vulnerability of these neurotransmitter systems to hypoxic insult. Similar decreases in acetylcholine synthesis have been reported following exposure of adult mice to KCN or $NaNO_2$, yielding methemoglobin levels of 30–80% (Gibson and Blass, 1976). Newby et al. (1978) reported that both hypoxia (8% O_2) and 1500 ppm carbon monoxide reduced the disappearance of DA from caudate nucleus and the olfactory region in subjects receiving the catecholamine synthesis inhibitor, α-methyl tyrosine. These data suggest a drop in DA utilization in the adult brain exposed to hypoxia. Similar experiments carried out in neonatal animals also indicate that neurotransmitter utilization may be disrupted by acute hypoxia or asphyxiation. However, only limited data are available on this point. Hedner et al. (1977a) reported that exposure to 12% O_2 for 30 minutes reduced accumulation of the catecholamine and serotonin precursors DOPA and 5-hydroxytryptophan in subjects administered an L-amino acid decarboxylase inhibitor. This experiment suggests that hypoxia reduces the rate of synthesis of these compounds, presumably by decreasing tyrosine and trytophan hydroxylase activity.

During a recovery period of up to 6 hours after hypoxia, evidence of a rebound elevation of DOPA levels was seen in the striatum of 4-day-old rats exposed to 6% O_2 for 30 minutes (Hedner and Lundborg, 1980). They also reported that hypoxic exposure (6% O_2 for 1–2 weeks) also slowed the rate of disappearance of DA from whole brain following α-methyl tyrosine treatment. Such findings are interpreted as indicating reduced utilization of the neurotransmitter.

Two reports of chronic consequences of neonatal asphyxia on catecholamine neurochemistry have appeared. Simon and Volicer (1975) in one of the most direct studies in this area asphyxiated neonatal rats and determined serotonin and catecholamine activity as incorporation of tritiated tryptophan and tyrosine at 5–6 weeks of age. They report an increase in norepinephrine synthesis in treated subjects. Shellenberger (1982) exposed 5-day-old rats to 4200 ppm CO for 2 hours and measured steady-state catecholamine and serotonin levels in the surviving subjects (75%) at ages 16–24 weeks. While several of the neurochemical changes observed appear to be due to the hypothermia and 'stress' associated with exposure, CO asphyxiation does appear to result in a clear reduction in striatal DA concentration per mg wet tissue.

Recently, Storm and Fechter (1983) reported preliminary evidence of enhanced norepinephrine levels in the cerebellum of 14–42-day-old rats prenatally exposed to 150 and 300 ppm CO. The significance of this effect in terms of cerebellar function or development of synaptic connections is uncertain.

5. *Cardiovascular consequences of CO exposure*

The study of cardiovascular and hematopoietic effects of CO exposure during early development is particularly interesting because of the possibility for adaptive changes with sustained exposure which might limit CO toxicity. Adaptation in the form of increased hematocrit, total hemoglobin and redistribution of blood flow have been described in the adult exposed to CO (Wilks et al., 1959; Theodore et al., 1977; Jones et al., 1971; Traystman et al., 1978). Prigge and Hochrainer (1977) exposed rats to 60, 125, 250 and 500 ppm CO prenatally for 21 days and examined the effects on a variety of fetal cardiovascular and hematopoietic measures (see Table 3). They reported significant reduction in hematocrit and hemoglobin in fetuses exposed to 250 and 500 ppm CO. A small increase in hematocrit was seen only in the 60-ppm exposure condition. All CO-treated groups showed elevated wet heart to body weight ratios, which reflected both decreased fetal body weights (seen at 125, 250 and 500 ppm) and an absolute increase in wet heart weight at all but the highest CO

TABLE III

EFFECTS OF PRENATAL CARBON MONOXIDE ON CARDIOVASCULAR DEVELOPMENT IN RAT

Exposure	HbCO (%)	Body weight	Wet heart weight	Heart/ body weight	Dry heart weight	Hematocrit	Total hemoglobin	Other	References
150 ppm CO, GD 1–21	15	–	↑	↑	↓	n.d.	n.d.	Nucleic acid protein unchanged. No significant differences at PD 4–21	Fechter et al. (1980)
230 ppm CO, GD 2–PD 21	24	↓	n.d.	↑PD5	n.d.	↑ PD5	↑ PD5		Hoffman and Campbell (1977)
60,125, 250, 500 ppm CO, GD 1–21	n.d.	↓	↑	↑	n.d.	↓,250–500 ppm	↓,250–500 ppm		Prigge and Hochrainer (1977)
157,166 200 ppm CO, GD 5–22	24.9% for 200 ppm	↓	↑ (ventricles)	↑	↑	–	–	↑ LDH M subunit ↑ DNA content	Penney et al. (1983)
200 ppm CO	27.8	↓	↑	↑	n.d.	↓	↓	No lasting effects of prenatal exposure	Penney et al. (1980)
30, 90 ppm CO	4.8–8.8	–	–	–	n.d.	–	–		Garvey and Longo (1978)

GD, gestational day; PD, postnatal day; n.d., not determined.

concentration. As noted by the authors, these results are of interest because the cardiomegaly observed cannot be attributed to increased blood viscosity, and thus the mechanism involved is uncertain.

Fechter et al (1980) proposed that edema might be responsible for the effects observed by Prigge and Hochrainer (1977). They showed that prenatal exposure to 150 ppm CO (15% HbCO) did produce elevated wet heart weight at birth, but that this was a transient effect not present at the neonatal age of 4 days, when subjects had been moved to a normal air environment. Since dry heart weight did not differ between groups at birth and because the dry/wet heart weight ratio was significantly depressed in CO neonates (see Table 4), the elevated wet heart weight was proposed to reflect edema. Supporting evidence in the form of slightly depressed protein and nucleic acid concentration but not content was also given.

These data have been disputed recently by Penney et al. (1983), who exposed pregnant rats to 157, 166 and 200 ppm CO from gestational days 5–22. They showed depressed red blood count, but elevated corpuscular hemoglobin and volume in treated subjects. While body weight was depressed, ventricular heart weight, ventricular heart weight to body weight ratio, placental weight, and its ratio to body weight were all elevated. In contrast to the findings of Fechter et al. (1980), Penney et al. (1982) showed elevation in ventricular dry heart weight and in DNA content (but not concentration) in subjects exposed to 157 and 200 ppm. Cardiac lactate dehydrogenase (LDH) M subunit, but not total LDH activity, was elevated by exposing fetuses to 200 ppm. Myoglobin concentration and content were also elevated. Cardiac hydroxyproline content, a measure of collagen, was elevated in fetal but not neonatal hearts of exposed rats. The discrepancies reported by Fechter et al. (1980) and Penney et al. (1983) are difficult to reconcile. They might reflect Penney's use of ventricles only in his heart measures, while Fechter et al. (1980) used the whole heart.

Alternatively, it might reflect differences in severity of the CO exposure despite what are nominally very similar CO concentrations used for exposure. Penney et al. (1983) reported maternal HbCO levels of 24.9% following 200 ppm exposure while

TABLE IV

BIRTHWEIGHT AND CARDIAC PARAMETERS IN 1-DAY-OLD RATS PRENATALLY EXPOSED TO AIR OR 150 ppm CARBON MONOXIDE

	Body weight (g)	Hematocrit	Wet heart (mg)	Dry heart (mg)	Dry/wet heart	Wet heart/ body weight
Air	5.92±0.42	39.9±5.8	21.4±3.4	6.0±1.2	0.28±0.05	0.36±0.07
Carbon monoxide	5.66±0.62	41.6±6.7	30.0±5.1	5.5±1.8	0.18±0.05	0.53±0.07
Student's *t*-test	1.2275	0.6	4.7702*	0.8	4.6569*	5.9569*
Degrees of freedom	21	18	21	21	21	21

Values are mean (±S.D.) * $P<0.002$.

we have not seen HbCO levels that high until subjects are exposed to 300 ppm CO. Thus, at a common CO concentration, we would expect the strain of rat used by Penney et al. (1983) to have higher HbCO levels than our subjects. Finally, Penney et al. (1983) have used individual subjects rather than litter means as their basic unit of analysis, and thus one might expect their statistical tests to be less conservative than those used by Fechter et al. (1980). In discussing the increased heart weight and DNA content of ventricles in CO-exposed neonates, Penney et al. (1983) attribute the effect to a possible increase in cardiac output and potentially increased blood volume based upon placental hypertrophy. These explanations are ad hoc and direct evidence clearly is needed. It should, finally, be noted that the increase in heart size and hematopoietic effects after prenatal CO exposure have been reported to be transitory (Penney et al., 1980).

VI. NEONATAL CARBON MONOXIDE EXPOSURE

Neonatal CO exposure (500 ppm for the first 35 days of life) has been shown to elevate hemoglobin and to enhance heart weight (Penney et al., 1974). In younger rats the right ventricle appears to show the largest increase in weight, although the left ventricle plus interventricular septum also significantly increases in weight (Penney et al., 1974). Neonatal CO exposure appears to induce a larger increase in heart weight than exposure later in life (Penney et al., 1974) and a far larger effect on the heart weight/body weight ratio than prenatal CO exposure alone (Penney et al., 1980). However, these findings are problematical in several respects. First, the increase in absolute heart weight tends to disappear after subjects are removed from the CO, while body weight remains significantly depressed into adulthood (Penney et al., 1980). As a result a significantly higher heart weight to body weight ratio is reported in adult subjects exposed neonatally to CO (Penney et al., 1980). Secondly, neither DNA nor hydroxyproline content is elevated by neonatal CO exposure lasting for 32 days (Penney et al., 1982) and cytochrome *c* and LDH M subunit were altered only during CO exposure (Penney et al., 1982). There is, then, an obvious need for functional studies to determine the significance of the rather long-lasting elevation in relative heart weight following neonatal CO exposure. Further, it would be useful to compare in one experiment the effects of hypoxia and CO exposure on neonatal heart cell proliferation using, for example, [^{3}H]thymidine incorporation with autoradiography. When such studies were conducted following neonatal exposure to 12–15% oxygen, evidence of enhanced cell proliferation was observed (Hollenberg et al., 1976).

VII. MATERNAL SMOKING AND FETAL DEVELOPMENT

The scientific literature bearing on the effects of in utero carbon monoxide exposure on development in humans is limited essentially to case reports of severe maternal carbon monoxide asphyxiation. Exposure levels and durations are not well documented and the number of cases is relatively small. There does exist an extensive epidemiological literature concerning the consequences of maternal cigarette smoking on the developing child. While it is not possible to attribute these consequences specifically to the carbon monoxide in cigarette smoke, similarities of findings in this literature, the experimental carbon monoxide literature and both epidemiological and experimental studies carried out at altitude strongly suggest that carbon monoxide exposure might be responsible for at least some of the findings. While the effects of maternal smoking on the fetus have been reviewed extensively elsewhere (US DHEW, 1979), a review of some of the most salient effects and their similarity to high altitude studies are presented here.

Literally dozens of reports conducted on an estimated half-million births have found a correlation between extent of maternal smoking and reduced birthweight (cf., US DHEW, 1979). This is probably the clearest association which can be drawn between maternal smoking and untoward developmental effects in the offspring. Decreased birthweight has also been associated with pregnancy at high altitude in epidemiologic reports conducted in Colorado (2744–3100 m) (McCullough et al., 1977; Moore et al., 1982) and in Peru (4600 m) (Kruger and Arias-Stella, 1970). Among women living at high altitude, the offspring of cigarette smokers showed even greater reduction in birthweight than did offspring of non-smokers (Moore et al., 1982). As noted above, reduced birthweight has also been reported in experimental investigations using rodents brought to high altitude during pregnancy.

Maternal cigarette smoking increases the frequency of premature births in a dose-dependent fashion, although mean gestation duration is only slightly decreased due to the overwhelming percentage of births of normal duration in both groups (Meyer, 1977). This increase in premature births cannot account for decreases in birthweights between groups. Rather, Butler and Alberman (1969) have shown that the offspring of cigarette smokers are lighter in weight at all gestational ages than are similarly aged offspring of non-smokers. Not only do the offspring of smokers weigh less at birth, but they are also shorter and have reduced head circumference (Kullander and Kallen, 1971). Findings similar to those of Kullander and Kallen (1971) have also been reported in children born at high altitude (Moore et al., 1982).

Maternal smoking is associated in a dose-dependent fashion both with increased perinatal mortality and with increased incidence of complications during delivery, including placenta previa, placenta abruptio and premature rupture of membranes (Meyer and Tonascia, 1977). Perinatal mortality due to maternal smoking tends to be associated with other risk factors, including low maternal hemoglobin levels, maternal age (over 35 and under 20), public vs. private hospital status and previous complications in pregnancy (Meyer et al., 1975). Thus, the finding of significant elevation in perinatal mortality in a particular epidemiological investigation reflects the presence of these other risk factors in the study population. Increased perinatal mortality has been reported to be associated with pregnancy at high altitude (McCullough et al., 1977). Rather little is known about the development of surviving offspring of cigarette smokers, although these obviously represent the bulk of cases.

Rantakallio (1978) studied mortality and morbidity among children of smokers and non-smokers up to the age of 5 years. In this study smoking and non-smoking pregnant women were matched on a variety of social and biological factors prior to birth. Rantakallio (1978) reported decreased birthweight in the offspring of smokers and increased mortality between the ages of 0 and 5 years. The relative risk of death among offspring of smokers was greatest in the heavier birthweight categories, perhaps suggesting that other life-threatening factors were responsible for the low birthweights of non-smokers' offspring who died. Hospital admissions were elevated among the offspring of cigarette smokers between 0 and 5 years of age for a wide variety of complaints, ranging from pulmonary to nervous system to skin disorders. The mechanisms responsible for elevating the occurrence of such a disparate group of disorders are unclear. Finally, Davie et al. (1972) have studied the development of children up to the age of 7 years as part of the British Perinatal Mortality Study. Offspring of cigarette smokers were reported to be significantly shorter (by 1 cm) and to show delays in reading attainment (4 months). Subjective ratings by teachers also indicated that these children showed poorer social adjustment than the offspring of non-smokers (Davie et al., 1972). That relatively subtle yet significant impairment of social and intellectual development is observed in children whose mothers smoked during pregnancy (and quite possibly during their early childhood) is an alarming finding which demands further study. Specifically, given the findings of learning and memory impairment in adult and juvenile rats prenatally exposed to CO, it is important both to replicate the findings of Davie et al. (1972) and to attempt to define more rigorously the agent(s) responsible.

VIII. CONCLUSIONS

Despite the fact that carbon monoxide has been recognized to be a potent toxicant for hundreds of years, there remain significant unanswered questions concerning the consequences of sub-lethal exposures. This is especially true in susceptible but rarely studied sub-populations such as the fetus and neonate. While profound effects have been demonstrated following CO asphyxiation, the threshold level at which biological changes of significance for the organism occur is unknown. Indeed, it is not clear what the most sensitive measure of CO toxicity is in the developing organism. This review has cited data which show that chronic prenatal exposures of at least 150 ppm CO (15% HbCO) do result in significant behavioral symptoms, which no doubt reflect disruption in CNS development. Both the nature of the insult to the brain and the lower dose at which this effect is seen remain to be elucidated.

This review has also stressed similarities between the consequences of CO exposure and exposure to other hypoxic conditions. Further study is needed to determine the extent of such similarities and to ascertain the mechanism of CO toxicity in the developing organism.

IX. ACKNOWLEDGEMENTS

This chapter is dedicated to the memory of Mary B. Meyer, Sc.M., teacher, colleague and friend, who contributed enormously to our knowledge of the consequences of maternal cigarette smoking on fetal development. This work was supported by Research Career Development Award No. ES 00125.

X. REFERENCES

Anders, M.W. and Sunram, J.M. (1982) Toxicol. Lett. 12, 231–234.

Astrup, P. (1972) Br. Med. J. 4, 447–452.

Astrup, P., Trolle, D., Olsen, H.M. and Kjeldsen, K. (1975) Arch. Environ. Hlth. 30, 15–16.

Beaudoing, A., Gachon, J., Butin, L.P. and Bost, M. (1969) Pediatrics 24, 539–553.

Brown, R. and Engel, J. (1973) J. Pharmac. Pharmacol. 25, 815–819.

Brown, R.M., Kehr, W. and Carlsson, A. (1974) Brain Res. 85, 491–509.

Butler, N.R. and Alberman,B.D. (1969) Perinatal Problems. The second report of the 1958 British Perinatal Mortality Survey, E. and S. Livingston Ltd., London.

Cole, P.V. (1975) Nature 255, 699–701.

Culver, B. and Norton, S. (1976) Expl. Neurol. 50, 80–98.

Davie, R., Butler, N. and Goldstein, H. (1972) From birth to 7: The second report of the National Child Development Study, with full statistical appendix, National Children's Bureau and Longman Group Ltd., London.

Davis, J. and Carlsson, A. (1973a) J. Neurochem. 20, 913–915.

Davis, J. and Carlsson, A. (1973b) J. Neurochem. 21, 783–790.

DiVincenzo, G.D. and Hamilton, M.L. (1975) Toxicol. Appl. Pharmacol. 32, 385–393.

DiVincenzo, G.D. and Kaplan, C.J. (1981) Toxicol. Appl. Pharmacol. 59, 130–140.

Fechter, L.D. and Annau, Z. (1977) Science 197, 680–682.

Fechter, L.D. and Annau, Z. (1980) Neurobehav. Toxicol. 2, 7–11.

Fechter, L.D. and Storm, J.E. (1984) Prog. Neuro-Psychopharm. Biol. Psychia., in press.

Fechter, L.D., Thakur, M., Miller, B., Annau, Z. and Srivastava, U. (1980) Toxicol. Appl. Pharmacol. 56, 370–375.

Garvey, D.J. and Longo, L.D. (1978) Biol. Reprod. 19, 8–14.

Gibson, G.E. and Blass, J.P. (1976) J. Neurochem. 27, 37–42.

Ginsberg, M.D. and Myers, R.E. (1974a) Acta. Obstet. Gynec. Scand. 53, 309–317.

Ginsberg, M.D. and Myers, R.E. (1974b) Arch. Neurol. 30, 202–208.

Ginsberg, M.D. and Myers, R.E. (1974c) Arch. Neurol. 30, 209–216.

Goldbaum, L.R., Orellano, T. and Dergal, E. (1976) Ann. Clin. Lab. Sci. 6, 372–376.

Gross, J., Burgoyne, R. and Rose, S. (1981) J. Neurochem. 37, 229–237.

Hardin, B.D. and Manson, J.M. (1980) Toxicol. Appl. Pharmacol. 52, 22–28.

Hedner, T. and Lundborg, P. (1980) Acta Physiol. Scand 109, 169–175.

Hender, T., Lundborg, P. and Engel, J. (1977a) Biol. Neonate 31, 122–126.

Hedner, T., Lundborg, P. and Engel, J. (1977b) Biol. Neonate 32, 229–236.

Hoffman, D.J. and Campbell, K.I. (1977) Toxicol. Lett. 1, 147–150.

Hollenberg, M., Honbo, N. and Samorodu, A.J. (1976) Am. J. Physiol. 1445-1450.

Jones, R.A., Strickland, J.A., Strunkard, J.A. and Siegel, J. (1971) Toxicol. Appl. Pharmacol. 19, 46–53.

Kahn, A., Rutledge, R.B., Davis, G.L., Altes, S.A., Gantner, G.E., Thornton, C.A. and Wallace, N.D. (1974) Arch. Environ. Hlth. 29, 127–135.

Kelley, F.C. and Pace, N. (1968) Am. J. Physiol. 214, 1168–1175.

Kruger, H. and Arias-Stella, J. (1970) Am. J. Obstet. Gynecol. 106, 586–591.

Kubic, U.L., Anders, M.W., Engel, R.R., Barlow, E.H. and Cauhey, W. S. (1974) Drug. Metab. Dispos. 2, 53–57.
Kullander, S. and Kallen, B. (1971) Acta. Obstet. Gynecol. Scand. 50, 83–94.
Linderholm, H. and Lundstrom, P. (1969) Acta. Obstet. Gynecol. Scand. 48, 362–370.
Longo, L.D. (1970) Ann. N. Y. Acad. Sci. 174, 313–339.
Longo, L.D. (1977) Am. J. Obstet. Gynecol. 129, 69–103.
Longo, L.D. and Hill, E.P. (1977) Am. J. Physiol. 232, H324–H330.
Mactutus., C.F. and Fechter, L.D. (1984a) Science 223, 409–411.
Mactutus., C.F. and Fechter, L.D. (1984b) Teratology, in press.
McCullough, R.F., Reeves, J.T. and Liljegren, R.L. (1977) Arch. Environ. Hlth. 32, 36–39.
Meyer, M.B. (1977) in The Epidemiology of Prematurity (Reed, D.M. and Stanley, F.J., eds.), pp. 81–104, Urban and Schwarzenberg, Baltimore.
Meyer, M.B. and Tonascia, J.A. (1977) Am. J. Obstet. Gynecol. 128, 494–502.
Meyer, M.B., Tonascia, J.A. and Buck, C. (1975) Am. J. Epidemol. 100, 443–452.
Myers, R.E. (1979) Adv. Neurol. 26, 195–223.
Moore, L.G., Rounds, S.S., Jahngen, D., Grover, R.F. and Reeves, J. T. (1982) J. Appl. Physiol. 52, 695–699.
National Research Council (1977) Carbon Monoxide Medical and Biologic Effects of Environmental Pollutants, Washington, DC.
Newby, M.B., Roberts, R.J. and Bhatnagar, R.K. (1978) J. Pharmacol. Exp. Therap. 206, 61–68.
Norton, S. and Culver, B. (1977) Brain Res. 132, 455–465.
Penney, D.G., Sakai, J. and Cook J. (1974) Growth 38, 321–328.
Penney, D.G., Baylerian, M.S. and Fanning, K.E. (1980) Toxicol. Appl. Pharmacol. 53, 271–278.
Penney, D.G., Baylerian., M.S., Thill, J.E., Fanning, C.M. and Yedavally, S. (1982) Am. J. Physiol. 243, H328–H339.
Penny, D.G., Baylerian, M.S., Thill, J.E., Yedavally, S. and Fanning, C.M. (1983) Am. J. Physiol. 244, H289–H297.
Prigge, E. and Hochrainer, D. (1977) Toxicol. Appl. Pharmacol. 42, 225–228.
Rantakallio, P. (1978) Early Human Dev. 2, 371–382.
Ratney, R.S., Wegman, D.H. and Elkins, H.B. (1974) Arch. Environ. Hlth. 28, 223–226.
Roughton, F.J.W. and Darling, R.C. (1944) Am. J. Physiol. 141, 17.
Schwetz, B.A., Leong, B.K.J. and Gehring, P.J. (1975) Toxicol. Appl. Pharmacol. 32, 84–96.
Schwetz, B.A., Smith, F.A., Leong, B.K.J. and Stalpes, R.E. (1979) Teratology 19, 385–392.
Shellenberger, M.K. (1982) Neuroscience 7, 667–671.
Simon, N. and Volicer, L. (1975) J. Neurochem. 26, 893–900.
Sjostrand, T. (1949) Scand. J. Clin. Lab. Invest. 1, 201–214.
Snider, S.R., Brown, R.M. and Carlsson, A. (1974) J. Neurol. Trans. 35, 283–291.
Stevens, J.L., Ratnayake, J.H. and Anders, M.W. (1980) Toxicol. Appl. Pharmacol. 55, 484–489.
Stewart, R.D. and Hake, C.L. (1976) J. Am. Med. Assoc. 235, 389–401.
Stewart, R.D., Hake, C.L., Wu, A., Stewart, T.A. and Kalbfleisch, J.H. (1976) Arch. Environ. Hlth. 280–285.
Storm, J.E. and Fechter, L.D. (1983) Soc. Neurosci. Abstr. 9, 669.
Theodore, J., O'Donnell, R.D. and Back, K.C. (1977) J. Occup. Med. 13, 242–225.
Traystman, R.J., Fitzgerald, R.S. and Loscutoff, S.C. (1978) Circ. Res. 42, 649–657.
US Department of Health Education and Welfare (1979) Smoking and Health: A Report of the Surgeon General, Ch. 8, Publication No. PHS79-50066.
Wallace, N.D., Davis, G.L., Rutledge, R.B. and Kahn, A. (1974) Arch. Environ. Hlth. 29, 127–135.
Wilks, S., Tomasherfski, J. and Clark, R. (1959) J. Appl. Physiol 14, 305–310.

S. Kacew and M.J. Reasor (eds), *Toxicology and the Newborn*
© 1984 Elsevier Science Publishers B.V.

Chapter 7

Developmental Consequences of Oxygen Toxicity

ROBERT J. ROBERTS[a] and LEE FRANK[b]

[a]*Departments of Pediatrics and Pharmacology, University of Iowa, College of Medicine, Iowa City, IA 52242 and* [b]*Department of Medicine, Pulmonary Division, University of Miami, School of Medicine, Miami, FL 33101, U.S.A.*

CONTENTS

I. LUNG DEVELOPMENT AND MATURATION

Immediately after birth, the newborn's lung must be prepared to assume independent respiratory function for the first time. Compared to the uterine environment in which it developed, the new world that greets the lung at birth is comparatively O_2-rich. In utero, the maternal placenta provides the respiratory needs of the fetus, the environment is warm, but hypoxic (p_{O_2} approximately 20–25 mmHg) relative to the extrauterine environment. In this protected setting the lung undergoes an orderly sequence of structural and biochemical changes — 'preparation for birth phenomena' — that will help assure a successful transition to independent respiratory function at the end of gestation. Problems will arise, however, if premature delivery ensues, so that a newborn with a lung ill-prepared for independent function enters a seemingly alien ex utero world.

1. Structural development

Because there are several excellent comprehensive reviews on the structural development of the lung, both in various animal species and in man (Hodson, 1977; Avery et al., 1981a; O'Hare and Sheridan, 1970; Polgar and Weng, 1979; Thurlbeck, 1975), we will describe only briefly certain aspects of this beautifully organized process, those that seem most relevant to pulmonary O_2 toxicity.

The lung bud arises from the gut (esophagus) in the primitive 1-month human embryo. Sequential divisions of the primitive lung bud (trachea) then give rise to the progressively smaller airways of the lung. Lung vascular development proceeds in step with airway development, branches of the future pulmonary artery and veins closely juxtaposed to the progressive divisions of the airways (Hislop and Reid, 1977). The lung parenchyma goes through several distinguishable morphologic stages, beginning from its origin as an undefined mesenchymal tissue. Precursors of the adult terminal air sacs or alveoli first take the form of glandular structures (human, approximately 4 months; rat, approximately 18 days), later evolve into a canalicular phase (human, approximately 4–5.5 months; rat, approximately 19–20 days), and then a saccular phase (human, approximately 6 months; rat, 21 days) (Meyrick and Reid, 1977; Farrell, 1982). The formation of distinct mature alveoli occurs postnatally in rats, mice, rabbits, etc., and predominantly postnatally in the human lung also (Thurlbeck, 1975; Kauffman et al., 1974; Polgar and Weng, 1979; Burri and Weibel, 1977). Alveolarization is complete in man some time after the 8th year of life (Thurlbeck, 1975; Avery et al., 1981a; Polgar and Weng, 1979).

With the formation of saccular lung structures, differentiation of the various cell types of the lung parenchyma is occurring. Although it has been traditional to state that the lung has 40 different cell types, the primary cell types of the alveolus are only four in number — the capillary endothelial cell, type I epithelial cell, type II epithelial cell and the interstitial cell.

As lung differentiation proceeds in late gestation, the maturational changes in the type II cell (or granular pneumocyte) are those most well studied, since they are of key importance to assure successful lung ventilatory function. The maturing type II cell develops lipid-containing inclusion bodies (the lamellar bodies), which represent storage sites for the alveolar surfactant. Many elegant studies now exist showing the uptake of lipid precursors into the mature type II cell, their transfer from endoplasmic reticulum to Golgi structures to the lamellar bodies and later secretion (by exocytosis) into the alveolar spaces (O'Hare and Sheridan, 1970; Battenburg and Van Golde, 1979; Engle et al., 1978).

2. *Biochemical/functional development*

Though not well defined as yet, there very likely are multiple enzyme/substrate concentration and activity changes in the lung which accompany structural maturation. This is presumed based on the more complete biochemical studies of enzymatic changes in the developing liver (Greengard, 1971, 1972). Some studies of lung biochemical changes with development are available, indicating (a) increased glycogen deposition followed by glycogen depletion with advancing maturation (O'Hare and Sheridan, 1970; Williams, 1977; Bourbon and Jost, 1982), (b) increased glucose uptake in the more mature lung in utero (Hamosh et al., 1978; Engle et al., 1978), (c) changes in hexose monophosphate shunt activity (Yeager and Hicks, 1972; Warshaw et al., 1980), (d) changes with maturation in cytochrome oxidase activity (Warshaw et al., 1980), (e) changes in developing lung collagen and elastin content (Bradley et al., 1974; Franzblau et al., 1977), and (f) differences in general protein-synthesis capacities as the lung matures (Bradley et al., 1974; Hamosh et al., 1978). The changes in phospholipid metabolism with advancing gestation and the activity changes in the enzymes involved in surfactant synthesis have been extensively studied. In all species examined, there occurs late in gestation a characteristic rise in the activity of these enzymes (choline kinase, choline phosphotransferase, phosphatidic acid phosphohydrolase, etc.), leading to an increased incorporation of lipid substrate (and glucose) into surfactant phospholipid. This results in increased lung tissue content (and later alveolar air space content) of the major surfactant component dipalmitoylphosphatidylcholine (lecithin) and of some important minor (percentage-wise) components — phosphatidylglycerol, phosphatidylinositol and phosphatidylserine. These same late gestational changes in surfactant synthesis have been identified in isolated type II cells maintained in tissue culture (Battenburg and Van Golde, 1979; Perelman et al., 1982; Avery et al., 1981a; King 1982).

The physiological importance of surfactant to normal lung function relates to the ability of the surfactant to lower surface tension between air and tissue interfaces. Lacking surfactant, the alveolar walls at the end of expiration would tend to collapse and stay closed because of high surface tension, resulting in closure of the alveolus and increasing the work of breathing required to reopen the closed air space. The film of surfactant lining the terminal air spaces and small airways in newborns tends to resist or decrease this tendency to close by effectively reducing the surface tension between the opposed walls. The partially collapsed terminal airspaces and small terminal airways can then be expanded again by minimal inspiratory effort (airway forces).

The consequences of premature birth (before approximately 20 days in rats (normal gestation = 21 days), before approximately 27 days in rabbit (31 days), or before approximately 34 weeks in humans (40 weeks)) include insufficient surfactant to stabilize terminal air spaces and airways and immaturity of the lung parenchyma. The resultant problems include diffuse lung atelectasis (alveolar closure without air filling) and ineffective gas exchange. In humans, these conditions are associated with the respiratory distress syndrome (RDS), previously named hyaline membrane disease (HMD) (Farrell and Avery, 1975; Clements and Tooley, 1977; Avery et al., 1981b; Hallman and Gluck, 1982). As might be expected, the degree of early respiratory difficulty and the severity of RDS/HMD bears a close relationship to the degree of immaturity of the newborn infant. The severity of RDS will also usually dictate the amount/duration of hyperoxic therapy needed to prevent the calamitous problems associated with hypoxemia in these sick, premature infants. In most studies reported, the incidence of severe O_2-induced lung toxicity will also be generally related to the degree of immaturity of the newborn infant. RDS affects approximately 50,000 infants in the U.S.A. each year. So the population liable to exposure to and to subsequent lung damage from high concentration O_2 therapy is indeed considerable (Farrell and Avery, 1975; Avery et al., 1981b).

II. OXYGEN TOXICITY

Those intrigued by biological paradoxes cannot but be impressed by the paradox of oxygen. Haugaard (1965) has summarized the quandary particularly well: "...although O_2 is necessary for the production of energy and survival of all aerobic cells, it is also a universal cell poison. It is only because cells in the course of evolution have developed special defense mechanisms against the toxic effect of O_2 that life as we know it has been able to flourish. In a sense, the study of O_2 toxicity is the study of ways in which organisms protect themselves against the oxidizing potential of molecular O_2". To the clinician who must use high levels of O_2 therapeutically, the frustrating problems related to this paradox are a source of constant concern.

1. Pathology of O_2 toxicity

The sequence of hyperoxic-induced changes in the lung has been well established in a variety of experimental animals of various species and ages (Kistler et al., 1967; Kapanci et al., 1969; Clark and Lambertsen, 1971; Balentine, 1977; Huber and Drath, 1981). It is useful to consider these changes in two phases: (a) acute or exudative changes and (b) chronic or proliferative changes (Table 1). A key point to keep in mind is that the cells of the gas-exchange region of the lung differ considerably in their susceptibility to O_2-induced injury. In order of sensitivity to O_2 toxicity, endothelial cell > type I epithelial cell > > > type II epithelial cell. One of the unknowns of O_2 toxicity research is why the capillary endothelial cell is the initial cell to show damage during exposure to elevated alveolar O_2 levels; another is why

TABLE 1

PATHOLOGY-PULMONARY O_2 TOXICITY

Acute/exudative	Chronic/proliferative
Edema	Absorption of exudates
Interstitial	
Perivascular	Thickening of alveolar wall
Peribronchiolar	Respiratory membrane of lung
Alveolar	Type II cell hyperplasia
Pleural effusion	Interstitial cell hyperplasia
Alveolar hemorrhage	Collagen, elastin deposition
Mononuclear cell influx	Lung fibrosis/emphysematous changes
Necrosis	
Endothelium	
Type I cells	

the type II cell is comparatively so resistant to hyper-oxidant stress, and is even able to undergo mitotic changes during O_2 exposure to regenerated destroyed type I epithelial cells and restore an intact epithelial lining (Kistler et al., 1967; Balentine, 1977; Huber and Drath, 1981).

With initial damage to the capillary endothelial lining by O_2, permeability changes may allow excess water and then protein-rich plasma fluid to leak into the interstitial space between the endothelial and epithelial lining layers of the gas-exchange region — perturbing Starling's equilibrium forces which normally govern and control fluid transfer between the capillary lumen and the interstitial space of the alveolar wall. With the progressive dissolution of the endothelial cell barrier, the plasma fluid leakage will exceed the capacity of the lymphatic channels to drain the normally thin interstitium, and interstitial swelling or edema results. The interstitial channels drain to larger lymphatic channels located more centrally in each lung lobule in a perivascular distribution. With progressive fluid leakage these areas will evidence very striking perivascular cuffs of edema fluid. The lung in adults appears to be much more susceptible to these events than the newborn lung.

As the type I cell of the alveolar lining undergoes progressive O_2-induced damage, its barrier function is compromised, and interstitial fluid is able to leak into the air spaces of the lung, producing progressive alveolar edema. Unless this process is halted, ineffective gas exchange will develop in the flooded alveoli.

Should O_2 exposure be stopped at this point or the animal manifest 'tolerance' to continued hyperoxia, a chronic or proliferative phase of O_2 toxicity can occur. Absorption of the exudative fluid takes place, so aeration of the alveolar spaces may be restored. However, other reparative changes usually do not result in a restoration of the normal respiratory membranes of the lung. While many of the destroyed capillaries may recanaliculize, others do not. The alveolar lining becomes re-populated at first with thick cuboidal type II cells which may differentiate gradually into new thin type I cells. The thin interstitial space is often permanently thickened and altered in composition due to proliferation of interstitial cells and fibroblasts and subsequent deposition of collagen and elastin in areas they were not present in before. The end result of these reparative efforts, plus the complete loss of some septal walls due to cell death, may be various degrees of lung fibrosis and emphysematous changes. Many of the restored septal walls, now thickened by a new type of epithelial lining and interstitial changes with new collagen and elastin deposition, are much less effective gas-exchange membranes. The major alteration of the pulmonary vascular bed may result in serious perfusion abnormalities. Thus, various degrees of permanent compromise of lung function and functional reserve may be the outcome in survivors of severe O_2 toxicity. Species' differences, age group differences and (little understood) individual variations will result in different spectra of permanent lung change in the survivors of O_2 toxicity (Kapanci et al., 1969; Balentine, 1977; Huber and Drath, 1981).

Detailed examination of the alterations in the lungs of human subjects treated with prolonged high levels of oxygen in inspired gas (FiO_2) suggests that a very similar sequence of pathologic changes occurs in man (Gould et al., 1972; Anderson et al., 1973; Bonikos et al., 1976; Huber and Drath, 1981; Churg et al., 1983).

Several recent studies have examined more closely other potential sequelae of prolonged O_2 exposure in experimental (newborn) animals. The effect of O_2 on the lung's synthetic abilities appears to be reflected in a striking inhibitory effect on newborn lung growth in hyperoxia and, specifically, an inhibition of the normal maturation of the lung structure from a saccularized to a well-alveolarized morphology (Bucher and Roberts, 1981a, b, 1982; Frank and Groseclose, 1982; Roberts et al., 1983a, b) (Fig. 1). To some extent the inhibition of alveolar development by O_2 has been shown to be a dose-related phenomenon of the O_2 exposure level tested (Bucher and Roberts, 1981a, b). Recently, early exposure to hyperoxia has been shown to alter also normal lung vascular (capillary) development (Roberts et al., 1983a, b). The end result of these growth-arresting effects as a feature of O_2 toxicity is a decreased development of the gas-exchange region in the neonatal lung. This type of O_2-induced lung developmental injury could seriously impair the total respiratory reserve and lung functional capacity, which would compromise its future ability to handle toxic, infectious and other stresses.

Several clinical studies suggest that the experimental findings just described may be extrapolatable to the growing lung of the premature human infant as well. Sobonya et al. (1983) reported that an infant dying at age 33 months with bronchopulmonary dysplasia (BPD) had only 10×10^6 alveoli in his lung compared to $(125–175) \times 10^6$ alveoli in the lungs of age-matched controls, and an internal surface area for respiratory exchange 2–3-fold less than in the normal infant. Other studies show persistent lung functional reserve deficits in human infants many months after long-term neonatal O_2 therapy and signs of BPD pathology (Fox, 1978; Bancalari et al., 1979; Edwards, 1979; Thurlbeck, 1979; Gerhardt et al., 1983). While some follow-up studies do not indicate persistent lung dysfunction, this may be explainable on the lesser original severity of pulmonary O_2 toxicity, the degree of prematurity at the

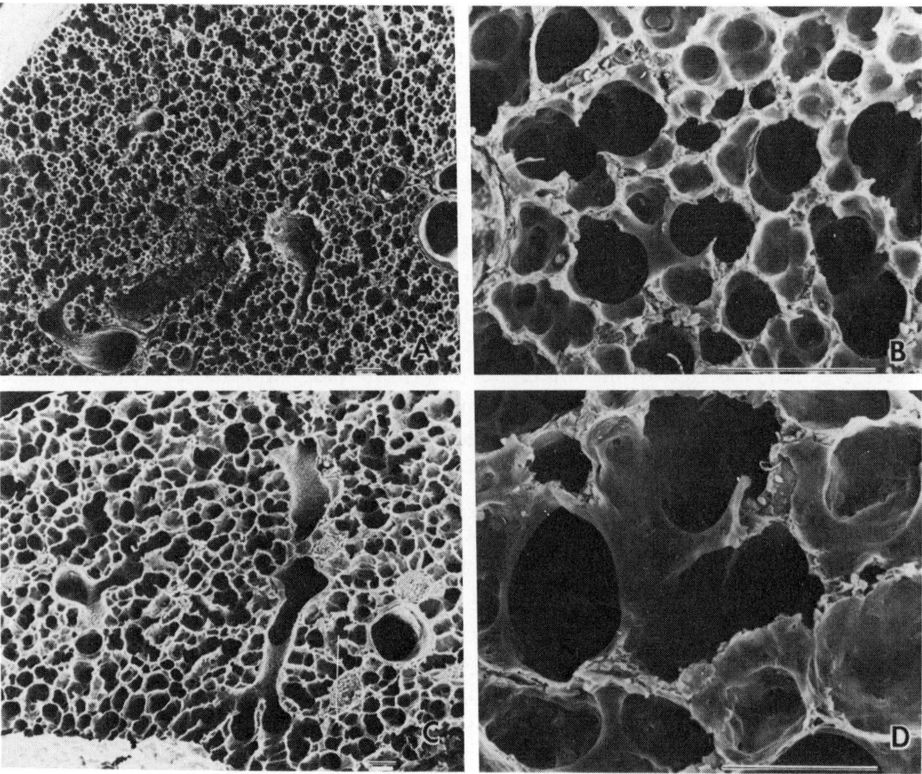

Figure 1. Scanning electron micrographs of fixed, inflated lungs from 6-day-old rats exposed to FiO_2: 21% (A and B) or >95% (C and D). Reference line at lower right corner in each frame is 100 μm in length. (From Roberts et al., 1983a, b.)

time of hyperoxic treatment, and/or individual differences in ability to compensate for early interference with lung development.

2. *O_2 toxicity in the newborn (bronchopulmonary dysplasia)*

In the 1940s and early 1950s, oxygen therapy was used in a rather cavalier fashion in the nursery. The concept of O_2 as a pharmacological agent was obviously unappreciated. The manual, 'Standards and Recommendations for Hospital Care of Newborn Infants' (American Academy of Pediatrics, 1948) even included the recommendation that "The premature is to be placed in 40–50% O_2 as soon as possible after birth, where it will remain anywhere from 12 hours to 1 month, depending upon the infant's size and condition" (James and Lanman, 1976). Later in the 1950s, the consequences of the misuse or overuse of elevated concentrations of O_2 became sadly apparent in the epidemic of blindness in premature infants reported from nurseries throughout the country. When the association of damage to the premature retina (so-called retrolental fibroplasia) due to elevated O_2 therapy became an inescapable conclusion, general use of O_2 therapy in all premature infants was sharply curtailed (James and Lanman, 1976).

This iatrogenic calamity resulted from several factors, including the lack of general knowledge about oxygen's toxic nature, specific knowledge of O_2's toxic action on the immature retina and, to reiterate, the failure to appreciate O_2 as a 'drug' and to apply appropriate pharmacological criteria with its use (dose-response considerations, risk-benefit concepts, appropriateness and duration of use, monitoring of blood levels, monitoring of early toxicity, etc.).

In 1967, Northway et al. reported for the first time on an association between treatment with elevated levels of O_2 and another side effect of O_2's toxic action, serious acute and chronic lung changes. These authors described the lung pathology seen after prolonged hyperoxic treatment in newborns and called the condition 'bronchopulmonary dysplasia' (BPD) (Northway et al., 1967). There followed multiple collaborating clinical reports on infants who required long-term O_2 therapy for severe hyaline membrane disease who, despite recovery from HMD, went on to succumb to O_2-induced lung pathological changes. The stages of development of BPD have been well described radiographically and pathologically (Northway and Rosan, 1969; Edwards, 1979; Avery et al., 1981c; Coalson et al., 1982; Escobedo et al., 1982). The incidence of BPD is difficult to determine exactly, because uniform criteria and definitions have not been established or agreed upon. Based on available information, it is estimated that 20–50% of premature infants requiring prolonged exposure to hyperoxia may develop signs of BPD. The incidence varies also in the infants born weighing over 1500 g (10–20%) and in those more prematurely born (birth weight under 1500 g), where the incidence is uniformly reported to be much higher (30–70%) (Tooley, 1979; Edwards et al., 1977; Saldanha et al., 1982; Smith et al., 1983). Those that do not succumb to the O_2 damage while still in the nursery may later show long-term disability, manifested by decreased respiratory reserve and repeated lower respiratory infections. Much controversy still exists as to whether BPD is primarily due to oxygen itself or is more a result of the mechanical ventilatory support used to deliver O_2 therapy, i.e., lung effects of high-pressure barotrauma. While additive effects from the use of high-pressure ventilation may contribute to the severity of BPD in a particular clinical situation, the experimental and clinical evidence (DeLemos et al., 1969; Nash et al., 1971; Wolfe and Sabiston, 1973; Coates et al., 1982; Roberts et al., 1983a, b) demonstrating lung pathology of O_2 toxicity analagous to that observed with BPD in the absence of high-pressure mechanical ventilation is hard to refute.

It is important to appreciate that O_2's damaging action will also affect the important normal clearance mechanism of the lung, which is vital to protection from the aerosol route of infection, for entrapment of environment debris that escapes the nasal filters, and for removal of normal turn-over products from the lower respiratory tract. The three principal components of this clearance-defense system — ciliated cells in the airways, mucous secretory cells and alveolar macrophages — are all subject to damage and altered function with hyperoxic exposure (Bonikos et al.,

1976; Boat et al., 1973; Raffin et al., 1972; Huber and Drath, 1981). This provides at least one reasonable explanation for why prolonged respiratory support with O_2 is so frequently complicated by pulmonary infection.

3. *Lung biochemical/functional changes with O_2 toxicity*

The importance of sufficient surfactant material to line the pulmonary airspaces and provide airway stability has been discussed previously. During O_2 exposure, surface tension changes and, often, diffuse atelectasis are know to occur, compounding the other pathological features of O_2 toxicity. Decreases in lung compliance (a physiological measure of surface tension and tissue elasticity) have been found in a variety of experimental animals and in man during exposure to hyperoxia (Burger and Mead, 1969; Clark and Lambertsen, 1971; Huber and Drath, 1981; Bucher and Roberts, 1981a, b). The mechanism for the alteration in lung compliance could involve direct (oxidative) effects on pulmonary tissue and surfactant, and/or inhibition of surfactant function by protein-rich edema fluid entering the pulmonary air spaces. Several studies have shown a decreased airway surfactant in O_2-ventilated lungs, and in O_2-exposed type II cells in culture (Gilder and McSherry, 1976; Gross and Smith, 1981; Huber and Drath, 1981; Ward and Roberts, 1984).

Serious gas-diffusion problems might be expected to result from the widespread damage to pulmonary capillaries, alveolar wall structure and lung edema. Marked reductions in diffusion capacity (in man and animals) have indeed been found in O_2-toxic subjects — and related to the pathological changes of atelectasis, widened respiratory membrane diffusion path, uneven ventilation-perfusion relationships ('shunting') and interference with normal capillary blood flow and disruption of pulmonary vascular development (Bucher and Roberts, 1981a, b; Huber and Drath, 1981; Roberts et al., 1983a, b). The clinical effects of these factors is to produce hypoxemia of varying severity, which in turn leads to the requirement for still higher levels of alveolar O_2 administration. Thus, a vicious cycle may be established which often terminates in death.

Important biochemical changes occur in O_2 toxicity due to damage by reactive molecular species against major cell components — proteins, lipids and nucleotides. Many critical cell enzymes, especially those containing essential sulfhydryl groups, are inactivated by hyperoxia exposure (Haugaard, 1968; Clark and Lambertsen, 1971; Frank and Massaro, 1980; Deneke and Fanburg, 1980; Halliwell, 1981). The consequences of such alterations are general depression of tissue metabolism and energy production. Interaction with lipid membrane components of the cell, causing lipid peroxidation of unsaturated fatty acid components, is another possibility. This would cause serious alterations in cell and cell organelle membrane integrity and function, including important cell metabolic activities and cell energy production (Haugaard, 1968; Frank and Massaro, 1980; Deneke and Fanburg, 1980; Mustafa and Tierney, 1978; Halliwell, 1981). And, finally, reactive species may interact with and cause scission of DNA, with later consequences on cell replicative and synthetic capacities (Frank and Massaro, 1980; Deneke and Fanburg, 1980; Halliwell, 1981).

Many studies have shown an overall depression of cell protein synthesis (in lung slices or in isolated type II cells or alveolar macrophages) and DNA synthesis during hyperoxic exposure (Haugaard, 1968; Mustafa and Tierney, 1978; Halliwell, 1981; Gacad and Massaro, 1973; Northway et al ., 1972). These combined insults seriously impair the ability to repair cell damage in the face of ongoing O_2 exposure.

It seems important to appreciate that the lung has some very important 'non-respiratory functions' which may be altered by O_2 toxicity. Many endogenous vasoactive compounds are normally metabolized and inactivated (or activated) by a single pass through the normal pulmonary circulation. Most prostaglandins and serotonin, for example, are removed nearly 100% by a single passage through the lung circulation, and angiotensin I is readily converted to the potent vasoactive angiotensin II form. The site of all these 'non-respiratory' functions is the endothelium — the very cells that are injured earliest by hyperoxic therapy. The systemic consequences of the loss of the O_2-toxic lung's metabolic activity on these endogenous hormones has simply not been well investigated, but, given their potential vasoactive effects, some systemic consequences almost certainly result from their failure to be cleared from the circulation by the O_2-damaged lung (Block and Fisher, 1977; Huber and Drath, 1981; Gillis and Greene, 1977).

4. O_2 toxicity and the developing eye (retrolental fibroplasia)

The other tissue that is subject to severe damage during oxygen exposure is the immature retina of the infant who is born prematurely. (Isolated studies which suggest O_2-induced damage to other organs besides the lung and eye can be found in the 1971 review of Clark and Lambertsen. Most of these studies, to our knowledge, have not been replicated conclusively since that review appeared.)

The peripheral retina is not completely vascularized in the human fetus until just before the end of the normal gestational period (James and Lanman, 1976; Silverman, 1977). The same delay in vascularization has been noted in the eye of the kitten, which is a frequently used model for O_2-induced retinal injury. The capillaries growing into the peripheral retina are believed to respond to O_2 tensions in the blood by sustained vasoconstriction. This leads to loss of oxygen and nutrition supply to the developing retinal cells, cell necrosis, and, in response to necrotic cell products, a secondary proliferation eventually of new capillaries into the area. The disorderly capillary proliferation, followed by contraction of this injured part of the retina, exerts increasing tension on the rest of the retina, with the outcome in severe cases being retinal detachment, dense scarring and blindness. This whole process is called retrolental fibroplasia (RLF). Although the correlation between degree of retinal damage and level of hyperoxia or duration of hyperoxic treatment is not strictly linear, the preponderance of clinical and experimental evidence indicates that RLF is a unique consequence of O_2 therapy in the very premature infant (James and Lanman, 1976; Silverman, 1977; Finer et al., 1982; Monaco, 1982/1983; Hittner et al., 1983).

III. DEFENSES AGAINST O_2 TOXICITY

In order to appreciate clearly what endogenous or exogenous defenses are available to help protect against O_2-induced tissue damage, one first needs to have an understanding of why O_2 is toxic. The so-called 'free radical theory of O_2 toxicity', which has become more firmly established and sophisticated over the past couple of decades, maintains that during normal metabolic processes in aerobic cells some O_2 is incompletely reduced so that very reactive species of O_2 result (Fig. 2). Most O_2 used by aerobic organisms is channelled through the mitochondrial respiratory chain of enzymes, producing high-energy compounds (ATP) for the cell and reducing two molecules of O_2 to two molecules of H_2O (four-electron reduction). Other O_2 used by the cell (by various oxygenase and other enzymes) results in two-electron reduction of O_2 to yield H_2O_2 as a product of the metabolic reaction. And finally, some enzymes (xanthine oxidase, ferrodoxin, some flavin enzymes) and some auto-oxidative processes (epinephrine, adrenochrome, hemoglobin, methemoglobin) involve only a single-electron reduction of O_2, with the production of O_2^- (superoxide anion). O_2^- is capable of interacting with H_2O_2 in the cell, in the presence of Fe^{2+}, producing a Fenton-type reaction (or as previously known, the Haber-Weiss reaction).

$$O_2^- + H_2O_2 \rightarrow OH^- + OH^{\cdot} + O_2$$

The O_2 metabolites O_2^-, H_2O_2, $OH^{\cdot}$ (hydroxyl free radical) and one other cellular O_2 product, singlet oxygen ($^1O_2$), are highly reactive species capable of cytotoxic interaction with all components of the cell (Fig. 2) (Fridovich, 1976; Halliwell, 1981; Frank and Massaro, 1980; Freeman and Crapo, 1982; Malmstrom, 1982). Under normoxic conditions the production of these unstable O_2 metabolites apparently does not exceed the detoxifying capability of the antioxidant defense systems of the cell listed in Figure 2. Superoxide dismutase (SOD) is a key protective enzyme, since by rapidly scavenging O_2^- it not only prevents damaging interaction of O_2^- with vital cell components, but also can prevent the reaction of O_2^- with H_2O_2 and the production of hydroxyl radical ($OH^{\cdot}$), which is chemically one of the most reactive free radicals known. Both catalase and glutathione peroxidase (GP) enzyme can detoxify $(2)H_2O_2$ by reducing it to $(2)H_2O$ + molecular O_2. In addition, GP functions to convert lipid peroxides, formed by the interaction of reactive O_2 metabolites with unsaturated lipids, into non-toxic lipid alcohol forms (Fridovich, 1976; Halliwell, 1981; Frank and Massaro, 1980; Freeman and Crapo, 1982).

Several other non-enzymatic antioxidant defenses are present in the cell, the most important of which is generally agreed to be alpha-tocopherol or vitamin E. Unlike the enzymatic defense systems, which are primarily soluble in the cytosol, vitamin E

Figure 2. Schematic representation of the source and generation of free radicals and reactive intermediates, and the cellular protective systems (enzymatic and nonenzymatic). The protective systems including vitamin E are believed to provide a protective environment from the cellular constituents by capturing or quenching the high-energy state of the toxic reactive molecular species. Additional discussion is provided in the text. (From Roberts, 1984.)

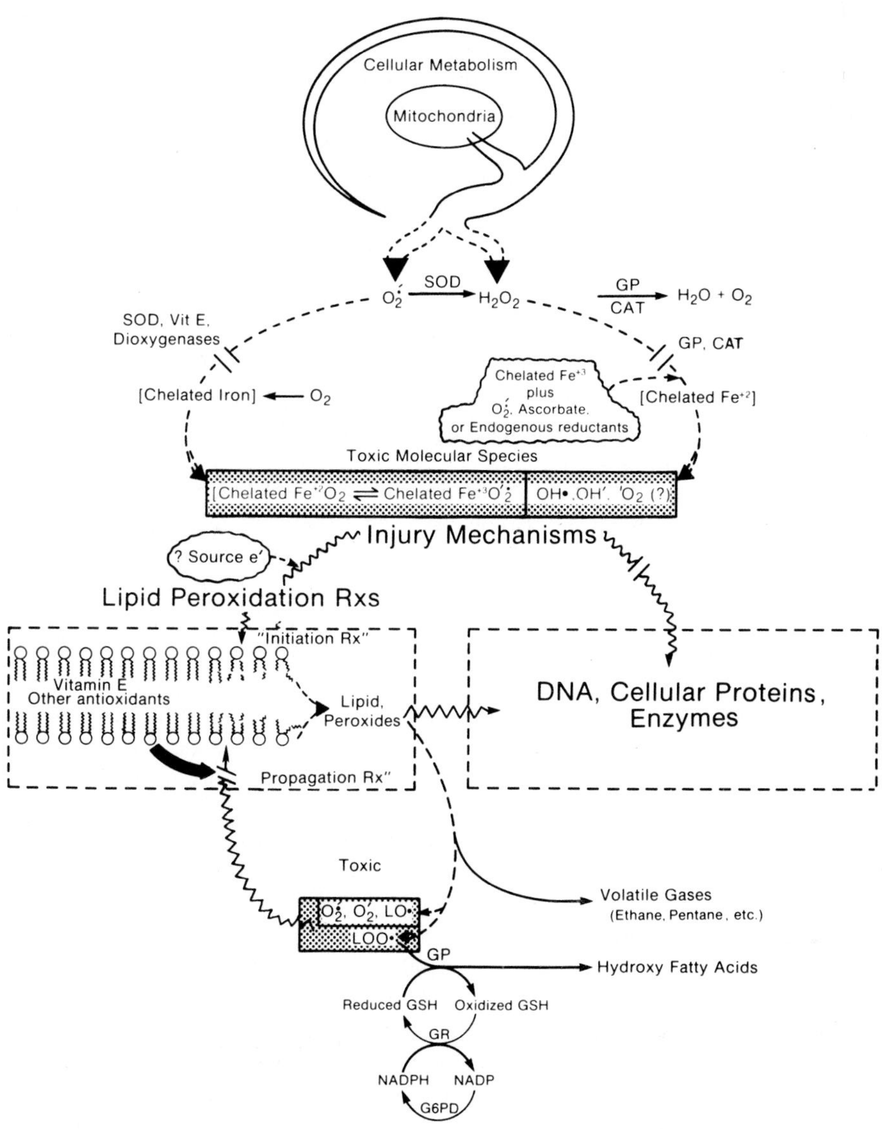

Toxic Molecular Species (⟿)

Superoxide radical ($O_2^{\dot{}}$)
Hydrogen peroxide (H_2O_2)
Hydroxyl radical (OH•)
Singlet oxygen ($'O_2$)
Peroxy radical (LOO•)
Alkoxy radical (LO•)

Protective Systems (⟶)

Superoxide dismutase (SOD)
Catalase (CAT)
Glutathione peroxidase (GP)
Glutathione reductase (GR)
Vitamin E (Vit E)
Dioxygenases
Other antioxidants (Vit A, ?)

is a lipid-phase antioxidant intercalated into lipid membranes and acting to donate reducing equivalents to interrupt chain reaction lipid peroxide damage in membranes (Horwitt, 1976; Mustafa and Tierney, 1978; Witting, 1980). The other substances in the cell which are capable of antioxidant activity are believed to be of lesser quantitative importance — some of these are cysteine, cysteamine and other thiol (SH)-containing substances, and ascorbic acid (vitamin C).

Again, under normoxic conditions these cooperative antioxidant systems seem to function quite effectively in policing the metabolic O_2 by-products of aerobic metabolism and preventing cell injury from reactive O_2 species. Under hyperoxic conditions, however, the production of the cytotoxic O_2 radicals has been shown to increase markedly (Fridovich, 1974; Freeman and Crapo, 1981; Freeman et al., 1982) and, in effect, overwhelm the normal complement of antioxidant defenses, with resultant O_2 free radical-induced cell injury. Unless the cell is able to increase its antioxidant armamentarium when under such oxidant stress, progressive cell damage and cell death may eventuate.

Over the past decade a variety of experimental models have been produced by many different laboratories to establish the association between relative resistance to hyperoxic lung toxicity and increased levels of the antioxidant enzymes (Mustafa and Tierney, 1978; Frank and Massaro, 1980; Deneke and Fanburg, 1980; Freeman and Crapo, 1982; Foreman and Fisher, 1982). Indirectly, these studies have provided experimental proof that O_2 toxicity may be mediated by the reactive O_2 metabolites ('O_2 free radicals') discussed above.

For at least 50 years, originating with the elegant studies of Smith et al. (1932) in rats (and the even earlier descriptive study by Binger and associates (1927) in reptiles), it has been recognized that very young animals are more resistant to O_2-induced lung damage and lethality than are older animals of the same species. Various hypotheses, mainly morphological ones, were proposed over the years to explain this age-related phenomenon. However, a biochemical basis has now been provided by the results of studies by Yam et al. (1978) and others. These studies reaffirmed the marked tolerance of neonatal animals of several species to hyperoxic exposure (100% of neonatal mice, rats and rabbits alive after 120 hours of $>95\%$ O_2 exposure) compared to the susceptibility to O_2 toxicity of parent/adult animals of these same species (nearly all adults dead by 60–120 hours of similar O_2 exposure). Additionally, these studies showed that unlike the adult animals, which demonstrated no increases in their lung antioxidant enzyme levels (SOD, catalase, GP) during hyperoxic exposure, the neonatal animals had rapid increases in all their antioxidant enzyme levels during hyperoxic challenge (Fig. 3) (Yam et al., 1978; Frank et al., 1979). This adaptive lung biochemical response to hyperoxia, as theoretically proposed above, would permit increased detoxifying capacity in the neonatal lungs and provide a sound biochemical explanation for the comparative resistance of immature animals versus adult animals to similar hyperoxic exposure. In a subsequent study, the importance of this antioxidant enzyme response to tolerance to O_2 toxicity was demonstrated by the use of an inhibitor of SOD activity — diethyldithiocarbamate (DDC). Young rats administered doses of DDC sufficient to prevent a

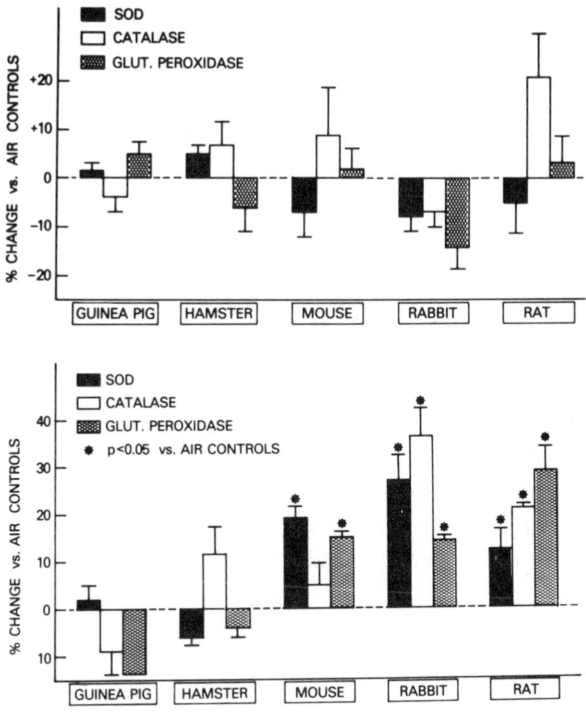

Figure 3. Top: antioxidant enzyme response to hyperoxia in adult animals. Adults of five species exposed to >95% O_2 for 24 hours; lung SOD (■), catalase (□) and glutathione peroxidase (▨) calculated per lung and expressed as percent change in enzyme activity compared to respective air control animals. (Reprinted, with permission, from Frank et al., 1979.) Bottom: antioxidant enzyme response to hyperoxia in neonatal animals. Neonates (1–5 days old) of five species exposed to >95% O_2 for 24 hours; lung SOD (■), catalase (□) and glutathione peroxidase (▨) calculated per lung and expressed as percent change in enzyme activity compared to respective air control pups. (Reprinted, with permission, from Frank et al., 1979.)

rise in SOD activity during exposure to >95% O_2 lost their tolerance to O_2 toxicity and incurred severe O_2-induced lung damage and died as readily as did adult rats in hyperoxia (Frank et al., 1978a, b).

Of interest in the studies of neonatal and adult animals described above was the finding that newborn guinea pigs behave in hyperoxia very similarly to adult guinea pigs, i.e., they show no tolerance to O_2 toxicity, and concomitantly show no significant response of their lung antioxidant enzyme system to high O_2 exposure (Frank et al., 1979). This exception seems to be explainable, however, by the fact that the guinea pig newborn, unlike the newborn rat, mouse and rabbit, is markedly precocious. The guinea pig lung undergoes nearly complete maturation while still in utero, and morphologically (and apparently biochemically) is quite similar at the time of birth to the adult guinea pig lung (Frank et al., 1979; Lechner and Sanchero, 1982; Sorokin et al., 1959). Thus, in O_2, the newborn guinea pig's lung appears

TABLE 2

AGENTS PRODUCING OXIDANT LUNG DAMAGE

Inhalants	X-irradiation
Hyperoxia	Drugs
Ozone	Bleomycin
Nitrogen dioxide	Adriamycin
Photochemical smog	Nitrofurantoin
Phosgene, others	Herbicide
	Paraquat

incapable of the type of adaptive protective response seen in the less mature lungs of the newborns of the other species tested.

Table 2 lists a variety of agents that are now believed to cause lung toxicity by means of an O_2 free radical mechanism similar to that proposed for hyperoxia (Frank, 1982). The evidence for this is from the work of biochemists, chemists, radiation physicists, etc., too numerous to mention individually. The methodology used in determining the presence of O_2 free radicals in these various toxic systems is a textbook of modern analytical techniques — nuclear magnetic resonance, stop-flow biochemical reactions, chemiluminescence, and so on. Three examples of the reactions that are believed to occur that generate O_2 free radicals with these hyper-oxidant agents are shown in Figure 4. The end-product of the irradiation event can be seen to be the generation in tissues of the same reactive O_2 metabolites that are the damaging species in O_2 toxicity (O_2^-, $OH^{\cdot}$, H_2O_2). Understanding this provides a theoretical basis for the long-standing observations that radiation damage is exacerbated under well-oxygenated conditions and, conversely, that hypoxic tumor cells, located usually in the center of a solid mass of tumor cells, are relatively undamaged by therapeutic irradiation (Quatiliana, 1977; Fowler et al., 1976; Adams, 1981; Miller et al., 1979).

As perhaps predicted from the contrasting responses of neonatal animals compared to adult animals in hyperoxia, experimental challenge with these other hyper-oxidant toxins also show age-related effects on the degree of lung toxicity and on survival. Young animals have been found to demonstrate significantly greater tolerance to the principle toxic components of photochemical smog, ozone (Stephens et al., 1978, 1982) and NO_2 (Stephens et al., 1978; Gregory and Hine, 1968); to paraquat (Smith and Rose, 1977); and to another lung edemagenic toxin with a possible free radical action, thiourea (Gregory and Hine, 1968). Whether neonatal tolerance to these other hyper-oxidant lung toxins is associated directly with adaptive changes in the antioxidant defense systems of the lung has thus far not been investigated, to our knowledge, though we would speculate that this might be the finding.

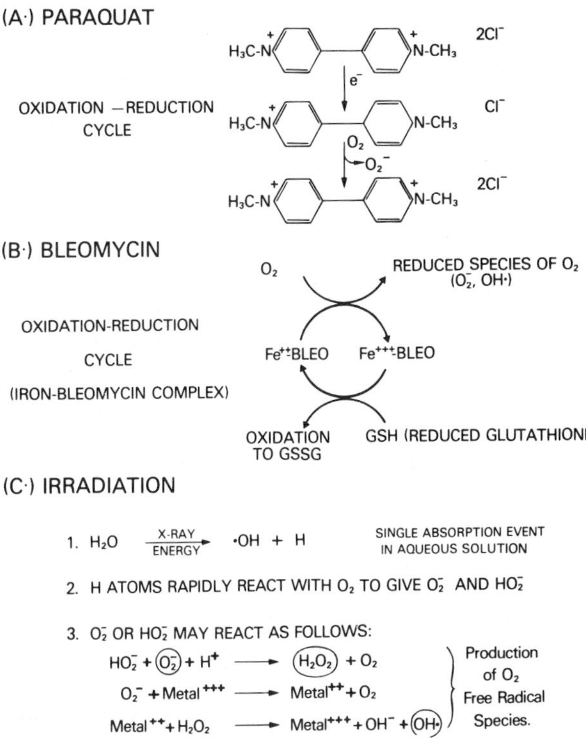

Figure 4. O_2 free radical production by lung toxins. A, Paraquat; B, bleomycin; C, irradiation. Repeated oxidation-reduction cycles of paraquat and iron-bleomycin complex in the lung result in production of large amounts of O_2 (and other reactive O_2 species). Lung irradiation produces bursts of reactive O_2 species in target tissues. (From Frank, 1982.)

IV. CLINICAL MEANS TO REDUCE THE EFFECT OF O_2 TOXICITY

In their comprehensive review of pulmonary O_2 toxicity, Clark and Lambertsen (1971) discussed a variety of experimental means found to have some effect in preventing or ameliorating the results of long-term, high-concentration O_2 exposure. However, after elucidating all these experimental manipulations, they arrived at the pessimistic conclusion that "In spite of these hopeful possibilities, it is likely that most of the agents listed...will have very limited clinical application".

A dozen years later, reviewing the list of experimental agents they discussed, we must reluctantly echo the conclusion of Clark and Lambertsen (1971). There is still, unfortunately, no pharmacological agent available to the clinician to help circumvent the toxic consequences to the lung of prolonged high O_2 therapy. However, there are a host of addenda we wish to add to these statements, both because we are constitutionally adverse to ending on a pessimistic note, and because there is truly cause for optimism in some newer pharmacological approaches to the problem of O_2 toxicity. These we will discuss in the subsections to follow.

1. Acceleration of maturation of the the lung

By far, the majority of infants who require prolonged hyperoxic therapy are those who are born too soon and develop the primary consequence of prematurity, RDS/HMD. The remediation of RDS/HMD does not lie in developing better postnatal methods of treatment, but the real cure is to prevent premature termination of pregnancy. Better obstetrical care beginning early in pregnancy has had some effect on reducing the incidence of prematurity (Avery et al., 1981b; Farrell and Avery, 1975). Some tocolytic agents (beta-adrenergic drugs, such as isoxsuprine and ritodrine, which reduce uterine muscle contractions) have been effective for short-term reversal of premature labor, but these agents must be carefully administered and undesirable side-effects on maternal cardiovascular function and on fetal blood flow and glucose levels are known complications (Boog et al., 1975; Bergman and Hedner, 1978; Epstein et al., 1979; Brazy and Pupkin, 1979).

An effective means, not of preventing prematurity per se, but of stimulating a rapid maturation of the fetal lung in obstetric conditions threatening premature delivery, is now available to the perinatologist. Multiple follow-up studies since the original reports of Liggins and Howie in 1972 have confirmed the finding in animals and in humans that prenatal administration of glucocorticoid hormone (cortisol, betamethasone, dexamethasone) can affect a premature maturation of the surfactant enzyme system in the fetal lung (Taeusch, 1975; Gluck, 1976; Ballard et al., 1979; Avery et al., 1981b). A late gestational rise in fetal plasma cortisol concentration may indeed be the normal physiologic control mechanism that switches on surfactant production in normal gestation (Farrell et al., 1977; Ballard, 1977; Farrell and Hamosh, 1978). Prenatal administration of betamethasone to the pregnant woman, if premature labor contractions can be quieted for at least 48 hours (by use of beta-adrenergic tocolytics, or by intravenous ethanol), has been found to be a highly successful means of reducing the incidence of severe RDS/HMD in prematurely born infants, presumably because the quantity of surfactant in their lungs is more sufficient than it would have been without this prenatal hormonal intervention (Liggins and Howie, 1972; Taeusch, 1975; Gluck, 1976; Taeusch and Avery, 1977; Ballard et al., 1979; Avery et al., 1981b). As a result, such an infant may be spared the need for the prolonged assisted ventilation and hyperoxic therapy that his premature gestational age, immature lung and surfactant deficiency would normally necessitate. Continued clinical studies are ongoing to find the best and safest means to achieve accelerated fetal lung maturation in threatened premature deliveries. These studies hope to evaluate the best hormonal agent to use (other hormones which reportedly will stimulate lung surfactant production prematurely include thyroxine, thyroid-releasing hormone, estrogen, prolactin and aminophylline) (Taeusch and Avery, 1977; Smith and Bogues, 1980; Avery et al., 1981a); the possible short-term and long-term side-effects of prenatal hormonal treatment in pharmacological dosages (since prenatal glucocorticoid in animals has a pronounced effect on growth of other organs, including the brain); and, ideally, how may premature labor itself be safely inhibited until such time as normal fetal lung maturation has occurred.

Some recent studies of normal developmental changes in the fetal lung may help to explain a clinical observation that has been remarked on by many who care for sick, premature infants requiring vigorous O_2 therapy. In addition, these studies may suggest perhaps a different approach to reducing the risk for serious O_2 toxicity in the prematurely born. These studies, first done in developing rats and more recently in fetal rabbits (Frank and Groseclose, 1982, 1983, 1984) indicate that normally there occurs a late gestational rise in the specific activity of the pulmonary antioxidant enzymes — SOD, catalase and GP. The data for rabbits (Fig. 5) show that SOD and catalase activity in the last 10–20% of gestation increase approximately 125% over the enzyme levels in the early 3rd trimester fetal lung, and GP activity increases approximately 200%. Of further interest is the finding that in the fetal rabbit the time course for this late fetal change in the protective antioxidant enzyme system closely parallels the (superimposed, Fig. 5) developmental pattern of late gestational change in the surfactant system. The maturation of both systems, therefore, may be viewed as important 'preparation for birth phenomena'. The activity of the surfactant system must be advanced enough in the newborn infant to provide sufficient phospholipid material to stabilize the airspace of the newly functional lung. What about the antioxidant enzyme system? Why might a pre-birth rise in lung activity be important to assure successful functioning of the newborn lung? The explanation perhaps is related to the fact that in utero the cells of the fetal lung experience a relative hypoxic environment (highest blood p_{O_2}, approximately 20–25 mmHg, and O_2 tension in fluid bathing the air spaces is very likely considerably lower) (Kirschbaum et al., 1967;

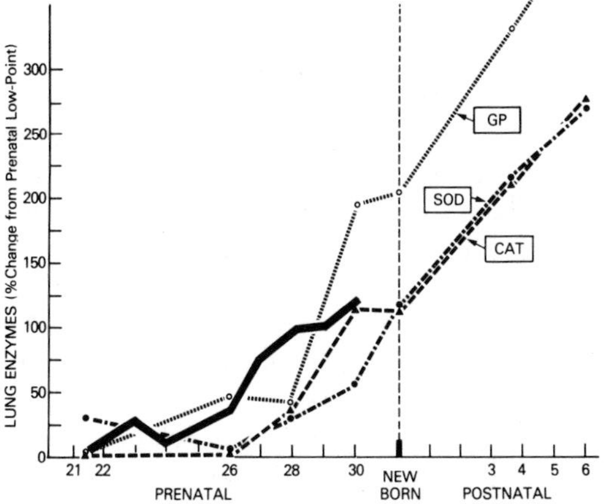

Figure 5. Antioxidant enzyme activity in lungs of fetal and neonatal rabbits expressed as percent increase in activity above the baseline value, which is the lowest activity measured over the gestational period tested. Mean values for SOD, catalase and GP show pattern of marked increases during the last few days of gestation (SOD and catalase increase approximately 110% and GP increases approximately 200%). Postnatally, all the antioxidant enzymes show continued elevations in activity. Also represented in the figure (thick solid-line curve) are the percent increases in lung lecithin concentration (mg/g dry weight), adapted from data of Farrell et al. (1977). (From Frank and Groseclose, 1983, 1984.)

DeJours, 1981). Yet, at birth, the lung will be expected to function immediately in a relatively O_2-rich world, with 21% alveolar O_2 and blood p_{O_2} ex utero >>> in utero. Thus, the late fetal elevation in levels of SOD, catalase and GP may be an important maturational phenomena to assure protection to the newly functional lung from potential O_2 toxicity due to the marked increase in O_2 concentration that it encounters at parturition.

The hormonal milieu of the fetus may control the late gestational rise in antioxidant enzymes. Erenberg et al. (1982) have demonstrated that thyroxin normalized pulmonary SOD activity in the athyrotic sheep fetus. If the enzyme activity changes are under the same type of hormonal control as the enzymes involved in surfactant production, then it may become possible to accelerate clinically the maturation of the antioxidant defense system in premature infants, much like the surfactant system is now stimulated with prenatal hormonal treatment. The implications of this recent information about prematurity and deficient maturation of the antioxidant defense system of the lung may be clinically quite relevant. The early respiratory difficulty the very premature infant experiences due to instability of airspaces and progressive atelectasis may be complicated by early effects of O_2 toxicity due to lung defenses inadequate to protect against the relative hyperoxia of a 21%-O_2 world. Whether or not ambient O_2 levels result in significant problems is unknown; however, it seems quite reasonable to predict that the less than full-term levels of lung SOD, catalase and GP activity will present potentially serious problems for the premature infant when he begins to require hyperoxic therapy with 40–100% O_2 often within a few hours after birth.

An important question, of course, is whether the developmental data in the fetal animal lung is extrapolatable to the human fetal lung. Does the human infant also require a full-term period of gestation to develop the levels of antioxidant enzymes in his lung which will best prepare him or her for the 21%-O_2 world about to be entered? The only human data available which provide some clue to the answer to this question are from a study by Autor et al. (1976). The SOD levels in the lungs of term infants (49 ± 6 units/mg DNA) were found to be significantly higher than the SOD activity in premature lungs (38 ± 4 units/mg DNA) and much higher than in 20–22-week fetal lungs (17 ± 1 units/mg DNA). Although the sample numbers available in this study were small, the data do suggest that human fetal lung SOD is lower in the earlier gestation period, and comparatively elevated in the term newborn versus the prematurely born, as in the case of rabbit and rat.

If one combines the deficiency of lung antioxidant enzyme system protection with the information that the newborn human infant is also relatively deficient in vitamin E compared to the adult (Gross et al., 1977; Johnson et al., 1974; Phelps, 1982), the compromised ability of the premature infant's lung to protect itself from hyperoxic stress is apparent.

While it is not possible to assess directly the lung antioxidant enzyme defense capacity in the premature and use this information perhaps for prognostic purposes, it may still be possible to get some clue to this information by blood analysis. This hypothesis is based on several studies in human infants in which the antioxidant enzymes were measured in term and premature infant red cells. All the values were found to be lower in the premature versus the term infants (Gross et al., 1967; Necheles et al., 1968; Amin et al., 1978). Additionally, serum levels of ceruloplasmin (a proposed scavenger of superoxide anion) are also reportedly reduced at birth in the prematurely born with RDS (Tyrala et al., 1982).

Two studies are also worthy of note, in which the changes in blood SOD levels during therapy for severe RDS/HMD were followed. Pooled together, the results of the serial SOD blood levels were as follows: 13/13 HMD infants who survived and did not develop any clinical signs of BPD or chronic O_2 toxicity showed increasing serial blood SOD levels; 11/11 infants who died despite intensive respiratory therapy for RDS/HMD showed either no change or decreasing serial blood SOD levels; and the same pattern of decreasing or unchanged SOD blood levels was found in the three infants who developed obvious clinical signs of BPD (Bonta et al., 1977; Bauer et al., 1982).

2. Pharmacological treatments to prevent O_2 toxicity

Knowledge about the mechanism(s) of action of a toxic process usually precedes the development of effective measures or agents to counter the process. Our understanding of the free radical theory of O_2 toxicity as it has evolved over the past decade or so has not only provided a rational perspective on the mechanism of O_2 toxicity at the molecular level, but also a direction for future therapeutic measures designed to circumvent O_2 toxicity. Interference with the initiation of O_2-induced toxic changes may come about with the use of agents that function to reinforce the endogenous antioxidant protective systems of the lung (and premature retina).

Where are we now? To date, the only pharmacologic agent that truly has graduated from experimental animal to clinical use is vitamin E. A large collection of experimental data indicates a peculiar aspect of vitamin E's protective ability. Animals made vitamin E-deficient are certainly much more susceptible to lung damage during hyper-oxidant exposure (Tierney et al., 1977; Bus et al., 1977; Mustafa and Tierney, 1978; Chow et al., 1981). However, supplemental vitamin E administered to animals on normal diets and replete with vitamin E produces no added protective action against toxicity due to hyperoxia, ozone, NO_2, paraquat, etc. (Schatte and Swansigner, 1976; Mustafa and Tierney, 1978; Yam and Roberts, 1979; Frank and Massaro, 1980; Deneke and Fanburg, 1980; Ward and Roberts, 1984). So, while administration of alpha-tocopherol to adequately nourished newborn infants or adult patients may be of little benefit in mitigating O_2's toxic action, alpha-tocopherol administration to newborn infants with RDS who do not receive nutritional sources of vitamin E may have a comparatively salutatory effect.

In fact, this has now been shown to be the case in RLF. Several controlled clinical studies have now indicated that vitamin E administration to prematurely born infants immediately after birth results in a reduced incidence of the more severe degrees of RLF. (While the overall incidence of RLF is not significantly changed, infants treated with vitamin E show significant reductions in the development of grade III and IV disease — the grades leading to severe retinal damage and blindness (Phelps, 1982; Finer et al., 1982; Monaco, 1982/1983; Hittner et al., 1983).)

A preliminary report of the efficacy of early vitamin E administration in reducing the occurrence of severe lung disease (BPD) (Ehrenkrantz et al., 1978) has, unfortunately, not been confirmed by subsequent larger clinical trials undertaken in several other neonatal intensive care units (including the larger follow-up study of the original group reporting preliminary evidence of success) (Ehrenkrantz et al., 1979; Saldanha et al., 1982; Finer et al., 1982; Hittner et al., 1981). It is possible, however, that if means were available to increase the lung complement of the antioxidant enzymes, that such therapy in combination with vitamin E treatment would have an additive, or even synergistic, protective action.

Clinical trials have just begun with a parenteral preparation of SOD, to test both the safety of its use in human infants and its possible efficacy as a protective agent versus O_2 toxicity (Rosenfeld et al., 1982, 1983). From a review of animal studies, one would have to take a sceptical view of SOD's possible protective effect against BPD (or RLF). The principle problem is that unmodified SOD, being a protein with a molecular weight of 32,000, essentially is unable to penetrate intracellularly, where the O_2 free radicals are being generated and where the antioxidant defensive system needs to be augmented (Petkau et al., 1975; Huber and Saifer, 1977). Very recently, there have been reports by Michelson et al. (1981) and Freeman et al. (1983) on the preparation of liposomal encapsulated SOD and catalase enzyme. Liposome encapsulation of proteins is a recognized pharmacological means known to 'fool' cells and facilitate transport of non-lipid drugs through the lipid membrane barrier and into the intracellular compartment. In preliminary studies with liposomal encapsulated SOD and catalase, it was reported that both lung endothelial cells in vitro and lung tissue in vivo will demonstrate increased SOD and catalase activity following treatment with these cleverly modified enzyme preparations (Michelson et al., 1981; Freeman et al., 1983). While there is still a fair amount of pharmacological and toxicological animal work that must be completed, the possible future clinical use of liposomal encapsulated antioxidant enzymes is certainly promising and exciting to contemplate.

We indicated scepticism above in referring to the present clinical testing for possible effectiveness of parenteral SOD in its unmodified form, since it fails to penetrate intracellularly into the lung. Perhaps we should modify this opinion, based principally on some recent work reported by Merritt (1982) in newborn guinea pigs exposed to hyperoxia. This study showed (as have previous studies in adult animals) that O_2 toxicity is associated with a substantial inflammatory influx of cells into the alveolar spaces of the lung (Fig. 6). Polymorphonuclear leukocytes and alveolar macrophages are known to respond to various stimuli, including cellular debris, which activates phagocytosis, with a release of potentially cytotoxic proteases and the release of O_2 free radicals (Cohen, 1979). Merritt (1982) and others have suggested that these products released extracellularly by inflammatory cells could provide additional toxic insult to the lung cells already suffering the consequences of intracellular O_2 free radical attack (Merritt, 1982; Carp and Janoff, 1979; Janoff et al., 1979; Fox et al., 1980).

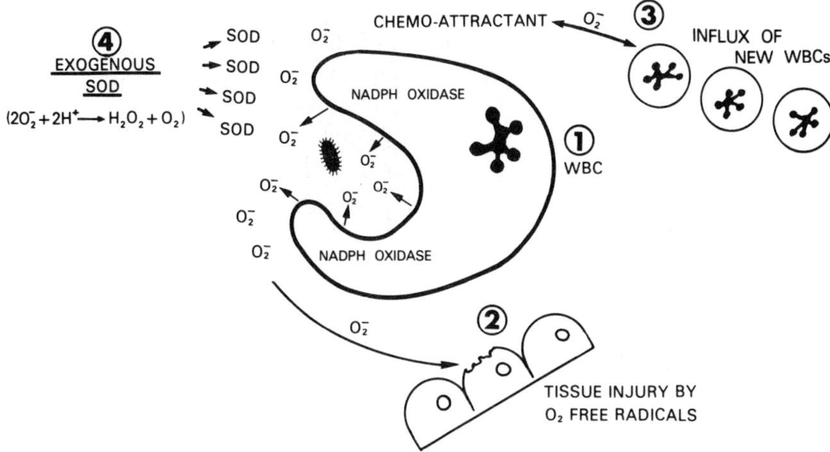

Figure 6. Proposed role of superoxide free-radical (O_2^-) and SOD in inflammation. (1) Activated white blood cells (WBCs) release large amounts of O_2^- when phagocytosis occurs. Most O_2^- released into forming phagosome, but O_2^- also escapes into extracellular space. (2) O_2^- released by WBCs capable of direct damage to tissues at inflammatory site. (3) O_2^- also acts as chemo-attractant to lure more WBCs to inflammation site. (4) Exogenous (parenteral) SOD, by detoxifying the released O_2^-, can prevent steps (2) and (3) from occurring. (From Frank, 1982.)

As it turns out, veterinarians have been using a product called Orgotein® for several years now to treat inflammatory conditions, e.g., in the joints of race horses. Orgotein® is SOD. Also, for several years now, clinical trials of Orgotein® have been under way, and promising results have been found in reducing tissue damage in certain chronic arthritic and other conditions in which inflammatory cell influx is a prominent feature of the pathology (Huber and Saifer, 1977; Huber et al., 1980; Meander-Huber, 1980; Flohe et al., 1980).

The point that needs to be emphasized is that although parenteral therapy with purified SOD enzyme will presumably not have any protective action against the primary toxic effect of O_2 within the cells of the lung, if the added insult produced by extracellular inflammatory cell products (specifically, superoxide anion) contributes significantly to the overall pathology of O_2 toxicity and the development of BPD, then exogenous SOD may be effective due to its reported extracellular action at inflammatory foci.

Another therapeutic tack different from all the above (exogenous antioxidants) would involve using pharmacological means to stimulate exogenous lung antioxidant defenses. As discussed earlier, if the factor(s) that control the normal developmental rise in lung SOD, catalase and GP activity were known (hormonal?), then prenatal treatment much like the current use of synthetic corticoids to try to hasten lung surfactant system enzyme maturation might be an important protective intervention. Experimentally, there is one pharmacological means of consistently stimulating marked elevations in lung antioxidant enzyme activity during O_2 exposure. This is by the administration of small doses of bacterial lipopolysaccharide, or endotoxin. Treatment of adult rats with 500 $\mu g/kg$ of endotoxin (approximately one-fiftieth of the LD_{50} for this species) has the dramatic effect of producing tolerance to O_2 toxicity (survival rate increased from under 25% in control rats to over 95% in endotoxin-treated animals) (Frank et al., 1978b, 1980; Frank and Roberts, 1979a, b; Frank, 1981b). In addition, recent evidence indicates that endotoxin treatment of adult rats in hyperoxia appears to overcome the normally seen inhibitory effect of high O_2 exposure on protein and nucleotide synthesis (Hass et al., 1982). This would permit pulmonary repair processes to take place during O_2 exposure, processes which are presumably severely limited in non-endotoxin-treated, O_2-exposed animal lungs.

If the exact mechanism of endotoxin's effect in stimulating the endogenous lung antioxidant enzyme defenses of the lung could be determined, it might be feasible to develop other pharmacological agents with similar activity but with less innate toxic potential than endotoxin itself. Alternatively, if ongoing studies to try to alter chemically the endotoxin molecule so that a preparation with much reduced toxic potential could be obtained — an 'endotoxoid' — which still maintains most of its stimulatory activity on lung SOD, catalase and GP activities during O_2 exposure, then such an agent would obviously have important clinical potential.

One final clinical intervention should be noted. This treatment modality is the end result of the massive amount of experimental work which has been done on the analysis of surfactant and its multiple components. Studies are currently being done to test the effects of either synthetic surfactant, bovine- or ovine-derived surfactant or surfactant isolated from human amniotic fluid administered by tracheal gavage to premature infants with RDS/HMD (Metcalfe et al., 1982; Glatz et al., 1982; Jobe et al., 1983). The aim of the studies is to try to provide the immature lungs with an exogenous supply of surfactant to make up for the deficient surfactant production which is making the work of breathing so arduous for them. The early reports indicate some transient success in lowering either the mechanical respiratory pressures required and/or the levels of O_2 required to maintain normoxic blood values. If this means of therapy reaches a sophisticated state in which ideal surfactant preparations, dosages, means of delivery, etc., are defined, then the result may be a marked reduction in the level and the duration of hyperoxic therapy required to manage the premature infant with RDS/HMD.

3. *Nutrition and O_2 toxicity*

In the clinical setting in which specific pharmacological means of treatment are not presently available, attention to every small detail of ideal supportive treatment is obligatory. When treating the seriously ill newborn, especially the fragile premature, attention to supportive factors such as maintenance of external heat control, replacement of insensitive fluid loss and provision of ideal nutritional needs may have surprisingly important influences on the period of morbidity or mortality. Unfortunately, with the concentrated attention demanded for careful monitoring of respiratory support in many of these sick infants, some supportive aspects of treatment, particularly adequate nutritional provision, are at times overlooked. Many premature infants requiring vigorous respiratory therapy with elevated levels of O_2 are inadequately nourished for the first several days of life or longer. Provision of ideal nutrition is usually complicated by the need to use parenteral routes of administration rather than oral. Nonetheless, it has now been shown in both experimental and clinical studies that failure to provide ideal caloric maintenance is a (preventable) factor which may have aggravating effects on O_2-induced lung toxicity (Polgar et al., 1966; Massaro, 1973; Hackney et al., 1977; Roberts, 1978; Gunn et al., 1978; Bucher and Roberts, 1981a, b; Frank and Groseclose, 1982).

One recent review of experimental studies on the influence of altered nutrition on O_2 tolerance/susceptibility has provided also a discussion of how specific nutritional factors in the human premature infant may influence resistance/susceptibility to O_2-induced lung problems (Roberts, 1978). Recently completed studies in newborn rats (Fig. 7) have found that hypocaloric intake will consistently reduce the tolerance of newborn rats to hyperoxic exposure during the first week of life (Bucher and Roberts, 1981a, b; Frank and Groseclose, 1982). Under-nutrition aggravates markedly the inhibitory effects of hyperoxia on the lung's ability to repair O_2-induced damage and shows additive effects with hyperoxia on lung growth potential (lung DNA decreased by a remarkable 65% in the undernourished pups in O_2). Measurement of lipid peroxidation by expired ethane and pentane also shows a marked increase in newborn rats with hypocaloric intake (Roberts et al., 1983a, b). Interestingly,

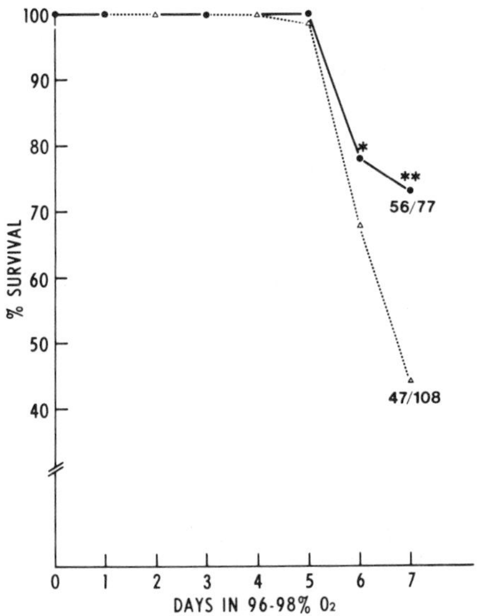

Figure 7. Survival rates for normally nourished (11 per litter, ●) and undernourished (18 per litter, △) rat pups exposed to 96–98% O_2 for first 7 days of life. Results are composite values from five exposure experiments. *Significant difference in survival rate at 6 days ($P<0.05$). **Significant difference at 7 days ($P<0.005$). (From Frank and Groseclose, 1982.)

hyperoxic exposure did not result in an increase in expired ethane or pentane, suggesting that lipid peroxidation may not be a critical event in oxygen toxicity. Clinically, it has been observed that respiratory-distressed infants who received a more normocaloric nutritional preparation parenterally did much better than a control group of similarly sick infants on O_2 whose nutrition consisted only of dextrose/electrolyte solutions early in life (Gunn et al., 1978).

It seems prudent to assume that undernourishment can have serious detrimental effects in newborn infants exposed to prolonged hyperoxic treatment and, therefore, early provision of normal nutrition should be a primary goal in their total clinical management.

V. SUMMARY

Although the consequences to the lung of prolonged exposure to high concentrations of O_2 are now well established, there are still, unfortunately, no pharmacological agents available to the clinician to help circumvent O_2-induced acute or chronic lung toxicity.

O_2-induced lung damage is a particularly tragic problem in the newborn, since many infants who require ventilatory support for surfactant deficiency and lung parenchymal immaturity (RDS/HMD) may show evidence for biochemical recovery from surfactant deficiency, but nonetheless still go on to suffer severe lung sequelae or death due to the damage incurred by their lungs during the period of hyperoxic therapy. Experimentally, exposure to high O_2 levels inhibits lung protein and DNA synthesis, airway surfactant and normal lung maturation, detrimental aspects of O_2 exposure that may explain some of the long-term sequelae of O_2 toxicity seen in human infants.

Premature infants require O_2 therapy principally because of the immaturity of their lung development and immaturity of the biochemical enzyme system involved with lung surfactant production. Additionally, premature newborns may have immature levels of their lung antioxidant enzymes and vitamin E, which would make their lungs particularly prone to early O_2-induced damage when high O_2 therapy is instituted.

The 'free radical theory' of O_2 toxicity provides a molecular basis to explain O_2's toxic action, and also provides important understanding of how best to approach pharmacologically the countering of O_2's toxic action. Means to augment the lungs' antioxidant defenses either with exogenous preparations of these agents (vitamin E, SOD, catalase) or with agents which stimulate the lungs' own endogenous defenses during O_2 exposure (endotoxin) are being tested currently in laboratory animals. Administration of pharmacological doses of alpha-tocopherol (vitamin E) already has been shown to have clinical effectiveness against O_2-induced retinal injury (RLF) in clinical trials in premature infants. The use of prenatal hormonal therapy to try to hasten maturation of the fetal lung in infants who are threatened with premature birth due to the early onset of labor has been successful in stimulating surfactant system production and lessening the incidence of RDS/HMD in these infants, thereby obviating their need for vigorous O_2 therapy.

Once the premature infant does require intensive ventilatory therapy and prolonged exposure to elevated concentrations of O_2, all means of supportive treatment become very important in helping to reduce the period of need for hyperoxic treatment. Attention to adequate nutritional needs (including vitamin E) plus ideal mechanical respirator management and pulmonary toilette could contribute to the overall reduction in the amount of O_2-induced injury that occurs in the immature infant's lung. Until more specific pharmacological treatment is available, these supportive factors may be vital in determining the degree of respiratory impairment resulting from exposure to toxic O_2.

VI. REFERENCES

Adams, G.E. (1981) Cancer 48, 696–707.

Amin, S., Chen, S.Y., Castro-Mangana, M., Maddaiah, V.T. and Collipp, P.J. (1978) Fed. Proc. 37, 758 (Abstract).

Anderson, W.R., Strickland, M.B., Tsai, S.H. and Haglin, J.J. (1973) Am. J. Pathol. 73, 327–348.

Autor, A.P., Frank, L. and Roberts, R.J. (1976) Ped. Res. 10, 154–158.

Avery, M.E., Fletcher, B.D. and Williams, R.G. (eds.) (1981a) The Lung and Its Disorders in the Newborn Infant, pp. 3–22, W.B. Saunders, Philadelphia.

Avery, M.E., Fletcher, B.D. and Williams, R.G. (eds.) (1981b) The Lung and Its Disorders in the Newborn Infant, pp. 222–262, W.B. Saunders, Philadelphia.

Avery, M.E., Fletcher, B.D. and Williams, R.G. (eds.) (1981c) The Lung and Its Disorders in the Newborn Infant, pp. 263–274, W.B. Saunders, Philadelphia.

Balentine, J.D. (1977) in Oxygen and Physiologic Function (Jobsis, J.J., ed.), pp. 311–378, Professional Information Library, Dallas, TX.

Ballard, P.L. (1977) in Development of the Lung (Hodson, W.A., ed.), pp. 419–442, Marcel Dekker, New York.

Ballard, R.A., Ballard, P.L., Granberg, J.P. and Sniderman, S. (1979) J. Ped. 94, 97–101.

Bancalari, E., Abdenour, G.E., Feller, R. and Gannon, J. (1979) J. Ped. 85, 819–823.

Battenburg, J.J. and Van Golde, M.G. (1979) in Reviews in Perinatal Medicine (Scarpelli, E.M. and Cosmi, E.V., eds.), Vol. 3, pp. 73–97, Raven Press, New York.

Bauer, C.R., Frank, L., White, A., Feller, R., Brennan, M.J. and Sultan, S. (1982) Ped. Res. 16, 277A (Abstract).

Bergman, B. and Hedner, T. (1978) Acta. Obstet. Gynecol. Scand. 57, 217–221.

Binger, C.A.L., Faulkner, J.M. and Moore, R.L. (1927) J. Exp. Med. 45, 849–864.

Block, E.R. and Fisher, A.B. (1977) J. Appl. Physiol. 42, 33–38.

Boat, T.F., Kleinerman, J.I., Fanaroff, A.A. and Matthews, L.W. (1973) Ped. Res. 7, 607–615.

Boog, C., BenBrahim, M. and Gandar, R. (1975) Br. J. Obstet. Gynecol. 82, 285–288.

Bonikos, D.S., Bensch, K.G., Northway, W.H., Jr. and Edwards, D.K. (1976) Human Pathol. 7, 643–666.

Bonta, B.W., Gawron, E.R. and Warshaw, J.B. (1977) Ped. Res. 11, 754–757.

Bourbon, J. and Jost, A. (1982) Ped. Res. 16, 50–56.

Bradley, K.H., McConnell, S.D. and Crystal, R.G. (1974) J. Biol. Chem. 249, 2674–2683.

Brazy, J.E. and Pupkin, M.J. (1979) J. Ped. 94, 444–448.

Bucher, J.R. and Roberts, R.J. (1981a) Ped. Res. 15, 999–1008.

Bucher, J.R. and Roberts, R.J. (1981b) J. Ped. 98, 806–811.

Bucher, J.R. and Roberts, R.J. (1982) Ped. Pharmacol. 2, 1–9.

Burger, E.J., Jr. and Mead, J. (1969) J. Appl. Physiol. 27, 191–197.
Burri, P.H. and Weibel, E.R. (1977) in Development of the Lung (Hodson, W.A., ed.), pp. 215–268, Marcel Dekker, New York.
Bus, J.S., Aust, S.D. and Gibson, J.E. (1977) in Biochemical Mechanisms of Paraquat Toxicity (Autor, A.P., ed.), pp. 157–172, Academic Press, New York.
Carp, H. and Janoff, A. (1979) J. Clin. Invest. 63, 793–797.
Chow, C.K., Plopper, C.G., Chiu, M. and Dungworth, D.L. (1981) Environ. Res. 24, 315–324.
Churg, A., Golden, J., Fligiel, S. and Hoff, J.C. (1983) Am. Rev. Respir. Dis. 127, 117–120.
Clark, J.M. and Lambertsen, C.J. (1971) Pharmacol. Rev. 23, 37–133.
Clements, J.A. and Tooley, W.H. (1977) in Development of the Lung (Hodson, W.A., ed.), pp. 349–366, Marcel Dekker, New York.
Coalson, J.J., Kuehl, T.J., Escobedo, M.B., Hilliard, J.L., Smith, F., Meredith, K., Null, D.M., Jr., Walsh, W., Johnson, D. and Robotham, J.L. (1982) Exp. Mol. Pathol. 37, 335–350.
Coates, A.L., Desmond, K., Willis, D. and Nogrady, B. (1982) Am. J. Dis. Child. 136, 892–895.
Cohen, A. (1979) Fed. Proc. 38, 2644–2647.
DeJours, P. (1981) in Principles of Comparative Respiratory Physiology, 2nd edn., pp. 147–171, Elsevier/North Holland, Amsterdam.
DeLemos, R., Wolfsdorf, J., Nachman, R., Block, A.J., Leiby, G., Wilkinson, H.A., Allen, T., Haller, A., Morgan, W. and Avery, M.E. (1969) Anesthesiology 30, 609–618.
Deneke, S.M. and Fanburg, B.L. (1980) N. Eng. J. Med. 303, 76–86.
Edwards, D.K. (1979) J. Ped. 85, 823–829.
Edwards, D.K., Dyer, W.M. and Northway, W.H., Jr. (1977) Pediatrics 59, 839–846.
Ehrenkrantz, R.A., Bonta, B.W., Ablow, R.C. and Warshaw, J.B. (1978) N. Eng. J. Med. 299, 564–569.
Ehrenkrantz, R.A., Ablow, R.C. and Warshaw, J.B. (1979) J. Ped. 95, 873–878.
Engle, M.J., Van Golde, L.M.G. and Wirtz, K.W.A. (1978) FEBS Lett. 86, 277–281.
Epstein, M.F., Nicholls, E. and Stubblefield, P.G. (1979) J. Ped. 94, 449–453.
Erenberg, A., Frank, L., Roberts, R.J. and Rhodes, M.D. (1982) Ped. Res. 16, 570, 572.
Escobedo, M.B., Hilliard, J.L., Smith, F., Meredith, K., Walsh, W., Johnson, D., Coalson, J.J., Kuehl, T.J., Null, D.M., Jr. and Robotham, J.L. (1982) Exp. Mol. Pathol. 37, 323–334.
Farrell, P.M. (1982) in Lung Development: Biological and Clinical Perspectives (Farrel, P.M., ed.), Vol. 1, pp. 3–25, Academic Press, New York.
Farrell, P.M. and Avery, M.E. (1975) Am. Rev. Respir. Dis. 111, 657–692.
Farrell, P.M. and Hamosh, M. (1978) Clin. Perinatol. 5, 197–229.
Farrell, P.M., Blackburn, W.R. and Adams, A.J. (1977) Ped. Res. 11, 770–773.
Finer, N.N., Schindler, R.F., Grant, G., Hill, G.B. and Peters, K. L. (1982) Lancet I, 1087–1091.
Flohe, L., Biehl, O., Hofer, H., Kadrnka, F., Kolbel, R. and Fuhl, W. (1980) in Biological and Clinical Aspects of Superoxide and Superoxide Dismutase (Bannister, W.H. and Bannister, J.V., eds), pp. 424–430, Elsevier/North Holland, New York.
Foreman, H.J. and Fisher, A.B. (1982) in Oxygen and Living Processes, An Interdisciplinary Approach (Gilbert, D.L., ed.), pp. 235–249, Springer-Verlag, New York.
Fowler, J., Adams, G. and Denekany, J. (1976) Cancer Treat. Rev. 3, 227–256.
Fox, R.B., Hoidal, J.R., Brown, D.M. and Repine, J.E. (1980) Am. Rev. Respir. Dis. 121, 340 (Abstract).
Fox, W.N. (1978) Ped. Ann. 7, 75–85.
Frank, L. (1981a) Biochem. Pharmacol. 30, 2319–2324.
Frank, L. (1981b) J. Appl. Physiol. 51, 577–583.
Frank, L. (1982) in Environmental Factors in Human Growth and Development (Banbury Report 11) (Hunt, V.R., Smith, M.K. and Worth, D., eds.), pp. 17–32, Cold Spring Harbor Laboratory, Cold Spring Harbor, NY.
Frank, L. and Groseclose, E.E. (1982) J. Appl. Physiol. 53, 1248–1255.
Frank, L. and Groseclose, E.E. (1983) Clin. Res. 31, 512A (Abstract).
Frank, L. and Groseclose, E.E. (1984) Ped. Res., 18, 240–243.
Frank, L. and Massaro, D. (1980) Am. J. Med. 69, 117–126.

Frank, L. and Roberts, R.J. (1979a) J. Appl. Physiol. 47, 577–581.
Frank, L. and Roberts, R.J. (1979b) Toxicol. Appl. Pharmacol. 50, 371–380.
Frank, L., Woods, D. and Roberts, R.J. (1978a) Biochem. Pharmacol. 27, 251–254.
Frank, L., Yam, J. and Roberts, R.J. (1978b) J. Clin. Invest. 61, 269–275.
Frank, L., Bucher, J.R. and Roberts, R.J. (1979) J. Appl. Physiol. 45, 699–704.
Frank, L., Summerville, J. and Massaro, D. (1980) J. Clin. Invest. 48, 505–510.
Franzblau, C., Hayes, J.A. and Snider, G.L. (1977) in Development of the Lung (Hodson, W.A., ed.), pp. 367–397, Marcel Dekker, New York.
Freeman, B.A. and Crapo, J.D. (1981) J. Biol. Chem. 256, 10986–10992.
Freeman, B.A. and Crapo, J.D. (1982) Lab. Invest. 47, 412–426.
Freeman, B.A., Topolosky, M.K. and Crapo, J.D. (1982) Arch. Biochem. Biophys. 216, 477–484.
Freeman, B.A., Turrens, J.F., Crapo, J.D. and Young, S.L. (1983) Am. Rev. Respir. Dis. 127, 273 (Abstract).
Fridovich, I. (1974) Adv. Enzymol. 41, 35–97.
Fridovich, I. (1976) in Free Radicals in Biology (Pryor, W.A., ed.), Vol. 1, pp. 239–277, Academic Press, New York.
Gacad, G. and Massaro, D. (1973) J. Clin. Invest. 52, 559–565.
Gerhardt, T., Tapia, J.L., Goldman, S.L., Hehre, D., Feller, R. and Bancalari, E. (1983) Ped. Res. 17, 376A (Abstract).
Gilder, H. and McSherry, C.K. (1976) Biochem. Biophys. Acta 441, 48–56.
Gillis, N.C. and Green, N.M. (1977) in Metabolic Functions of the Lung (Bakhle, Y.S. and Vane, J.R., eds.), pp. 173–193, Marcel Dekker, New York.
Glatz, T., Ikegami, M. and Jobe, A. (1982) Ped. Res. 16, 711-715.
Gluck, L. (1976) Am. J. Dis. Child. 130, 976–978.
Gould, V.E., Tosco, R., Wheelis, R.F., Gould, N.S. and Kapanci, Y. (1972) Lab. Invest. 26, 499–508.
Greengard, O. (1971) Essays Biochem. 7, 159–205.
Greengard, O. (1972) Clin. Pharmacol. Ther. 14, 721–726.
Gregory, A.R. and Hine, C.H. (1968) Proc. Soc. Exp. Biol. Med. 128, 693–695.
Gross, N.J. and Smith, D.M. (1981) J. Apl. Physiol. 51, 1198–1203.
Gross, R.T., Bracci, R., Rudolph, N., Schroeder, E. and Kochen, J. A. (1967) Blood 29, 481–493.
Gross, S.J., Landaw, S.A. and Oski, F. (1977) Pediatrics 59, 995–997.
Gunn, T., Reamon, G., Outerbridge, F.W. and Colle, E. (1978) J. Ped. 92, 608–613.
Hackney, J.J., Evans, M.J., Bils, R.F., Spier, C.E. and Lones, M.P. (1977) Exp. Mol. Pathol. 25, 350–358.
Halliwell, B. (1981) in Age Pigments (Sohal, R.S., ed.), pp. 1–62, Elsevier/North Holland, New York.
Hallman, M. and Gluck, L. (1982) Ped. Clin. North Am. 29, 1057–1075.
Hamosh, M., Schechter, Y. and Hamosh, P. (1978) Ped. Res. 12, 95–100.
Hass, M., Frank, L. and Massaro, D. (1982) J. Biol. Chem. 257, 9379–9383.
Haugaard, N. (1965) Ann. N.Y. Acad. Sci. 117, 736–744.
Haugaard, N. (1968) Physiol. Rev. 48, 311–373.
Hislop, A. and Reid, L.M. (1977) in Development of the Lung (Hodson, W.A., ed.), pp. 37–86, Marcel Dekker, New York.
Hittner, H.M., Godio, L.B., Rudolph, A.J., Adams, J.M., Garcia-Pratts, J.A., Friedman, Z., Kautz, J.A. and Monaco, W.A. (1981) N. Eng. J. Med. 305, 1365–1371.
Hittner, H.M., Godio, L.B., Speer, M.E., Rudolph, A.J., Taylor, M. M., Blifeld, C. and Kretzer, F.L. (1983) Pediatrics 71, 423–432.
Hodson, W.A. (ed.) (1977) Development of the Lung. Vol. 6, in series Lung Biology in Health and Disease, Marcel Dekker, New York.
Horwitt, M.K. (1976) Am. J. Clin. Nutr. 29, 569–578.
Huber, G.L. and Drath, D.B. (1981) in Oxygen and Living Processes. An Interdisciplinary Approach (Gilbert, D.L., ed.), pp. 273–324, Springer-Verlag, New York.
Huber, W. and Saifer, M.G.P. (1977) in Superoxide and Superoxide Dismutases (Michelson, A.M., McCord, J.M. and Fridovich, I., eds.), pp. 517–536, Academic Press, New York.
Huber, W., Saifer, M.G.P. and Williams, L.D. (1980) in Biological and Clinical Aspects of Superoxide and

Superoxide Dismutase (Bannister, W.H. and Bannister, J.V., eds.), pp. 395–407, Elsevier/North Holland, New York.

James, L.S. and Lanman, J.T. (1976) Pediatrics 57 (Suppl.), 589–642.

Janoff, A., White, R., Carp, H., Havel, S., Dearing, R. and Lee, D. (1979) Am. J. Pathol. 97, 111–136.

Jobe, A.H., Jacobs, H.C., Ikegami, M. and Jones, S.J. (1983) Ped. Res. 17, 319A (Abstract).

Johnson, L., Schaffer, D. and Boggs, T.R., Jr. (1974) Am. J. Clin. Nutr. 27, 1158–1173.

Kapanci, Y., Weibel, E.R., Kaplan, H.P. and Robinson, F.R. (1969) Lab. Invest. 20, 101, 118.

Kauffman, S.L., Burri, P.H. and Weibel, E.R. (1974) Anat. Record 180, 63–76.

King, R.K. (1982) J. Appl. Physiol. 53, 1–8.

Kirschbaum, T.H., Lucas, W.E., DeHaven, J.C. and Assail, N.S. (1967) Am. J. Obstet. Gynecol. 98, 429.

Kistler, G.S., Cladwell, P.R.B. and Weibel, E.R. (1967) J. Cell Biol. 32, 605–628.

Liggins, G.C. and Howie, R.N. (1972) Pediatrics 50, 515–525.

Lechner, A.J. and Sanchero, N. (1982) Am. J. Anat. 163, 235–246.

Malmstrom, B.G. (1982) Annu. Rev. Biochem. 51, 21–59.

Massaro, D. (1973) Proc. Soc. Exp. Biol. Med. 143, 602–603.

Meander-Huber, K.B. (1980) in Biological and Clinical Aspects of Superoxide and Superoxide Dismutase (Bannister, W.H. and Bannister, J.V., eds.), pp. 408–423, Elsevier/North Holland, New York.

Merritt, T.A. (1982) Ped. Res. 16, 798–805.

Metcalfe, I.L., Burgoyne, R. and Enhorning, G. (1982) Ped. Res. 16, 834–839.

Meyrick, B. and Reid, L.M. (1977) in Development of the Lung (Hodson, W.A., ed.), pp. 135–214, Marcel Dekker, New York.

Michelson, A.M., Puget, K. and Durosay, P. (1981) Mol. Physiol. 1, 85–96.

Miller, B.C., Fielden, E.M. and Steel, J.J. (1979) Int. J. Radiat. Biol. 36, 177–180.

Monaco, W.A. (1982/1983) Current Eye Res. 2, 123–139.

Mustafa, M.G. and Tierney, D.F. (1978) Am. Rev. Respir. Dis. 118, 1061–1090.

Nash, G., Bowen, J.A. and Langlinais, P.C. (1971) Arch. Pathol. 21, 234–240.

Necheles, T.D., Boles, T.A. and Allen, D.M. (1968) J. Ped. 72, 319–323.

Northway, W.H., Jr. and Rosan, R.C. (1969) Hosp. Pract. Jan., 59–67.

Northway, W.H., Jr., Rosan, R.C. and Porter, D.Y. (1967) N. Eng. J. Med. 276, 357–368.

Northway, W.H., Jr., Petriceks, R. and Shahinian, L. (1972) Pediatrics 49, 67–72.

O'Hare, J.H. and Sheridan, M.N. (1970) Am. J. Anat. 127, 181–206.

Perelman, R.H., Engle, M.J., Kemnitz, J.W., Kotas, R.V. and Farrell, P.M. (1982) J. Appl. Physiol. 53, 230–233.

Petkau, A., Kelly, K., Chelack, W.S., Pleskach, S.D. Meeker, B.E. and Brady, C.M. (1975) Biochem. Biophys. Res. Commun. 65, 886–893.

Phelps, D. (1982) Ped. Clin. North. Am. 29, 1233–1240.

Polgar, G. and Weng, R.T. (1979) Am. Rev. Respir. Dis. 120, 625–695.

Polgar, G., Antagnoli, W., Ferrigan, L.W., Martin, E.A. and Gregg, W.P. (1966) Am. J. Med. Sci. 112, 580–587.

Quatiliana, M. (1977) Int. J. Radiat. Oncol. Biol. Phys. 5, 1069–1076.

Raffin, T.A., Braun, D., Simon, L.M., Theodore, J. and Robin, E.D. (1972) Clin. Res. 25, 422A (Abstract).

Roberts, R.J. (1978) Adv. Pharmacol. Ther. 8, 53–64.

Roberts, R.J., Weesner, K.M. and Bucher, J.R. (1983a) Ped. Res. 17, 368–375.

Roberts, R.J. Rendak, I. and Bucher, J.R. (1983b) Dev. Pharmacol. Ther. 6, 170–178.

Roberts, R.J. (1984) Drug Therapy in Infants, Ch. 9. W.B. Saunders, Philadelphia.

Rosenfeld, W., Evans, M., Jhaveri, R., Moanie, H., Vohra, K., Georgatos, E. and Salazar, J.D. (1982) Dev. Pharmacol. Ther. 5, 151–161.

Rosenfeld, W., Evan, H., Concepcion, L., Jhaveri, R., Schaeffer, H. and Friedman, A. (1983) Ped. Res. 17, 154A (Abstract).

Saldanha, R.L., Cepeda, E.E. and Poland, R.L. (1982) J. Ped. 101, 89–93.

Schatte, C. and Swansigner, A. (1976) Aviat. Space Environ. Med. 47, 147–150.

Silverman, W.A. (1977) Sci. Am. 236, 100–107.

Smith, B.T. and Bogues, W.G. (1980) Pharmacol. Ther. 9, 51–74.

Smith, D.W., Stevenson, D.K., Sunshine, P., Northway, W.H. and Ariagno, R.K. (1983) Ped. Res. 17, 390A (Abstract).

Smith, F.J.C., Bennett, G.A., Heim, J.W., Thompson, R.M. and Drinker, C.K. (1932) J. Exp. Med. 56, 79–93.

Smith, L.L. and Rose, M.S. (1977) in Biochemical Mechanisms of Paraquat Toxicity (Autor, A.P., ed.), pp. 187–199, Academic Press, New York.

Sobonya, R.E., Logvinoff, M.M., Taussig, L.M. and Theriault, A. (1983) Ped. Res. 16, 969–972.

Sorokin, S., Padykula, H.A. and Herman, E. (1959) Dev. Biol. 1, 125–150.

Stephens, R.J., Sloan, M.F., Groth, D.G., Negi, D.S. and Lunman, K. D. (1978) Am. J. Pathol. 93, 183–199.

Stephens, R.J., Tallent, C., Hart, C. and Negi, D.S. (1982) Exp. Mol. Pathol. 37, 1–14.

Taeusch, H.W. (1975) J. Ped. 87, 617–623.

Taeusch, H.W., Jr. and Avery, M.E. (1977) in Development of the Lung (Hodson, W.A., ed.), pp. 399–418, Marcel Dekker, New York.

Thurlbeck, W.M. (1975) Am. Rev. Respir. Dis. 111, 803–844.

Thurlbeck, W.M. (1979) J. Ped. 85, 842–843.

Tierney, D.F., Ayers, L. and Kasuyama, R.S. (1977) Am. Rev. Respir. Dis. 115, 59–65.

Tooley, W.H. (1979) J. Ped. 851–855.

Tyrala, E.E., Manser, J.I. and Tran, N. (1982) Ped. Res. 16, 180A (Abstract).

Ward, J. and Roberts, R.J. (1984) Ped. Res. 18, 329–334.

Warshaw, J.B., Terry, M.L. and Ranis, M.B. (1980) Ped. Res. 14, 296–299.

Williams, M.C. (1977) Fed. Proc. 36, 2653–2659.

Witting, L.A. (1980) in Free Radicals in Biology (Pryor, W.A., ed.), Vol. IV, pp. 295–319, Academic Press, New York.

Wolfe, W.C. and Sabiston, D.C., Jr. (1973) Surg. Gynec. Obstet. 137, 763–768.

Yam, J. and Roberts, R.J. (1979) Toxicol. Appl. Pharmacol. 47, 367–373.

Yam, J., Frank, L. and Roberts, R.J. (1978) Ped. Res. 12, 115–119.

Yeager, H., Jr. and Hicks, P.S. (1972) Proc. Soc. Exp. Biol. Med. 141, 1–3.

S. Kacew and M.J. Reasor (eds), *Toxicology and the Newborn*
© 1984 Elsevier Science Publishers B.V.

Chapter 8

Developmental Toxicology of Methylmercury

LOUIS W. CHANG

Departments of Pathology and Pharmacology/Toxicology, University of Arkansas for Medical Sciences, Little Rock, AR 72205, U.S.A.

CONTENTS

I. INTRODUCTION

Since the outbreak of methylmercury poisoning in Minamata Bay, Japan during the early 1950s, methylmercury has been recognized as a hazardous environmental pollutant, and organomercury intoxication has been referred to as Minamata disease (Kurland et al., 1960; Takeuchi, 1968). Besides the recent massive outbreak of methylmercury poisoning in Iraq (Amin-Zaki et al., 1974a; Bakir et al., 1973), an alarmingly high mercury content was also found in the waters of some parts of Canada and the United States (Takeuchi et al., 1978), which suggest strongly that methylmercury poisoning is still a realistic and serious problem affecting our environment and health.

The toxic effects of methylmercury on adult organisms (human as well as animals) have been investigated extensively, and were presented in several excellent reviews (Takeuchi, 1968; Chang, 1977, 1979, 1980, 1982) demonstrating toxic damage to various organ systems of the exposed animals. Other studies have indicated that the fetus accumulates more mercury than the maternal tissues, and thus presents a much higher toxic risk than the mother (Suzuki et al., 1967; Yang et al., 1972; Null et al., 1973; Garcia et al., 1974; Reynolds and Pitkin, 1975; King et al., 1976; Fujita and Takabatake, 1977). Indeed, an alarming finding of the Minamata Bay episode was the high vulnerability of the fetus toward methylmercury toxicity. The congenitally affected children displayed a progressive neurologic disturbance resembling cerebral palsy, ataxia and mental retardation. Of the first 120 patients with confirmed methylmercury poisoning in Minamata, 19 were infants showing symptoms of 'fetal Minamata disease'. By 1976, 40 cases of fetal Minamata disease had been positively identified by attending physicians in Japan (Harada, 1976).

Despite the extensive investigations and increased conceptual development on the understanding of pathogenetic mechanisms of methylmercury poisoning in adult systems (Chang, 1979), comprehensive summaries and concepts on the developmental toxicity of methylmercury are still relatively few. Earlier reviews on this subject have been made by this author (Reuhl and Chang, 1979; Chang et al., 1980). Despite that most of the information still remains unchanged, it is this author's hope that the present review will provide appropriate modifications and updating of those previously published.

II. HUMAN STUDIES

1. *Clinical observations*

Studies of patients prenatally exposed to methylmercury confirmed that the developing human nervous system is highly vulnerable to the deleterious effects of this toxicant (Takeuchi, 1968, 1977; Takeuchi et al., 1978; Matsumoto et al., 1964; Harada, 1968, 1976). The signs and symptoms resulting from 'fetal Minamata disease' have been well documented (Takeuchi, 1968; Snyder, 1971; Amin-Zaki et al.,

TABLE 1

PREVALENCE OF SYMPTOMS IN 22 CASES OF PRENATAL METHYLMERCURY INTOXICATION IN MINAMATA

Symptoms	Prevalence (%)
Mental disturbance	100
Ataxia	100
Impairment of gait	100
Disturbance in speech	100
Disturbance in chewing and swallowing	100
Brisk and increased tendon reflex	82
Pathologic reflexes	54
Involuntary movement	73
Salivation	77
Forced laughing	27

Visual fields and hearing of the victims were not examined. Data are from Harada (1968).

1974a; Harada, 1968, 1976, 1977). In the Japanese cases, the major neurological signs included mental disturbance, mental retardation, impairment of gait, speech and visual ability. Both spastic and flaccid paralysis and delayed developmental mileposts, such as grasping, crawling and standing, were frequently observed. The major symptomology of these patients are summarized in Table I. The expression of fetal injury varied widely between individuals, ranging from barely detectable mental and/or physical deficits to complete physical incapacitation and profound mental retardation (Harada, 1968, 1976). The type and severity of the nervous system injury was variable. This was probably influenced by the duration and intensity of exposure as well as the gestational stage during which the exposure occurred (Takeuchi, 1977).

The first signs of neurologic injury in the Minamata cases began to appear in infants weeks to months after birth (Harada, 1976, 1977). Lethargy, delayed movement, failure to follow visual stimuli, uncoordinated sucking or swallowing, and convulsions were observed. Persisting or prolonged primitive reflexes, and marked impairment of coordination were consistent findings thoughout infancy or childhood. Although blindness was present in five of 15 patients in the Iraqi episode (Amin-Zaki et al., 1976) and in the single case reported by Snyder (1971), blindness was not observed among the 40 congenital Minamata cases when initially studied, but constriction of visual fields was noted when the patients were tested in later years (Harada, 1976). This discrepancy may be the result of much more acute exposure conditions in the Iraqi incident.

Motor defects, chiefly ataxia and mental disturbances, became more severe as the infants matured. 100% of the Japanese fetal Minamata disease patients developed mental or neurological changes (Harada, 1976). In the most severely affected cases, the patients became profoundly retarded.

2. *Placental and mammary transfer*

Methylmercury crosses the placental barrier readily and reaches the developing fetus. Levels of methylmercury in the fetal system may eventually exceed those in the mother. Blood analysis from maternal-infant pairs exposed to methylmercury revealed as much as 28% greater concentration of methylmercury in the infant's blood as compared to that of the mother (Tejning, 1968). Elevated ratios of umbilical cord blood-mercury versus maternal blood-mercury levels were also observed in normal obstetrical patients (Fujita and Takabatake, 1977; Suzuki et al., 1971; Pitkin et al., 1976). The mechanisms accounting for the high level of methylmercury accumulation in the fetal blood are not clear. Blood analysis failed to detect any major differences in mercury binding or release between adult or fetal erythrocytes (White and Rothstein, 1973).

The elevated infant-maternal blood-mercury ratio was found to be maintained for a considerable time after birth (Amin-Zaki et al., 1974a,b). Maternal nursing was believed to contribute to maintaining high blood-mercury levels in the infant (Pitkin et al., 1976; Fujita and Takabatake, 1977). The half-time of clearance in blood of human nonlactating females was found to be approximately 75 days, and only 42 days in lactating females (Greenwood et al., 1978). This finding was also observed in mice.

The exact mechanism responsible for the increased blood clearance of mercury in lactating females is still not clear. Since loss of methylmercury via milk accounts for only 3% of the reduction in body burden, this loss of mercury in milk cannot account for the significant change in blood-mercury half-life. It is possible that increased food intake by lactating females could enhance biliary excretion and the altered hormonal status of the lactating female may also influence the rate of methylmercury removal from the blood.

3. *Neuropathology*

The main body of literature of human fetal methylmercury poisoning was based on the autopsy examinations in the Minamata Bay area (Matsumoto et al., 1964), and two cases from Iraq (Choi et al., 1978). Peripheral nerve examination of biopsy material was reported later (Takeuchi et al., 1978).

(a) Japanese cases

The brains appeared to be symmetrically atrophic, with brain weights one-half to one-third of the age-matched controls. Coronal sections of the brains revealed reduction in the size of the corpus callosum and generalized thinning of the cortex. Cerebral white matter appeared poorly developed, and the basal ganglia were small.

Microscopical examination revealed widespread neuronal involvement throughout the brain. This was in marked contrast to the infantile and adult forms of methylmercury poisoning, which showed considerable anatomic selectivity (Fig. 1). Disruption of the cerebral and cerebellum cytoarchitecture was striking. Resting

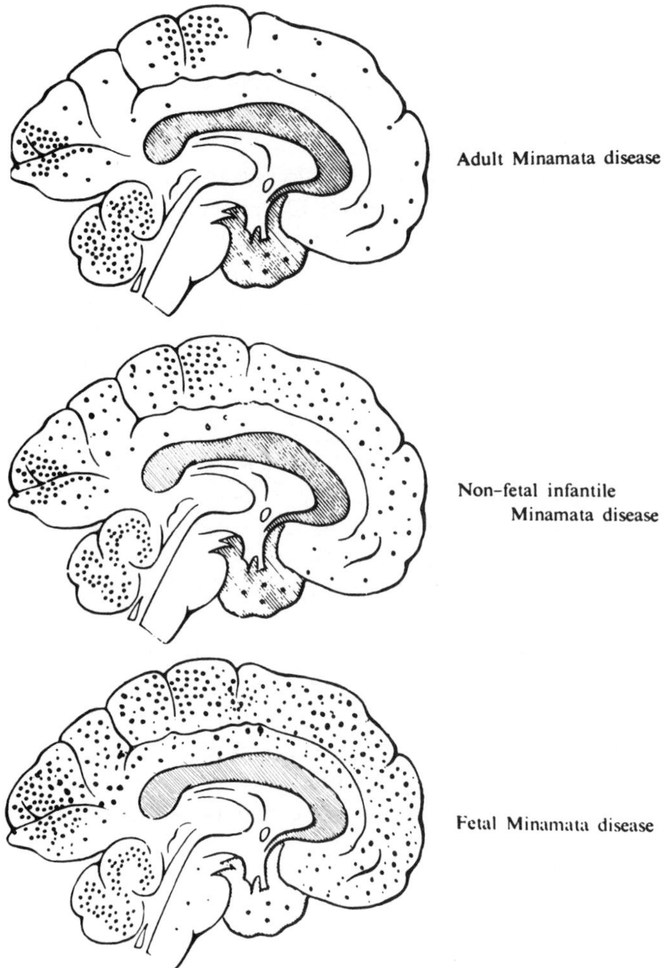

Figure 1. Diagramatic representation of lesion distribution in adult, infantile and fetal Minamata disease. (After Takeuchi, 1968.)

matrix cells lined the periventricular region, and atypical neurons, described as hypoplastic and dysplastic, were identified in the cortex. Extensive neuronal loss, involving primarily the granule and small pyramidal cells, occurred throughout the cerebrum. Although no active demyelination was noted, the white matter was poorly myelinated. Such microscopic findings were characteristic for prenatal methylmercury poisoning and could be used to differentiate the fetal from the infantile form of the disease.

As a rule, the cerebellum was affected significantly. The cerebellar hemispheres and vermis were atrophic, with a thinning of both the granular and molecular layers

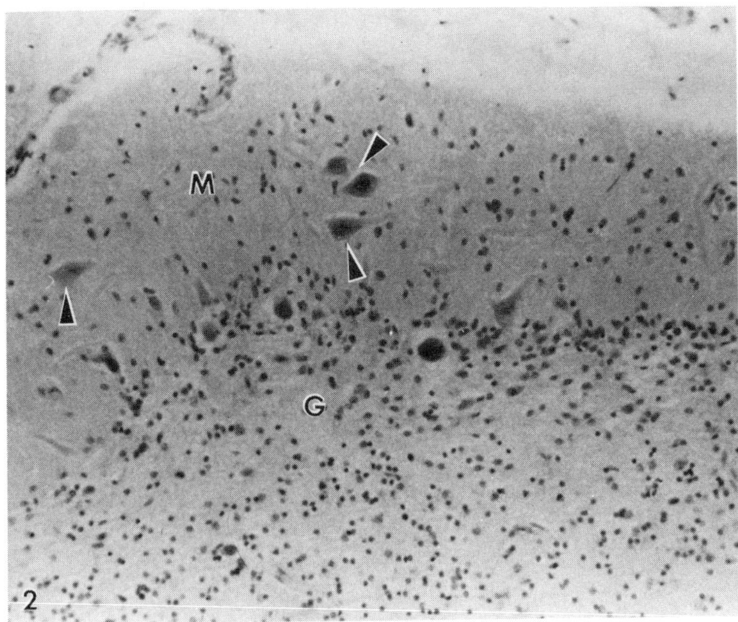

Figure 2. Cerebellum, fetal Minamata patient. Extensive loss of neurons in the granule cell layer (G) with atopic Purkinje cells (arrows) in the molecular layer (M). H and E. ×450.

(Fig. 2). Granule cell loss was most pronounced in the culmen and declive of monticulus, but was not only limited to the depth of the sulci, as in adult methylmercury poisoning. Atopic and disoriented Purkinje cells demonstrated dendritic swelling, and degeneration could also be demonstrated (Fig. 2), indicating migratory and maturation disturbance in these neurons. Poor development of the Purkinje dendritic processes was evident (Fig. 3). Basket cells and parallel fiber degeneration were also found. As in the cerebrum, the cerebellar white matter was poorly developed, without active demyelination. Except for the poor myelination of pyramidal and corticospinal tracts, no remarkable pathology was found in the spinal cord.

Little was known about the influence of congenital methylmercury exposure on the peripheral nervous system. Recently, Takeuchi et al. (1978) reported light and electron microscopic findings in sural nerve biopsy material taken from three patients with documented congenital methylmercury poisoning. Major findings consisted of poorly developed myelinated fibers and incomplete myelination of some axons.

(b) Iraqi cases

The brains of both infants were described as smaller than normal. Abnormal gyral patterns were seen in the frontal, parietal, temporal and occipital lobes. Cut sections revealed a heterotopic gray in the white matter of the brain. White matter of both cerebrum and cerebellum appeared to be reduced, but corpus callosum and basal ganglia were grossly normal.

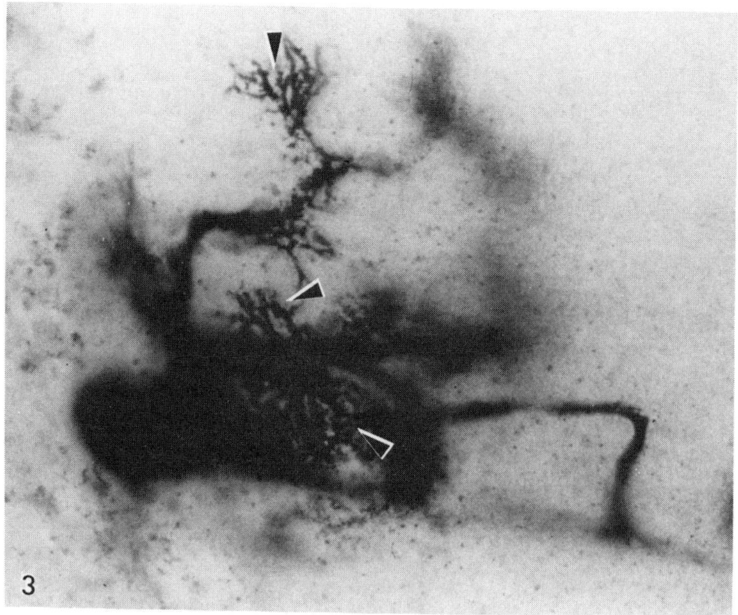

Figure 3. Cerebellum, fetal Minamata patient. Poorly developed, shrunken dendritic aberration (arrows) was observed. Golgi stain. × 1,000.

Miscroscopically, these brains were characterized by a marked disruption of the cytoarchitecture. Many nests of heterotopic neurons were seen in the white matter of the cerebrum and cerebellum. The normal pattern of the cerebral cortex was disrupted by irregular aggregates or vertical columns of neurons. In some areas the cortical layers were described as having an 'undulating' pattern, and in these areas the overlying gyri were poorly developed. Large numbers of plump, gemistocytic astrocytes were noted in the white matter of both cerebrum and cerebellum; however, no reactive proliferation of microglia was observed. The cerebellum also contained multiple heterotopic neurons in the white matter. These neurons appeared to be both granule and Purkinje cells. Unlike the Japanese cases, there was no neuronal necrosis in either cerebellum or cerebrum.

Both Japanese and Iraqi cases are characterized by a reduction of brain size and major disturbances in the cellular architecture. The multiple nests of heterotopic neurons indicate that interference with normal neuronal migration underlies methylmercury's effect on the developing nervous system. These changes in cytoarchitecture appear to be permanent and would disrupt the normal synaptic circuitry in the brain. Such defective synaptic communication could underlie some of the behavioral or electrophysiological defects reported in these victims.

III. ANIMAL STUDIES

Most of the experimental work can be divided into four general areas: placental and mammary transfer of methylmercury, biochemistry, teratology/pathology, and behavioral toxicology.

1. Placental and mammary transfer

The mammalian placenta provides the developing fetus with a stable physical environment by regulating transport of materials from the mother to the fetus. Under normal situations, the placenta is quite efficient in preventing undesirable substances from entering the fetal bloodstream while permitting the passage of essential nutrients and trace metals. Methylmercury, however, is capable of passing through the 'placental barrier' readily. Pharmacokinetic and tissue distribution studies have documented transplacental tissue passage of methylmercury in mice (Suzuki et al., 1967; Childs, 1973; Olson and Massaro, 1977a), rats (Yang et al., 1972; Casterline and Williams, 1972; Null et al., 1973; Mansour et al., 1973, 1974; Yamaguchi and Nunotani, 1974; Garcia et al., 1974; King et al., 1976), hamsters (Gale and Hanlow, 1976), guinea pigs (Kelman and Sasser, 1977) and rhesus monkeys (Reynolds and Pitkin, 1975). Inorganic and aryl mercurials may also cross the placenta, but do so to a much smaller extent (Mansour et al., 1973, 1974; Garrett et al., 1972; Suzuki et al., 1967).

The amount of methylmercury which accumulates in the fetus appeared to be greatly influenced by the administered dose, the period of gestation at which it was given, and the time interval between the dose administration and sample analysis. Following a single administration of methylmercury, the fetal mercury level took several days before reaching a peak (Yang et al., 1972). Elimination of methylmercury from the fetus occurred slowly, resulting in a heavier tissue concentration in the fetus than in the maternal animal.

As in the adult form of Minamata disease, the kidney, liver, and brain were preferential sites of deposition for methylmercury. Methylmercury could be detected in the fetal brain as early as 10 minutes following intravenous administration (Reynolds and Pitkin, 1975). Continuing deposition from blood-bound mercury and redistribution of methylmercury from other organs both contributed to the continued increase in brain mercury 1 day later. Levels of mercury in the fetus as well as the rate of accumulation have been related to the amount of mercury given.

Null and co-workers (1973) compared the levels of methylmercury in the brains of the fetuses and their mothers as well as in the non-pregnant female rats exposed to equal levels of mercury. The concentration of mercury in the fetal brain was found to be at least twice that of their mothers. Evidence also indicated that the rate of mercury transfer was much greater in the direction from the mother toward the fetus than in the reverse direction (Reynolds and Pitkin, 1975), allowing the 'trapping' of mercury in the fetal tissue.

Transfer of methylmercury from the lactating mother to her offspring was documented both in humans and in experimental animals (Amin-Zaki et al., 1974b; Greenwood et al., 1978; Pitkin et al., 1976; Fujita and Takabatake, 1977; Garcia et al., 1974; Yang et al., 1973; Mansour et al., 1973). Neurological lesions characteristic of methylmercury poisoning were also induced successfully in animals exposed to mercury via mother's milk only (Deshimaru, 1969). Yang et al. (1973) calculated that it would be necessary to feed a lactating female rat approximately 17–25 mg of methylmercury before neurological problems in the pups could be induced. Such calculations were based on the assumption that only about 1% of the dose will pass from the lactating mother to the offspring during a 21-day weaning period. This postulation correlated well with the findings of Deshimaru (1969), who found neurological lesions in neonates which had been nursed by mothers treated with 14–16 mg of methylmercury over a period of 18 days.

2. *Biochemical studies*

Although the biochemical alterations in the nervous system of adult animals following methylmercury intoxication have been investigated by numerous laboratories (Omata et al., 1978; Farris and Smith, 1975; Brubaker et al., 1973; Verity et al., 1977; Cavanagh and Chen, 1971; Yoshino et al., 1966; Chang et al., 1972a, b, 1973), only few investigations have been performed on animals exposed to methylmercury in utero.

By means of enzyme histochemistry, Khera and Nera (1971) observed an inhibition of DPN-diaphorase, succinic dehydrogenase, cytochrome oxidase and ATPase in mice exposed prenatally to methylmercury. These changes were most prominent in early postnatal life. However, only cytochrome oxidase was still suppressed when animals were examined on postnatal day 7. All enzymatic activity returned to normal after day 14, indicating that the depression of the enzyme activity was only transient. The activities of choline acetyltransferase, cholinesterase, and acetylcholine esterase were not altered significantly following in utero administration of methylmercury to either mice or hamsters (Spyker et al., 1972).

Alterations in lipid metabolism following prenatal methylmercury administration have also been reported (Menon et al., 1979). Inhibition of the incorporation of the label from (D, L)-3-hydroxy[3-^{14}C]butyrate into the total extractable brain lipid was observed in brain slices from prenatally treated rats during the period of active myelination. A reduction of incorporation of 3-hydroxybutyrate into cholesterol, free fatty acids, phosphatidylcholine and phosphatidylserine on day 14 was also observed, while incorporation of the label into sphingomyelin was increased greatly at this time. These data indicated inhibition of the steps between the uptake of 3-hydroxybutyrate and its conversion to lipids. It was also thought that there was a further defect either in the conversion of cytidine diphosphatecholine to phosphatidylcholine or in myelination. Abnormal myelin profiles have been observed in peripheral nerves of humans (Takeuchi et al., 1978) and rodent cerebellum (Chang, unpublished data) following in utero methylmercury exposure.

Exposure to methylmercury during early postnatal life would also result in lasting biochemical changes in the brains of developing animals. Taylor and DiStefano (1976) investigated the influence of methylmercury on biogenic amines in neonatal rat pups. A dose of 5 mg/kg methylmercury on days 5, 6 and 7 postpartum resulted in a decrease in serotonin, 5-hydroxyindole acetic acid and norepinephrine in animals on day 8. From day 8 to day 15, however, levels of biogenic amines steadily increased and surpassed control levels. After day 15, brain serotonin (5-hydroxytryptophan) levels remained elevated until the experiment was terminated on day 60. The significance of these findings is not understood fully. It is possible that alterations in biogenic amines may induce behavioral changes in young methylmercury-intoxicated animals, and it is unknown as yet whether in utero exposure to organomercurials will yield similar findings.

Studies utilizing whole fetuses have revealed significant decreases in total fetal protein and DNA content following administration of methylmercury. Olson and Massaro (1977b) reported that injection of 5 mg/kg on day 12 of gestation was followed by a maximal reduction of fetal protein levels 48 hours after mercury administration, while fetal DNA levels were maximally decreased 72 hours post-injection, suggesting that altered protein synthesis could result in a decreased rate of cell growth and an increased cell cycle time by reducing DNA levels. Such a mechanism might explain the retarded growth in mercury-treated animals and may underlie the developmental malformations reported, as well as the delayed limb regeneration seen in mercury-treated amphibians (Chang et al., 1976).

The transport of amino acids across the placenta of mercury-treated animals was examined by Olson and Massaro (1977b). A reduction in placental amino acid treatment and in the levels of alanine, valine, methionine, leucine and isoleucine were found in the fetus 12 hours after methylmercury had been given to the mother on the 12th day of gestation. Such reduction of placental transport and reduced fetal amino acid levels may explain the decreased protein synthesis in the fetus.

Damage to other organ systems may also contribute to the development of neuropathologic lesions. Snell et al. (1977) investigated alterations in carbohydrate metabolism in the offspring of rats treated with a subcutaneous injection of either 4 or 8 mg/kg methylmercury on gestational day 9. Biochemical analysis showed a decrease in plasma glucose and in liver glycogen concentrations and hepatic glucose-6-phosphatase activity. Impaired glycogen mobilization was also observed within the first few hours of life, and was associated with a severe protracted hypoglycemia which may have resulted from a lowered hepatic glucose-6-phosphatase activity in fetal animals, limiting the production of free glucose from glycogen-derived glucose phosphate and/or from defective glycogen mobilization at birth. The extent to which the protracted hypoglycemia at birth contributes to central nervous system (CNS) dysfunction or injury is unclear. However, since the CNS is highly sensitive to alterations in glucose concentrations, it is conceivable that severe hypoglycemia occurring during a highly sensitive period of brain development could contribute to both the observed clinical and behavioral alterations (Snell et al., 1977).

Fetal hepatic mitochondria have been shown to be sensitive to methylmercury exposure. Fowler and Woods (1977) exposed female rats to drinking water containing methylmercury prior to and during pregnancy. Besides a significant reduction of amino acid uptake in the mercury-exposed pups, a decrease in the structural proteins within the mitochondria was also noted. Enzyme studies confirmed that the mitochondrial enzymes, such as monoamine oxidase, cytochrome oxidase and ALA-synthetase, were all reduced in a dose-related fashion. A reduction in the volume density of the mitochondria was also found. In addition, mitochondrial respiratory control was lost in animals exposed to 3 ppm mercury and the state 3 respiration function was suppressed completely in animals treated with 5–10 ppm mercury (Fowler and Woods, 1977). Alterations of mitochondrial enzymes have been observed in brains of adult animals (Yoshino et al., 1966). These findings support the morphological observations of Chang and Hartmann (1972) who, by means of electron microscope histochemical techniques, demonstrated the close association of mercury with the mitochondria in the nervous system.

The effects of fetal exposure to methylmercury on biochemical systems may not appear until later in the animal's life. Robbins et al. (1978) observed a decrease in the hepatic cytochrome *P*-450-dependent systems of methylmercury-treated male rats after 7 months of life; these changes were not observed in the earlier life of the animals. It is interesting to note that while a significant reduction in hepatic cytochrome *P*-450, NADPH-cytochrome *c* reductase, ethylmorphine-*N*-demethylase and benzo(*a*)pyrene hydroxylase was observed in male rats, these enzyme levels remained normal in the female animals. This finding indicated a sex-related difference in toxicity.

3. Methylmercury-induced teratology and developmental pathology

The effects of methylmercury on the developing organism have been studied with various animal models. At high doses, the compound is embryo-lethal, but at lower doses various teratology (malformation) and pathological lesions could be induced in the developing organism.

Early experiments by Chang and co-workers demonstrated a definite developmental change in tadpoles which had been exposed to various concentrations of methylmercury (Chang et al., 1974). It was found that when tadpoles were injected with a minute amount of methylmercury, swelling of the hind limbs and defective metamorphosis occurred (Fig. 4). Total arrest of metamorphosis occurred in tadpoles raised in water containing low concentrations of methylmercury. Teratogenic effects of methylmercury were also observed in chick embryos exposed to the toxicant. Microphthalmia (small eye development) and exencephaly (extrusion of brain matter) were the most frequent malformations observed (Fig. 5). Although these animal models did not have the placental barrier system, as in mammalian systems, nevertheless, data obtained were important and clearly demonstrated the teratogenicity of methylmercury.

The impact of methylmercury on the mammalian system has been studied fairly extensively. It appeared that the sensitivity of both the mother and the fetus to the toxic effect of methylmercury could be influenced by various factors, such as the

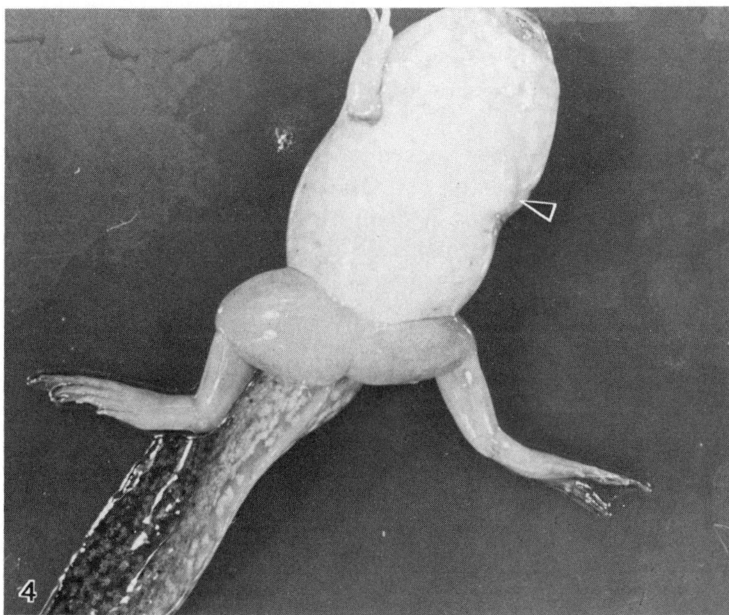

Figure 4. *Rana pipiens* tadpole, injected with 0.025 mg methylmercury. Edematous swelling of the hind limbs and failure of development of one of the forelimbs (arrow) were observed. × 1.2.

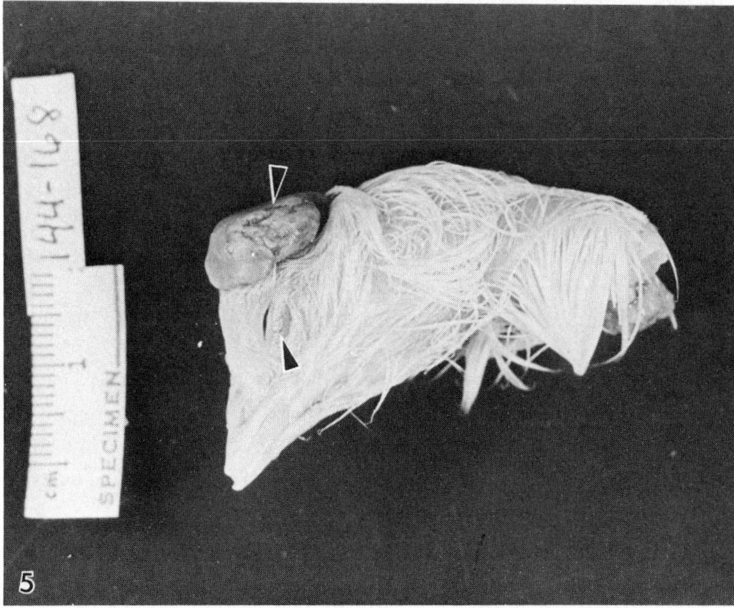

Figure 5. Head of chick embryo exposed to 0.05 mg of methylmercury. Microphthalmia (small eye development; lower arrow) and exencephaly (protrusion of brain matter; upper arrow) were observed. × 1. 5.

species/strain of animals employed (Spyker et al., 1972; Su and Okita, 1976b), duration of exposure during pregnancy (Harris et al., 1972), the dose of mercury administered (Spyker et al., 1972; Harris et al., 1972) and the route of exposure (Lown et al., 1977).

Intrauterine death is a frequent result of congenital organomercurial intoxication. When given during developmentally sensitive periods, particularly during the days of rapid organogenesis, relatively low levels of methylmercury can produce a high fetal mortality rate. Harris et al. (1972), using golden hamsters, reported that a single intraperitoneal injection of 8 mg/kg methylmercury on the 8th gestational day resulted in a 42% incidence of fetal death and a 36% incidence of grossly malformed pups. The same dose administered on day 4 of gestation resulted in only 5% mortality and 8% malformations, while administration on day 10 caused 30% intrauterine death but no gross malformations.

Strains within a species frequently show a marked variation in susceptibility to methylmercury. Spyker and Smithberg (1972) compared the incidence of intrauterine death in two strains of mice (129 Sv/S1 and A/J), and found that a single intraperitoneal administration of 8 mg/kg to pregnant 129 Sv/S1 mice between fetal days 9 and 13 resulted in over 80% of the fetal implants being resorbed. The same dose produced significantly lower lethality (less than 40% of the implants were resorbed) in the A/J strain, with a much higher percentage of the A/J offspring being malformed. Su and Okita (1976b) also found a marked difference in methylmercury sensitivity among C57BL, CD and 129 Sv/S1 strains of mice treated subcutaneously with several doses of methylmercury on day 10 of gestation.

Congenital malformations are another frequent manifestation of methylmercury's impact on developing organisms. The most common malformations produced in experimental animals have been cleft palate (Spyker and Smithberg, 1972; Harris et al., 1972; Olson and Massaro, 1977b; Su and Okita, 1976b), limb defects (Harris et al., 1972) and brain and facial malformations (Spyker and Smithberg, 1972; Gilani, 1975). While the precise mechanism by which methylmercury induces cleft palate is unknown, it has been suggested that the inhibitory effect on protein synthesis might disrupt the regulatory processes controlling closure of the palate (Olson and Massaro, 1977b).

The neuropathological lesions resulting from experimental fetal methylmercury poisoning were reported initially in the Japanese literature (Moriyama, 1967; Tatetsu et al., 1968), and are summarized in a comprehensive review by Murakami (1972). The most severe methylmercury-induced congenital abnormalities are exencephaly and encephalocele (Spyker and Smithberg, 1972; Gilani, 1975). Hydrocephalus had also been reported by several authors (Harris et al., 1972; Murakami, 1972). The type or cause of the hydrocephalus was not described.

Light microscopic studies of the CNS of congenitally treated animals have revealed a variety of pathologic findings. Loss of neurons and cytoarchitectural changes have been reported in the brains of rat pups exposed to 5 mg/kg methylmercury on gestational days 0–12 (Murakami, 1972). Cystic changes, small hemorrhages and destruction in the cortex and white matter were also observed (Tatetsu et al., 1968;

Fuyuta et al., 1978). In the cerebellum, the lesions involved primarily the granule cell layers. Delayed migration of the external granular cell layer was observed in mice following exposure to 1 mg/kg on gestational days 6–17 (Khera and Tabacova, 1973). Alterations of cerebral and cerebellar architecture, with hypoplastic and atrophic neurons and incomplete granular cell layer formation, were found in cats following chronic methylmercury poisoning during gestation (Harada, 1977; Khera, 1973). If the kitten survived, marked ataxis usually appeared. Atopic neurons, dendritic swelling of the Purkinje cells and degeneration of the granule cells were also observed in our laboratory (Reuhl et al., 1981a,b).

Recently, Chang and co-workers reported ultrastructural evidence of cellular damage in the brains of mice, rats and hamster fed low doses of methylmercury during gestation (Chang et al., 1977a,b; Reuhl et al., 1981a,b). In the cerebellum, both Purkinje and granular cell neurons contained abnormal accumulations of lysosomes. Disorientation and shortening of the rough endoplasmic reticulum was seen in Purkinje cells. Occasional nerve cells and their processes contained dilated saccules resembling smooth endoplasmic reticulum, aggregates of tubular structures (Fig. 6), and segmentally incomplete myelination of axons (Fig. 7) was encountered frequently. Large cytosegresomes (Fig. 8), dendritic degeneration (Fig. 9), focal cytoplasmic degradation (Fig. 10) and neuronal necrosis (Fig. 11) were common. Follow-up studies indicate that such toxic changes may persist into adult life. Abnormalities of myelin formation, with accumulation of large myelin ovoids,

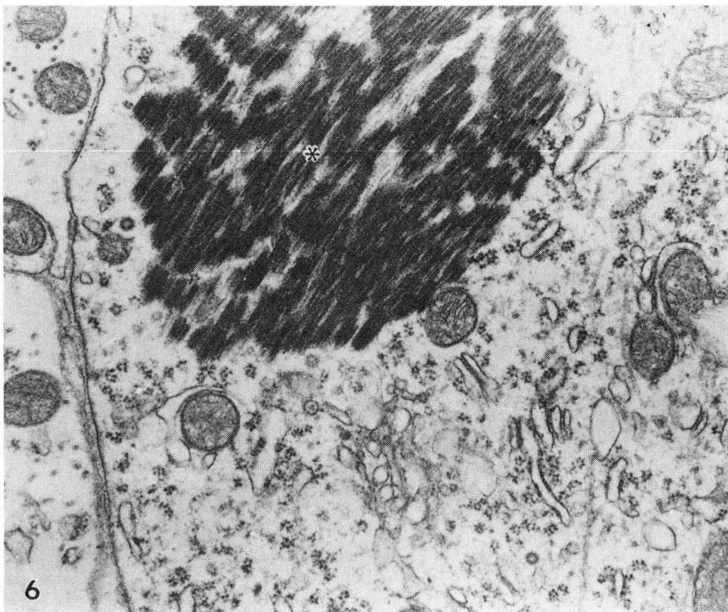

Figure 6. Cerebellum, hamster, prenatally exposed to methylmercury. Accumulation of dense filamentous or tubular structure (*) in a Purkinje neuron. × 50,000.

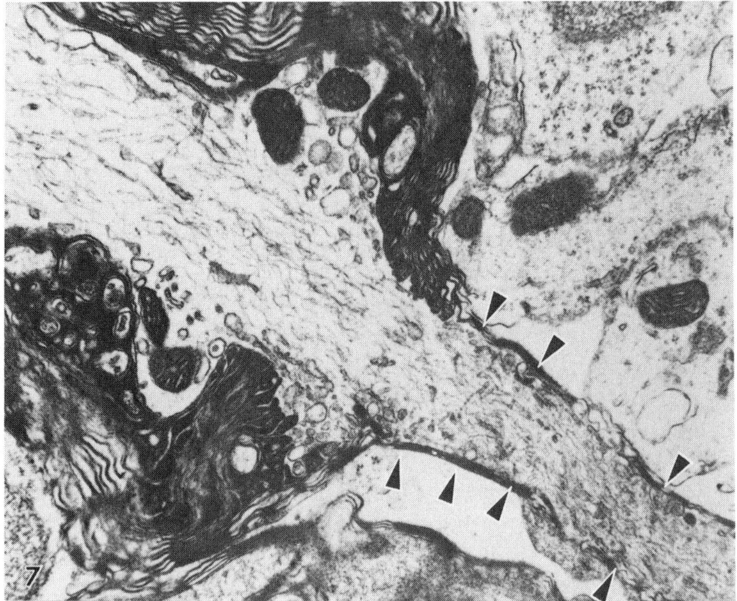

Figure 7. Cerebellum, mouse, prenatally exposed to methylmercury. Segmental thinning of the myelin sheath (arrows) in a nerve fiber is demonstrated. ×25,000. (From Chang et al., 1977b.)

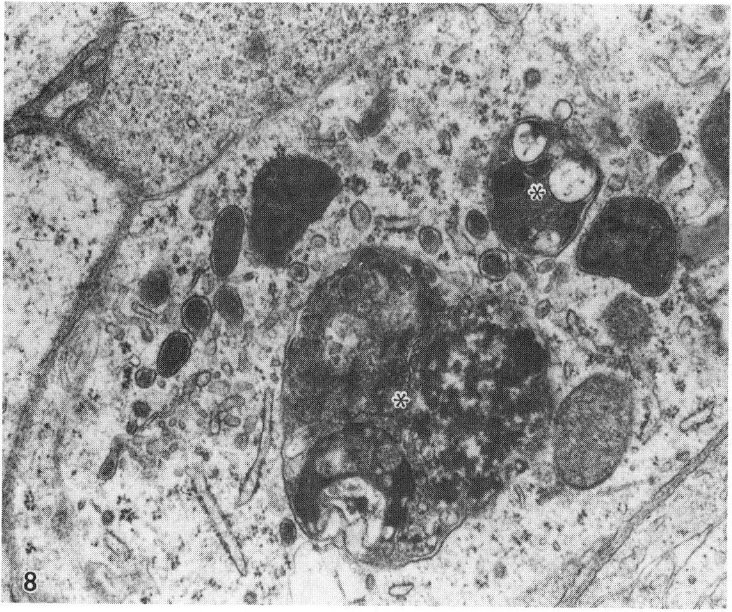

Figure 8. Cerebellum, hamster, prenatally exposed to methylmercury. Accumulation of lysosomes and large cytosegresomes (*) in a cell. ×30,000.

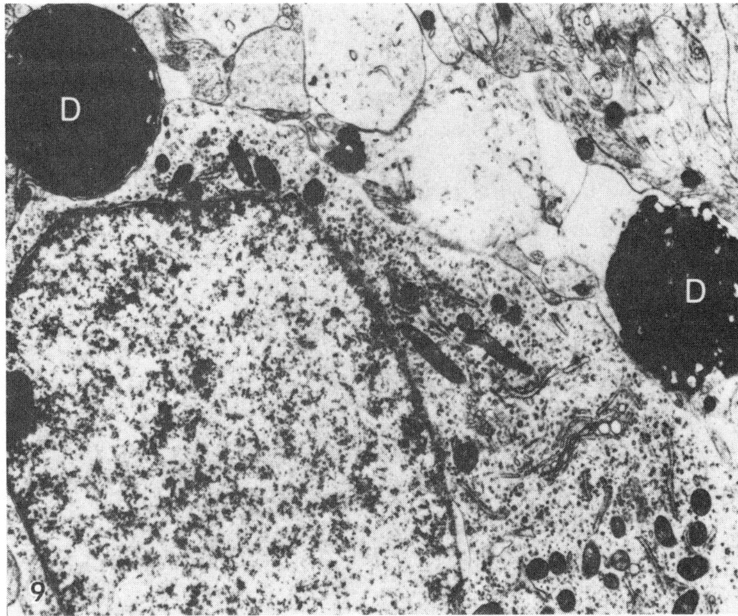

Figure 9. Cerebellum, hamster, prenatally exposed to methylmercury. Degenerating dendrites (D) appeared to be filled with cellular debris. ×25,000. (From Reuhl et al., 1981a.)

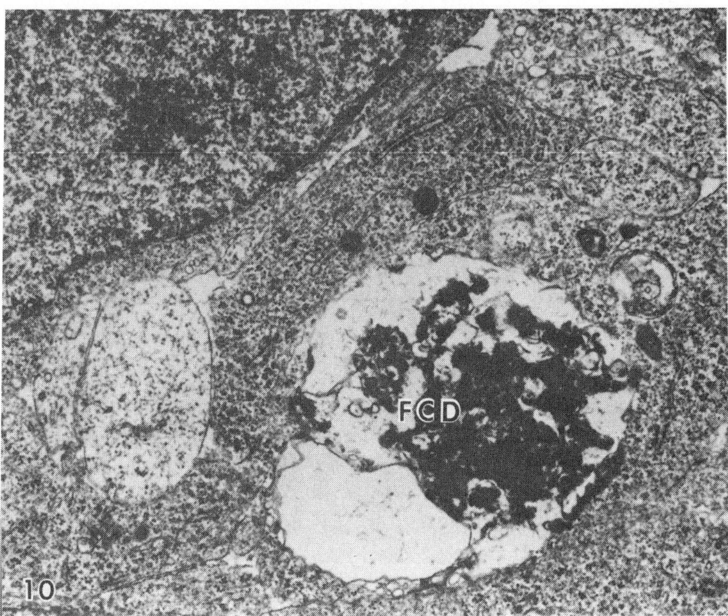

Figure 10. Cerebellum, rat, prenatally exposed to methylmercury. Large area of focal cytoplasmic degradation (FCD) was observed within a nerve cell. ×20,000. (From Chang et al., 1977a.)

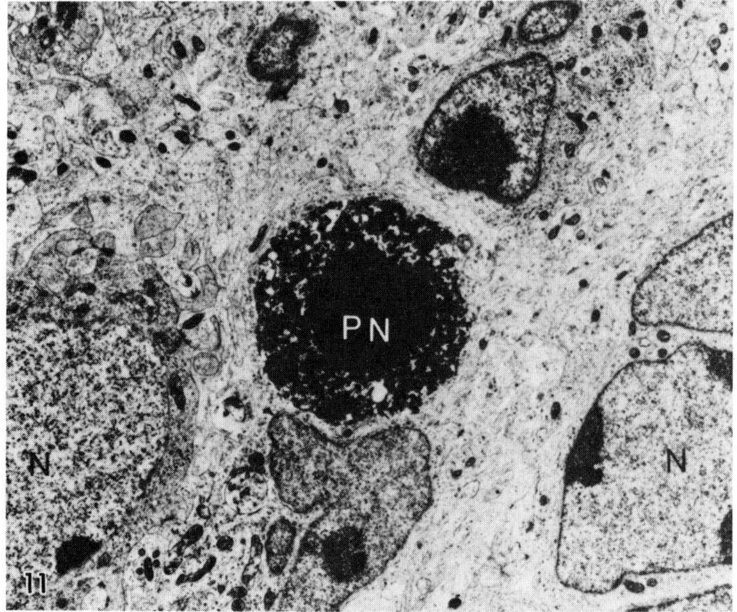

Figure 11. Cerebellum, hamster, prenatally exposed to methylmercury. A pyknotic neuron (PN) is demonstrated. × 15,000. (From Reuhl et al., 1981a.)

degenerating axons (Fig. 12) and abnormal synaptic formation (Figs. 13 and 14), could still be demonstrated in the adult animals.

4. *Behavioral changes*

Behavioral studies of offspring from mercury-treated animals have shown behavioral deviations before any classical neurological symptoms appear (Spyker et al., 1972). Su and Okita (1976a) exposed mice to various amounts of methylmercury prenatally and also revealed abnormalities manifested by prolonged center-square latency, decreased ambulatory and exploratory activity, lower frequency of grooming and urination, and increased backing movements when compared to the controls. The treated offspring were also found to be abnormally sensitive to the induction of convulsions by fluorothyl.

Hughes and Annau (1976) conducted extensive tests on the offspring of mice treated with various doses of methylmercury on day 8 of gestation. Little change was found in motor skills in the animals. However, definite differences from controls were detected in passive avoidance task and in the number of consecutive avoidances in the shuttle box, indicating that the deficit was one of learning rather than of motor impairment. Unlike Spyker et al. (1972) and Su and Okita (1976a), the authors noted no differences in the results of open-field tests. Differences in strain or experimental procedure may account for this discrepancy.

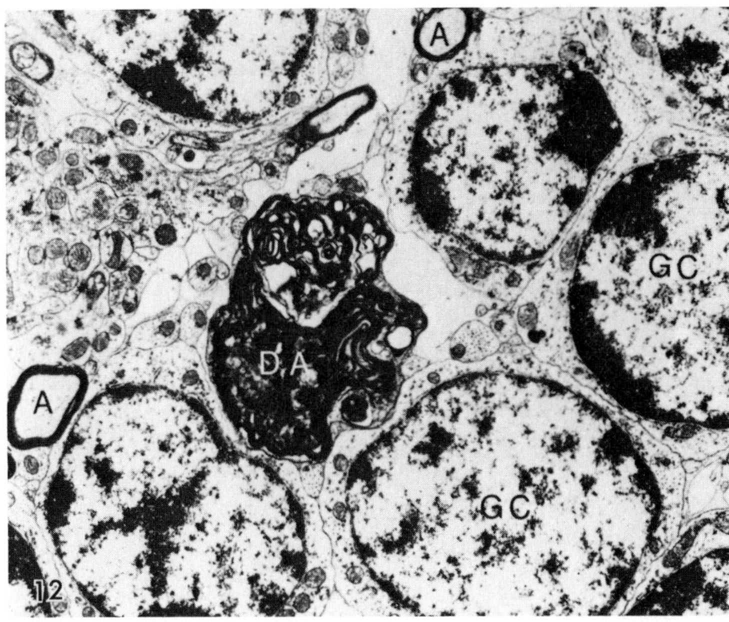

Figure 12. Cerebellum, hamster, prenatally exposed to methylmercury. A degenerated axon (DA) was seen among the granule cells (GC). A, axon. ×15,000. (From Reuhl et al., 1981b.)

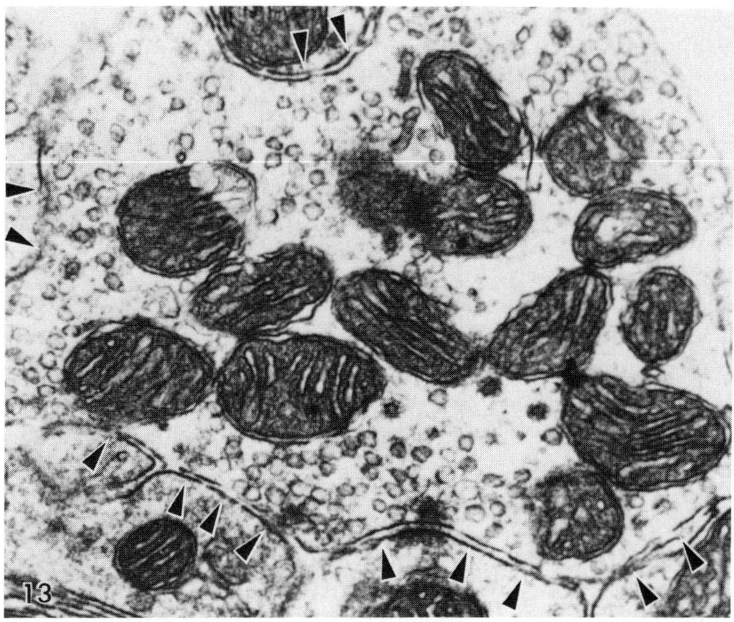

Figure 13. Cerebellum, mouse, prenatally exposed to methylmercury. A large mossy fiber terminal showing reduction or total lack of postsynaptic density (arrows) in the synaptic junctions. ×55,000. (From Chang et al., 1977b.)

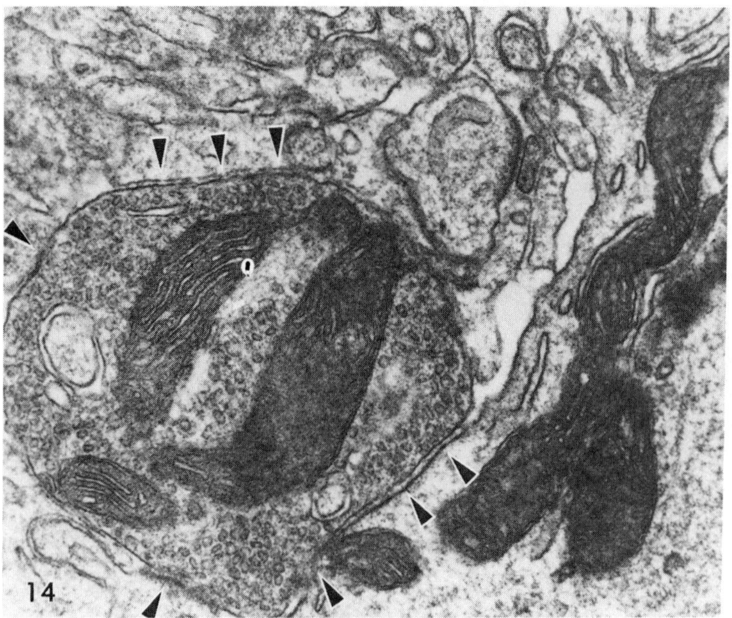

Figure 14. Cerebellum, mouse, prenatally exposed to methylmercury. A large synaptic terminal displaying no postsynaptic density (arrows). ×55,000. (From Chang et al., 1977b).

Musch et al. (1978) used operant conditioning procedures to test rats which had been exposed to methylmercury on various days of gestation. Test results showed that significant differences between experimental and control groups appeared with increasing demand on performance. The reduction of successful performance was dose-related and reflected a decreased learning rate among the treated animals. Using the same experimental technique, Bornhausen et al. (1980) also demonstrated that even at 0.01 mg/kg there were residual effects of prenatal mercury exposure.

Since methylmercury has been reported to be excreted in mother's milk and to cause neurologic and behavioral changes in suckling rat pups (Deshimaru, 1969), it is of some importance to attempt to differentiate the effects of congenital exposure from those of exposure during infancy. Brown et al. (1972) tested water-escape T-maze performance in mice and found that there was a qualitative difference in sensitivity to methylmercury between prenatal and postnatal exposure, and that the fetal brain is more sensitive than the neonatal brain. Similar findings were reported by Zenick et al. (1972).

Recent studies by Eccles and Annau (1982a,b) examined the effect of two doses (5 and 8 mg/kg) of methylmercury chloride administered at two different stages of gestation in rats. Mercury exposure altered the neonatal development of locomotor activity in the rats both as a function of dose and time of administration. 5 mg/kg administered on day 8 of gestation significantly elevated activity on day 4, whereas 8 mg/kg administered on day 8 elevated activity on postnatal days 8 and 15. Mercury administration on day 15 of gestation at both doses resulted in enhanced activity on postnatal days 8 and 15. These behavioral alterations occurred without any signs of maternal or neonatal toxicity.

In the two-way avoidance task the animals were trained to a criterion of ten consecutive avoidances, extinguished and retrained to the original criterion. Methylmercury administered on day 8 of gestation did not alter significantly avoidance training. During retraining, however, the animal exposed to 8 mg/kg required significantly more trials to criterion than controls. When given on day 15 of gestation, both doses of mercury prolonged training and retraining severely.

These studies again point to the importance of developmental stage in the study of the prenatal administration of neurotoxic agents. The variability in the results obtained by different laboratories may be due, at least in part, to mercury affecting different developing cell populations, and thereby altering behavior differentially.

IV. CONCLUSIVE REMARKS

Methylmercury, besides being a neurotoxicant to the adult animal, is also a potent embryotoxicant, inducing pathological and functional changes in the developing nervous system. Since the fetal tissues, especially the brain, are known to concentrate mercury to higher levels than the mother, the fetus is at much greater risk than the mother, even when the mother is exposed to a low level of mercury.

Methylmercury is known to cross the placenta very readily, exerting both direct toxic insults and metabolic disturbances to the fetus. These actions subsequently precipitate a cascade of pathological events leading to both morphological and behavioral changes in the tissues and animals. A proposed cascade of pathological consequences induced by methylmercury in the developing nervous system is constructed and presented in Diagram 1. It must be borne in mind that this proposed scheme of events merely represents a 'scientific logic' on the impact of methylmercury on the fetal organism. Needless to say, it may be overly simplified, but it is the hope of this author that it will help to put the various findings (biochemical, morphological, and behavioral) to date in their proper perspectives and in a meaningful correlated fashion. Future work in this area is still very much needed and will certainly provide new information to our presently proposed 'mechanism'.

It must also be emphasized that the nervous system is not the only system vulnerable to methylmercury toxicity. Effects of methylmercury on the hepatic, renal and immune systems, in newborns as well as in adult animals, have been reported. These findings are still very limited and are summarized in recent reviews (Chang, 1979; Chang and Reuhl, 1983); therefore, they will not be included in the present presentation.

V. ACKNOWLEDGMENTS

The author wishes to express his gratitude towards Mrs. Laurie McDonald for her excellent effort in helping to complete this manuscript. Portions of the materials and

DIAGRAM 1

SCHEMATIC POSTULATION OF EFFECTS OF METHYLMERCURY ON THE DEVELOPING NERVOUS SYSTEM

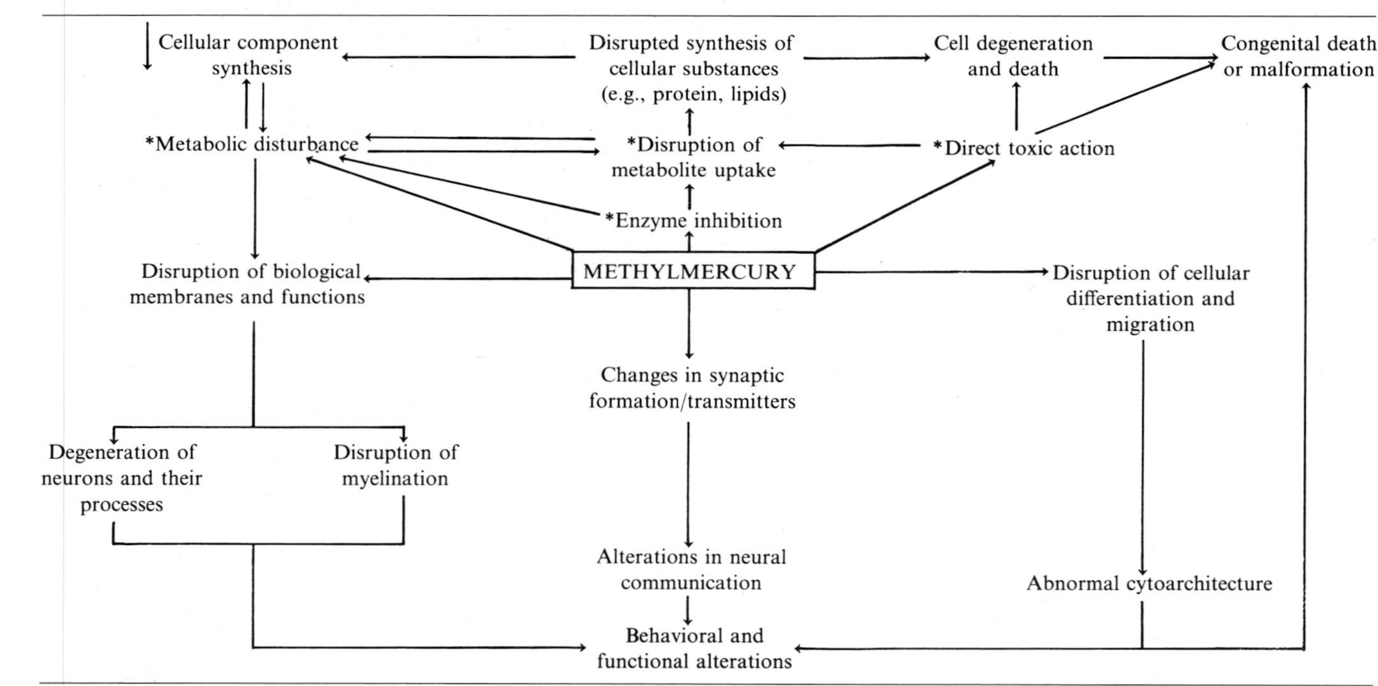

*Occur at placental and/or fetal level.

illustrations have been published by the same author, by Academic Press (Environmental Research) and by Elsevier Biomedical Press. Their courtesy in giving permission to reuse some of these materials is deeply appreciated.

VI. REFERENCES

Amin-Zaki, L., Elhassani, S., Majeed, M.A., Clarkson, T. W., Doherty, R.A. and Greenwood, M.R. (1974a) Pediatrics 54, 587–595.

Amin-Zaki, L., Elhassani, S., Majeed, M.A., Clarkson, T.W., Doherty, R.A. and Greenwood, M.R. (1974b) J. Ped. 85, 81–84.

Amin-Zaki, L., Elhassani, S., Majeed, M.A., Clarkson, T.W., Doherty, R.A., Greenwood, M.R. and Giovanoli-Jakubczak, T. (1976) Am. J. Dis. Child. 130, 1070–1076.

Bakir, F., Damluji, S.F., Amin-Zaki, L., Murtadha, M., Khalidi, A., Al-Rawi, N.Y., Tikriti, S., Dhahir, H.I., Clarkson, T.W., Smith, J. C. and Doherty, R.A. (1973) Science 181, 230–241.

Bornhausen, M., Musch, H.R. and Greim, H. (1980) Toxicol. Appl. Pharmacol. 56, 305–310.

Brown, R.V., Zenick, H., Cox, V. Jr. and Fahim, M.S. (1972) Fed. Proc. 31, 1970.

Brubaker, P.E., Klein, R., Herman, S.P., Lucier, G.W., Alexander, L. T. and Long, M.D. (1973) Exp. Mol. Pathol. 18, 253–280.

Casterline, J.L. Jr. and Williams, C.H. (1972) Bull. Environ. Contam. Toxicol. 7, 292–295.

Cavanagh, J.B. and Chen, F.C.K. (1971) Acta Neuropathol. 19, 216–224.

Chang, L.W. (1977) Environ. Res. 14, 329–379.

Chang, L.W. (1979) in Biogeochemistry of Mercury (Nriagu, J.O., ed.), pp. 518–580, Elsevier Science Publishers, New York.

Chang, L.W. (1980) in Experimental and Clinical Neurotoxicology (Spencer, P.S. and Schaumberg, H.H., eds.), pp. 508–526, Williams and Wilkins, Baltimore.

Chang, L.W. (1982) in Mechanisms of Neurotoxic Substances (K.N. Prasad and A. Vernadakis, eds.), pp. 51–66, Raven Press, New York.

Chang, L.W. and Hartmann, H.A. (1972) Exp. Neurol. 35, 122–137.

Chang, L.W. and Reuhl, K.R. (1983) in Trace Elements and Health (J. Rose, ed.), Ch. 6, pp. 132–149, Butterworth, London.

Chang, L.W., Desnoyers, P.A. and Hartmann, H.A. (1972a) J. Neuropathol. Exp. Neurol. 31, 489–501.

Chang, L.W., Martin, A.H. and Hartmann, H.A. (1972b) Exp. Neurol. 37, 62–67.

Chang, L.W., Desnoyers, P.A. and Hartmann, H.A. (1973) Acta Neuropath. 23, 77–83.

Chang, L.W., Reuhl, K.R. and Dudley, A.W. Jr. (1974) Environ. Res. 8, 82–91.

Chang, L.W., Mak, L.L. and Martin, A.H. (1976) Environ. Res. 11, 305–309.

Chang, L.W., Reuhl, K.R. and Spyker, J.M. (1977a) Environ. Res. 13, 171–185.

Chang, L.W., Reuhl, K.R. and Lee, G.W. (1977b) Environ. Res. 14, 414–423

Chang, L.W., Pounds, J.G., Reuhl, K.R. and Wade, P.R. (1980) in Advances in Pharmacology and Chemotheraphy (Farattini, S., Goldin, A., Hawking, F., Kopin, I.J. and Schnitzer, R.J., eds.), Vol. 17, pp. 195–231, Academic Press, New York.

Childs, E.A. (1973) Arch. Environ. Hlth. 27, 50–52.

Choi, B.H., Lapham, L.W., Amin-Zaki, L. and Saleem, T. (1978) J. Neuropath. Exp. Neurol. 37, 719–733.

Deshimaru, M. (1969) Seishin Shinkeigaku Zasshi 71, 506.

Eccles, C.U. and Annau, Z. (1982a) Neurobehav. Toxicol. Teratol. 4, 371–376.

Eccles, C.U. and Annau, Z. (1982b) Neurobehav. Toxicol. Teratol. 4, 377–382.

Farris, F.F. and Smith, J.C. (1975) Bull. Environ. Contam. Toxicol. 13, 451–455.

Fowler, B.A. and Woods, J.S. (1977) Lab. Invest. 36, 122–130.

Fujita, M. and Takabatake, E. (1977) Bull. Environ. Contam. Toxicol. 18, 205–209.

Fuyuta, M., Fujimoto, T. and Hirata, S. (1978) Teratology 18, 353–366.

Gale, T.F. and Hanlow, D.P. (1976) Environ. Res. 12, 26–31.

Garcia, J.D., Yang, M.G., Wang, H.C. and Belo, P.S. (1974) Proc. Soc. Exp. Biol. Med. 147, 224–231.
Garrett, N.E., Garrett, R.J. and Archdeacon, J.W. (1972) Toxicol. Appl. Pharmacol. 22, 649–654.
Gilani, S.H. (1975) Environ. Res. 9, 128–134.
Greenwood, M.R., Clarkson, T.W., Doherty, R.A., Gates, A.H., Amin-Zaki, L., Elhassani, S. and Majeed, M.A. (1978) Environ. Res. 16, 48–54.
Harada, Y. (1968) in Minamata Disease (Organic Mercury Poisoning) (Kutsuna, M., ed.), pp. 92–121, Study group of Minamata disease, Kumamoto University, Japan.
Harada, Y. (1976) Bull. Inst. Constitutional Med., Kumamoto Univ. Suppl. 25, 1–60.
Harada, Y. (1977) in Minamata Disease–Methylmercury Poisoning in Minamata and Niigata, Japan (Tsubaki, T. and Irukayama, K., eds.), Elsevier Scientific Publ. Co., New York.
Harris, S.B., Wilson, J.G. and Printz, R.H. (1972) Teratology 6, 139–142.
Hughes, J.A. and Annau, Z. (1976) Pharmacol. Biochem. Behav. 4, 385–391.
Kelman, B.J. and Sasser, L.B. (1977) Toxicol. Appl. Pharmacol. 39, 119–127.
Khera, K.S. (1973) Teratology 8, 293–304.
Khera, K.S. and Nera, E.A. (1971) Teratology 14, 233.
Khera, K.S. and Tabacova, S.A. (1973) Food Cosmet. Toxicol. 11, 245–254.
King, R.B., Robkin, M.A. and Shephard, T.H. (1976) Teratology 13, 275–280.
Kurland, L.T., Faro, S.N. and Siedler, H. (1960) World Neurol. 1, 370–395.
Lown, B.A., Morganti, J.B., Stineman, C.H. and Massaro, E.J. (1977) Gen. Pharm. 8, 97–101.
Mansour, M.M., Dyer, N.C., Hoffman, L.H., Schulert, A.R. and Brill, A.B. (1973) Environ. Res. 6, 479–484.
Mansour, M.M., Dyer, N.C., Hoffman, L.H., Davies, J. and Brill, A.B. (1974) Am. J. Obstet. Gynecol. 119, 557–562.
Matsumoto, H., Koya, G. and Takeuchi, T. (1964) J. Neuropath. Exp. Neurol. 24, 563–574.
Menon, N., Lopez, R.R. and Kark, R.A.P. (1978) Society for Neuroscience. Abstracts of 8th Annual Meetings. A. 1020, November.
Moriyama, H. (1967) J. Kumamoto Med. Soc. 41, 506.
Murakami, U. (1972) Adv. Exp. Med. Biol. 27, 301–336.
Musch, H.R., Bornhausen, M., Kriegel, H. and Griem, H. (1978) Arch. Toxicol. 40, 103–108.
Null, D.H., Gartside, P.S. and Wei, E. (1973) Life Sci. 12, 65–72.
Olson, F.C. and Massaro, E.J. (1977a) Toxicol. Appl. Pharmacol. 39, 263–273.
Olson, F.C. and Massaro, E.J. (1977b) Teratology 16, 187–194.
Omata, S., Sakimura, K., Tsubaki, H. and Sugano, H. (1978) Toxicol. Appl. Pharmacol. 44, 367–378.
Pitkin, R.M., Bahns, J.A., Filer, L.J. Jr. and Reynolds, W.A. (1976) Proc. Soc. Exp. Biol. Med. 151, 565–567.
Reuhl, K.R. and Chang, L.W. (1979) Neurotoxicology 1, 21–55.
Reuhl, K.R., Chang, L.W. and Townsend, J.W. (1981a) Environ. Res. 26, 281–306.
Reuhl, K.R., Chang, L.W. and Townsend, J.W. (1981b) Environ. Res. 26, 307–327.
Reynolds, W.A. and Pitkin, R.M. (1975) Proc. Soc. Exp. Biol. Med. 148, 523–526.
Robbins, M.S., Hughes, J.A., Sparber, S.B. and Mannering, G.J. (1978) Life Sci. 22, 287–294.
Snell, K., Ashby, S.L. and Barton, S.J. (1977) Toxicology 8, 277–283.
Snyder, R.D. (1971) N. Engl. J. Med. 284, 1014–1016.
Spyker, J.M. and Smithberg, M. (1972) Teratology 5, 181–190.
Spyker, J.M., Sparber, S.B. and Goldberg, A.M. (1972) Science 177, 621–623.
Su, M.Q. and Okita, G.T. (1976a) Toxicol. Appl. Pharmacol. 38, 195–205.
Su, M.Q. and Okita, G.T. (1976b) Toxicol. Appl. Pharmacol. 38, 207–216.
Suzuki, T., Matsumoto, N., Miyama, T. and Katsunuma, H. (1967) Ind. Hlth. 5, 149–155.
Suzuki, T., Miyama, T. and Katsunuma, H. (1971) Bull. Environ. Contam. Toxicol. 5, 502–508.
Takeuchi, T. (1968) in Minamata Disease (Organic Mercury Poisoning) (Kutsuna, M., ed.), pp. 141–228, Study group of Minamata disease, Kumamoto University, Japan.
Takeuchi, T. (1977) Pediatrician 6, 69–87.
Takeuchi, T., Eto, K., Oyanag, S. and Miyajima, H. (1978) Virchows Arch. B. Cell Pathol. 27, 137–154.

Tatetsu, S., Takagi, M. and Miyakawa, T. (1968) Psychiat. Neurol. Jpn. 70, 162.
Taylor, L.L. and DiStefano, V. (1976) Toxicol. Appl. Pharmacol. 38, 489–497.
Tejning, S. (1968) Report No. 680529, University Clinic, Lund, Sweden.
Verity, M.A., Brown, W.J., Cheung, M. and Czer, G. (1977) J. Neurochem. 29, 673–679.
White, J.F. and Rothstein, A. (1973) Toxicol. Appl. Pharmacol. 26, 370–384.
Yamaguchi, S. and Nunotani, H. (1974) Environ. Physiol. Biochem. 4, 7–15.
Yang, M.G., Krawford, K.S., Garcia, J.D., Wang, J.H. and Lei, K.Y. (1972) Proc. Soc. Exp. Med. Biol. 141, 1004–1007.
Yang, M.G., Wang, J.H., Garcia, J.D., Post, E. and Lei, K.Y. (1973) Proc. Soc. Exp. Med. Biol. 142, 723–726.
Yoshino, Y., Mozai, T. and Nakao, K. (1966) J. Neurochem. 13, 1223–1231.
Zenick, H., Wright, D.C. and Brown, R.V. (1972) Fed. Proc. 32, 3563.

S. Kacew and M.J. Reasor (eds), *Toxicology and the Newborn*
© 1984 Elsevier Science Publishers B.V.

Chapter 9

The Toxicity of Cadmium in the Newborn

JOHN U. BELL

Departments of Preventive Medicine and Pharmacology and Therapeutics, University of Florida, Gainesville, FL 32610, U.S.A.

CONTENTS

I. INTRODUCTION

The thalidomide episode of the early 1960s illustrated, with frightening impact, the sensitivity of the developing organism to chemical exposure. Prior to that time, it was widely assumed that the embryo and fetus were protected from such toxicity by the so-called 'placental barrier'. Research conducted during the past two decades, however, indicates that the mammalian placenta is not a particularly effective barrier to the passage of a variety of foreign chemicals.

An extensive literature exists concerning the toxicity of cadmium to man, following occupational exposure. However, in recent years there has been an increasing number of reports which suggest that, under appropriate conditions, cadmium may pose a threat to members of the general population as well. In the Toyama area of Japan, inadvertent contamination of river water with cadmium led to elevated levels of the metal in crops and ultimately to the emergence, in local inhabitants, of a condition known as 'Itai-Itai disease' (Tsuchiya, 1969). There is evidence that the metal tends to accumulate in man throughout his lifetime, with estimates of its biological half-life ranging from 9 to 30 years (Friberg et al., 1974). Unfortunately, there is a relative paucity of knowledge concerning the effects of this acknowledged toxicant in the developing mammal. In this chapter, the available literature on the subject is reviewed and those areas in need of additional investigation are documented.

II. PLACENTAL TRANSFER OF CADMIUM

1. *Animal studies*

As early as 1964, it was demonstrated that the pregnant animal was extremely sensitive to the toxicity of cadmium. Parizek (1964) reported that a single subcutaneous injection of cadmium salt, injected at a dose of 4.5 mg cadmium/kg late in gestation, produced massive degeneration of placental tissue within 24 hours. Removal of the fetuses prior to administration of cadmium did not prevent the placental damage. In a study conducted in mice, Chiquoine (1965) found that administration of a single injection of cadmium chloride (6.7 mg/kg) between gestational days 6 and 17 caused intrauterine death of the embryos/fetuses and localized placental necrosis. Webb (1970) also confirmed the placental necrosis in rats injected with cadmium chloride (2.5 mg/kg) on days 11, 15, 17 and 18 of pregnancy. Interestingly, it appeared from that study that preexisting maternal stores of cadmium were not mobilized during pregnancy to produce toxicity.

In addition to these and other reports which document placental toxicity, cadmium has been implicated as a teratogen in a variety of animal species, including hamsters (Ferm, 1971; Gale and Ferm, 1974), rats (Barr, 1972, 1973; Chernoff, 1973) and mice (Chiquoine, 1965; Layton, 1979). A critically important factor concerning teratology studies with cadmium is to determine if the lesions observed result from a direct action of the metal on the embryo or from an indirect action mediated through the maternal-fetal unit. To exert a direct effect, significant amounts of cadmium have to pass from the maternal circulation into the embryo-fetal circulation through the so-called placental barrier.

Until the mid-1960s, researchers felt that the mammalian placenta protected the developing embryo/fetus from exposure to maternal cadmium. For example, Berlin and Ullberg (1963) administered radioactively labeled cadmium intravenously to pregnant mice and, using autoradiographic techniques, were unable to detect the metal in the fetuses, despite demonstrating placental localization of the metal. Subsequent studies have shown, however, that cadmium can cross the placenta and reach the embryo/fetus. Ferm et al. (1969) administered a single dose of radioactively labeled cadmium sulfate (7.9 mg cadmium/kg) to pregnant hamsters on day 8 of gestation. Examination of the placental and fetal tissues on day 9 disclosed cadmium concentrations higher than those found in maternal blood. Of interest, the appearance of cadmium in the embryo at this time coincides with the period during which cadmium is teratogenic in the hamster embryo. By day 12, the fetal cadmium concentration had dropped to a level one-sixtieth of that measured on day 9. The authors suggested that the decreased concentrations might result either from an active removal of cadmium via the developing yolk sac or from an increased resistance to the placental passage of the cadmium as the pregnancy progressed.

In investigations using the rat, Lucis et al. (1972) injected pregnant females with a solution containing both ^{65}Zn and ^{109}Cd. Examination of the neonates revealed that the cadmium was detectable only in the liver, brain and intestinal tract, with the bulk of the metal located in the liver and the intestinal tract. The authors proposed the existence of a fetal enterohepatic cycle which might play a role in the sequestration or excretion of cadmium. Wolkowski (1974) administered radioactively labeled cadmium chloride to two strains of pregnant mice, one strain which was referred to as 'cadmium-resistant' and the other 'cadmium-sensitive'. Cadmium was detected in the embryos of both strains as early as 30 minutes after maternal administration. Interestingly, the 'cadmium-sensitive' mice were found to have higher levels of cadmium bound to a 10,000 molecular weight protein localized in the cytosol of the embryos than the 'cadmium-resistant' mice. Cadmium in the latter appeared to be bound preferentially to a higher molecular weight protein localized in the placental tissue, thus affording a degree of protection from the toxic metal. A study conducted by Sonawane et al. (1975) investigated the influence of age and dose on the placental transfer of cadmium in the rat. Radioactively labeled cadmium chloride at doses of 0.1, 0.4 and 1.6 mg cadmium/kg was administered as a single injection on days 12, 15 and 20 of gestation. The rats were killed 24 hours later. Cadmium concentrations were measured in the fetus and placenta, as well as in maternal liver and blood. It was found that the placental transfer of cadmium increased with increasing gestational age as well as with increasing dose. Although cadmium was shown to cross the placenta, the amounts which actually reached the fetus, when expressed as percent of the injected dose, were relatively small. For example, fetuses of mice treated on gestational day 12 accumulated only 0.0001, 0.0028 and 0.0095% of the low, medium and high doses, respectively.

Ahokas and Dilts (1979) investigated the placental transfer of cadmium after the oral administration to pregnant rats of a single dose of 100 μg of the metal on days 6, 10, 14 and 17 of gestation. 24 hours later, the rats were killed and various tissues were evaluated for cadmium content. Levels of cadmium in the embryo were highest prior to the formation of a functional placenta on day 10–11. After placental formation, fetal levels were decreased; however, the accumulation of cadmium by placental tissue was observed to increase with increasing gestational age. The authors concluded that the (rat) embryo only accumulates significant amounts of cadmium during early organogenesis and that during the last third of gestation the placenta effectively protects the fetus from exposure. Although the quantities of cadmium reaching the fetal rat late in gestation, following maternal exposure, are relatively small, they apparently are related to maternal dose. 48 hours after the subcutaneous injection of cadmium chloride (0.25, 0.50 and 1.00 mg cadmium/kg body weight) to pregnant rats on day 19 of gestation, cadmium was found in the cytosol of fetal liver (Waalkes and Bell, 1980a). The low, medium and high maternal dosages yielded cytosolic cadmium levels of 13.4, 30.5 and 106.9 pgatoms/ml in the fetal liver, approximately 1000-fold lower than levels found in the maternal liver. In a similar study utilizing the pregnant rabbit, Waalkes et al. (1982) confirmed the placental transfer of cadmium late in gestation. In agreement with the findings of the rat study, there was a proportional relationship between the dose of cadmium administered and the levels detected in the fetal hepatic cytosol. However, the levels found in the hepatic cytosol of the fetal rabbit were only 100-fold lower than levels found in the comparable maternal compartment.

The placental transfer of cadmium in the guinea pig has been studied using a very sophisticated perfusion technique which involves isolation of the fetal side of the placental circulation in situ (Kelman and Walter, 1977; Kelman, 1979). It was suggested by these authors that the reason very little cadmium reaches the fetus following a single intravenous injection to the mother is because the metal is removed quickly from the maternal circulation into the liver and kidneys, where it probably becomes incorporated into metalloproteins. With this model, radioactive cadmium clearance from the maternal circulation was found to be approximately 0.36 ml/minute at a perfusion rate of 2.5 ml/minute, which was more than twice the clearance rate for methylmercury. Clearance of cadmium from the fetal to maternal circulation, measured in that same guinea pig model, was found to be only 0.063 ml/minute, or 17% of the maternal to fetal clearance. Kelman (1979) concluded that maternal to fetal clearance of cadmium appeared to be a 'flow-limited process', whereas fetal to maternal clearance appeared to be a 'membrane-limited process'. These data suggest the possibility that placental transfer of cadmium may be bidirectional. A recent report by Garcia and Lee (1981) lends support to that possibility. In their study, they administered $^{115m}CdCl_2$ to pregnant rats on day 9 of gestation. Small but measurable amounts of cadmium were detected in embryonic tissue within 24 hours of administration; however, levels of the metal fell rapidly after that time. By gestational day 20, cadmium was not detectable in fetal tissues at all.

2. *Human studies*

Although obviously it has not been possible to conduct similar studies on the placental transfer of cadmium in humans, a considerable amount of literature does exist on the subject. The data are primarily epidemiological in nature and have relied on the measurement of cadmium in fetal tissue, obtained during autopsy, in placental tissue and in neonatal umbilical cord blood.

Karp and Robertson (1977) determined cadmium levels in human placentas from three different cities in the United States and found an average value of 0.037 μg/g wet weight. Significant differences in cadmium levels were found among the cities studied. Similar levels of placental cadmium (0.003–0.038 μg/g wet weight) were found in a study which involved 70 women in a rural region of Belgium (Hubermont et al., 1978). In addition, they determined that cord blood cadmium levels ranged from 0.01 to 0.43 μg/100 ml. In a study conducted in Japan, Chaube et al. (1973) measured tissue cadmium levels in embryos and fetuses from terminated pregnancies and detected cadmium in 57% of first trimester terminations. In second trimester specimens, they determined that liver, kidney and brain levels were 113, 50 and 140 ppb, respectively. Undoubtedly, the most extensive epidemiological study concerning the placental transfer of cadmium in humans was conducted during 1975 and 1976 in Belgium, utilizing data from over 500 pregnant women (Lauwerys et al., 1978; Buchet et al., 1978; Roels et al., 1978). Their findings included the following: a comparison of cadmium concentrations in maternal and newborn blood disclosed that the median level was 50% lower in the newborns, indicating that the human placenta does interfere with the passage of cadmium; both cadmium and carboxyhemoglobin levels were found to be significantly higher in cord blood obtained from mothers who smoked than in cord blood obtained from non-smoking mothers; placental tissue obtained from mothers who smoked contained 25% more cadmium than did placental tissue from non-smokers; and placental tissue was found to concentrate cadmium to levels approximately 10-fold higher than maternal blood.

From both the human and animal studies, it is apparent that the placenta does provide the embryo and fetus with a certain degree of protection against cadmium. What should be equally apparent from the studies just discussed, however, is that this protection appears to be somewhat dependent both on the species and on the stage of gestation. Clearly, the potential does exist for the neonate to begin extrauterine life with a measurable body burden of cadmium. To date, the significance of such an exposure has not been explored adequately.

III. CADMIUM TRANSFER IN THE MILK

As pointed out above, the neonate may be born with detectable cadmium levels derived from its mother as a consequence of placental transfer of the metal. Another potential source of cadmium for the neonate is maternal milk during the period of lactation. Unfortunately, a survey of the literature provides very limited information on this subject.

Lucis et al. (1972) found that administration of carrier-free ^{109}Cd and ^{65}Zn to maternal rats on the day of parturition resulted in the excretion of both metals in the milk. Although the concentration of cadmium was fairly low, the metal was detectable in milk throughout the period of nursing. When the nursing neonates were analyzed for cadmium, continuously increasing amounts of the label were detected in the gastrointestinal tract, with lesser amounts found in the liver and the brain. Of interest, the authors reported that there appeared to be an accumulation of cadmium in mammary tissue, with levels detectable even after lactation ceased. Although the nature of cadmium binding in mammary tissue is not yet fully understood, the authors point out that binding of the metal to macromolecules within that tissue could limit its transfer into the milk, and thus provide the neonate with a degree of protection. In a similar study conducted using mice, more than 60% of a cadmium dose, administered intravenously 24 hours before parturition, reached the neonates via the mothers' milk (Tanaka et al., 1972). When unexposed neonatal mice were nursed by cadmium-treated females, they were found to accumulate 0.05% of the maternal dose within 24 hours, and a maximum of 0.3% during 14 days of nursing.

In a study using nursing human volunteers, the cadmium content of colostrum was determined to be 22–25 ppb (Schulte-Lobbert and Bohn, 1977). However, when transitional and mature milk were examined, cadmium levels had decreased to approximately 10 ppb (a reduction of 50–60%). Other values reported for cadmium in human milk are 20–42 ppb (Murthy and Rhea, 1971) and 28–95 ppb (Maruna et al., 1976).

Although somewhat limited in number, the existing reports do indicate that maternal milk can be a source of cadmium for the nursing neonate. The question that remains to be answered is whether or not the levels of cadmium which can accumulate in the neonate from this source will cause toxicity.

IV. PHARMACOKINETICS OF CADMIUM IN THE NEONATE

1. *Absorption*

There are numerous reports in the literature suggesting that the accumulation of cadmium in the human body is proportional to age. It has been postulated that cadmium levels increase more than 200-fold during the first 3 years of life and that during this period man accumulates nearly 30% of his total lifetime body burden. There is certainly convincing evidence to indicate that cadmium can be passed from mother to nursing neonate via the milk (see above). What is poorly understood at this time is the effect of exposure of the developing organism to this toxic metal. Lucis et al. (1972) reported that newborns from rats which had been exposed to cadmium during pregnancy only had measurable levels of the metal in brain, gastrointestinal tract and liver. In an attempt to explain these findings, they suggested the presence in the fetus of an enterohepatic system which presumably was responsible for the movement of maternally derived cadmium from the fetal liver to the gut.

In order to investigate neonatal absorption from the gastrointestinal tract, Sasser and Jarboe (1977) administered radioactively labeled cadmium chloride by gavage to rat pups 2 and 24 hours after birth. A control group of 6-week-old animals was also included in the study. Pups dosed at 2 hours of age and killed 24 hours later had absorbed approximately 8% of the administered dose, or roughly six times more cadmium during the same time period than pups which had been dosed when they were 24 hours old. After that initial 24-hour period, the absorption of cadmium was similar in both age groups; however, over 60% of the administered label still remained in the gastrointestinal tract 15 days after dosing. In contrast, the disappearance of cadmium from the gut of 6-week-old rats was very rapid, with less than 2% of the original dose remaining after 4 days. Only 0.5% of the administered dose was actually absorbed during that time. Using autoradiographic techniques, the authors were able to determine that a considerable portion of the cadmium label had adhered to the brush border and surface epithelium of the gut. Cadmium was also localized in diffuse lymphatic tissue in the intestinal wall. No satisfactory explanation was given for the marked absorption of cadmium during the initial 24 hours following birth. It was of interest that the rate of cadmium loss from the gastrointestinal tract increased significantly when the diet was changed from milk to solid chow, when the rats reached 17 days of age.

The influence of age and dietary composition on the intestinal absorption of cadmium was investigated further by Kello and Kostial (1977). They used rats of different ages (1, 3, 6 and 52 weeks old) fed either milk or a standard rat chow and then monitored whole-body retention of orally administered cadmium chloride. Whole-body retention of cadmium was found to be highest in newborn rats. Within each dietary group, cadmium retention declined with age; however, those rats on the milk diet were found to retain more cadmium than did age-matched animals receiving rat food. A comparison of results obtained 6 days after the administration of labeled cadmium indicated that the newborn animals showed an 80 times higher retention of cadmium than adult rats receiving solid food. To prove that the dietary effect was mediated at the level of gastrointestinal absorption, the authors determined that the whole-body retention of cadmium following a single intraperitoneal injection was the same in both milk-fed and control 6-week-old rats. It was suggested that the observed effect of diet on cadmium absorption might be caused by an as yet unidentified cadmium-binding ligand in the milk. Further investigations are needed to clarify this point.

Unfortunately, we are faced with the situation where most of the available literature concerning cadmium absorption in the neonate deals with laboratory animals. Again, the majority of the human data is epidemiological in nature, relying heavily on the measurement of cadmium levels in autopsy material as it becomes available. One such study was conducted in the Cincinnati area and included tissues from 107 individuals. Neonates (0–1 month old) were found to have hepatic, renal and hair cadmium levels of 0.01, 0.05 and 0.45 μg/g wet weight, respectively, whereas older neonates (1–23 months old) had cadmium levels of 0.05, 0.13 and 3.30 μg/g wet weight, respectively (Gross et al., 1976). An obvious difficulty associated with metal analysis in the human neonate is not being able to determine with certainty if the cadmium being measured has resulted from placental transfer or from postnatal ingestion and subsequent absorption of the metal.

2. Distribution

When animals are exposed to cadmium, either acutely or chronically, the metal can be found in nearly every tissue of the body. Generally, the age of the animal and the route of exposure will influence markedly both tissue levels and tissue distribution of cadmium. The influence of age on the distribution of cadmium was evaluated by Wong and Klaassen (1980). They injected male rats (4, 21 and 70 days old) with a single intravenous dose of cadmium chloride and measured tissue levels of the metal after 2 hours and at 1, 2, 7 and 21 days. Within 2 hours of treatment, cadmium concentrations were significantly higher in liver, spleen, bone, testes, brain and muscle of the 4-day-old rat than in comparable tissues in the adult. Of particular interest was the determination of 5-fold higher cadmium concentrations in the brains of treated 4-day-old rats, when compared with treated adults. No significant differences were found in the concentration of cadmium in the brains of treated adults and treated 21-day-old rats. Based on these results, the authors suggested that in the neonatal rat the blood-brain barrier is not yet mature, permitting cadmium to accumulate in the brain. However, prior to the animal reaching 21 days of age, the blood-brain barrier becomes a functional reality.

A similar situation was observed with the so-called blood-testes barrier. 2 hours after exposure to cadmium, the testicular concentration of the metal in 4-day-old rats was 5-fold higher than in exposed adults. Testicular cadmium concentrations in 21-day-old rats were only 50% higher than those measured in the adult, indicating that the blood-testes barrier, virtually nonexistent in the neonate, is fairly well developed by day 21.

In the week following cadmium exposure on day 4, there were decreases in both the content and concentration of hepatic cadmium. In renal tissue, even though the concentration of cadmium decreased during that same period, the content did not change. These data suggest that there is a redistribution of cadmium away from the neonatal liver, but not from the kidney. The inability of the neonatal kidney to accumulate cadmium may be a reflection of renal immaturity. Administration of cadmium by the intravenous route resulted in significant levels of the metal in intestinal tissue within 2 hours. The cadmium content of intestinal tissue from treated adult and 21-day-old rats fell dramatically within 48 hours; however, in the treated 4-day-old rats, the intestinal cadmium content remained constant over a 1-week period. Since the cadmium was administered parenterally, interpretation of this finding becomes somewhat difficult.

Pietrzak-Flis et al. (1978) evaluated the distribution of cadmium in neonatal rats following chronic oral administration. They found that the accumulation of cadmium in renal tissue of 1–15-day-old rats was not as rapid as that observed in liver tissue. This was a somewhat unexpected finding, since 21-day-old rats exposed to dietary cadmium from day 15 had renal levels twice those found in the liver. As an explanation of their findings, the authors suggested that the kidney might be able to accumulate cadmium more efficiently during that period of development than earlier. Alternatively, the relatively high renal cadmium levels may result from a redistribution of the metal from liver tissue as the neonate matures.

V. CADMIUM-METALLOTHIONEIN INTERACTIONS IN THE NEONATE

1. *Metallothionein in the developing mammal*

Although metallothionein has been the subject of numerous investigations since its discovery in equine renal cortex over 20 years ago (see the following reviews: Cherian and Goyer, 1978; Nordberg and Kojima, 1979; Webb and Cain, 1982), it has been during only the last 5 years that researchers have attempted to unravel the role of this unique protein in the developing mammal. Reports from a number of laboratories, including our own, have presented convincing evidence that a variety of perinatal tissues contain a protein (or proteins) with characteristics very similar to the metallothionein induced in hepatic tissue following exposure of adult rats to cadmium. To date, metallothioneins have been detected in hepatic tissue from the human fetus (Riordan and Richards, 1980), the term fetal rabbit (Waalkes and Bell, 1980b), the perinatal rat (Bell, 1979a, b; Wong and Klaassen, 1979; Kern et al., 1981) and the fetal sheep (Bremner et al., 1977; Bell, 1979c). In addition, metallothionein-like proteins have also been identified in the kidney (Brady and Webb, 1981; Panemangalore et al., 1983), intestine (Johnson and Evans, 1980) and testes (Brady and Webb, 1981) of the perinatal rat.

Gel-filtration techniques indicate that neonatal hepatic metallothionein has a low molecular weight (8,000–10,000) and, like adult metallothionein, exists in two forms which can be separated using anion-exchange chromatography. Wong and Klaassen (1979) noted that the amino acid composition of metallothionein from neonatal rat liver was similar to that of zinc-induced metallothionein in that they found a high half-cystine content and a virtual absence of aromatic amino acid residues. In most reports to date, zinc is the primary metal bound to perinatal metallothionein, although it is not uncommon to find both copper and zinc. At birth, more than 50% of the total body zinc in the fetal rat is present in the liver (Oh and Whanger, 1979), and more than 95% of the cytosolic zinc is associated with metallothionein (Kern et al., 1981).

In an investigation of the postnatal development of hepatic metallothionein in the laboratory rat (Fig. 1), we found that the metallothionein concentration increased from term through postnatal day 7, and then progressively declined until levels were barely detectable by day 28 (Bell, 1979b). This developmental pattern was confirmed by a number of other laboratories (Wong and Klaassen, 1979; Kern et al., 1981). If the data are expressed in terms of total hepatic content rather than concentration, we find that the total amount of metallothionein in rat liver remains relatively constant during the first 3–4 weeks of life, despite an 8–10-fold increase in liver weight. Of interest relative to a biological role for metallothionein in the perinatal mammal was

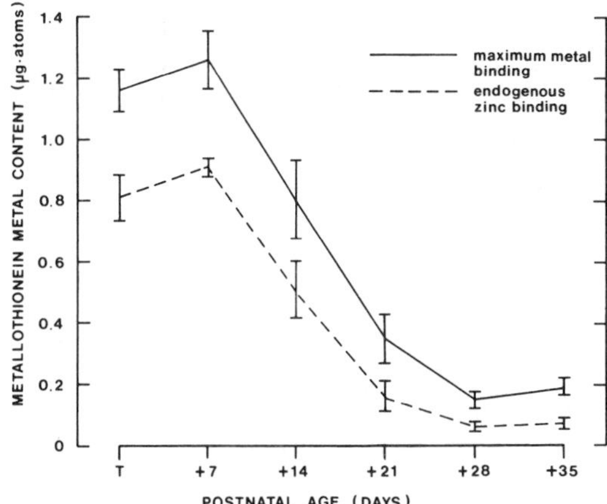

Figure 1. The effect of development on hepatic metallothionein concentrations in the rat. Metallothionein was determined using the cadmium saturation method described by Probst et al. (1977). The solid line represents metallothionein, the broken line represents the normal levels of zinc associated with the protein at various stages of development.

the observation that the cytosolic zinc concentrations paralleled the metallothionein concentrations. As was stated earlier, the major metal binding to metallothionein in perinatal rat liver is zinc. Based on data generated using immunohistochemical methods, Panemangalore et al. (1983) suggested that during the first few days following birth rat hepatic metallothionein has a nuclear localization. As the neonatal rat matures, the protein is translocated from the nucleus into the cytoplasm. The authors suggest that this nuclear localization of the protein in neonatal liver may be related to the increased requirement for zinc in the synthesis of nucleic acids and proteins during development.

A number of other tissues in the perinatal rat have been reported to contain metallothionein. An example is the kidney, where the primary metal bound to metallothionein is zinc, although the protein apparently also binds low levels of copper (Brady and Webb, 1981). At least until weaning, renal concentrations of metallothionien remain fairly constant (Wong and Klaassen, 1979). Perinatal rat testes also contain a zinc thionein, with little or no associated copper. Although the concentration of thionein-bound zinc is initially quite low, it increases to high levels by postnatal day 15 (Brady and Webb, 1981). There is fairly convincing evidence for the existence of a zinc- and copper-containing metallothionein in the distal portion of the small intestine of 5-day-old rat pups (Johnson and Evans, 1980). The authors suggested that the protein may play a role in the regulation of copper, and possibly zinc, transport across the intestinal mucosa.

2. *Cadmium-metallothionein interactions*

Since in the adult, at least, metallothionein has been proposed to play a role in the mediation of cadmium toxicity (Leber and Miya, 1976; Probst et al., 1977; Webb,

1972), it is not unreasonable to suggest a similar involvement in the neonate.

Based on our observation that the neonatal rat contains relatively high levels of hepatic metallothionein compared to older rats, we conducted an experiment in which we compared the response of the 5-day-old rat with the response of the 26-day-old rat, following administration of a single subcutaneous dose of cadmium chloride (Bell, 1980). Cadmium doses of 1, 2, 3 and 6 mg/kg body weight were selected. Within 48 hours, the 26-day-old animals had responded to the cadmium exposure in much the same manner as adults. There was a dose-related increase in hepatic metallothionein levels (Fig. 2) and binding of both cadmium and zinc (Fig. 3). The ratio of zinc to cadmium was found to remain fairly constant, suggesting that the accumulation of the two metals was related. The response of the 5-day-old rat was quite different. Despite the presence of relatively high levels of hepatic metallothionein, the binding of administered cadmium, measured 48 hours after treatment, was not significantly different from that measured in the 28-day-old rat. An exception was noted with the highest dose of cadmium (6 mg/kg), which resulted in higher levels of metallothionein-bound cadmium in the younger animals. It was interesting to note that the binding of cadmium at the lower doses (1, 2 and 3 mg/kg) in the neonate occurred without any increase in metallothionein levels, whereas at the 6 mg/kg dose there was a significant increase measured. Despite our findings that preexisting hepatic metallothionien can bind cadmium in the neonatal rat and that synthesis of the protein can occur, the highest cadmium dose (6 mg/kg) proved to be more toxic in the neonate than in the 26-day-old rats. At that dose, 30% of the 5-day-old rats died within 48 hours, compared to only 4% of the 26-day-old animals.

In a similar study, Wong and Klaassen (1980) confirmed that the presence of high concentrations of metallothionein in the livers of neonatal rats did not protect them from the lethal effects of cadmium. They also determined that the intravenous administration of a 1 mg/kg dose of cadmium to 10-week-old rats caused a 700%

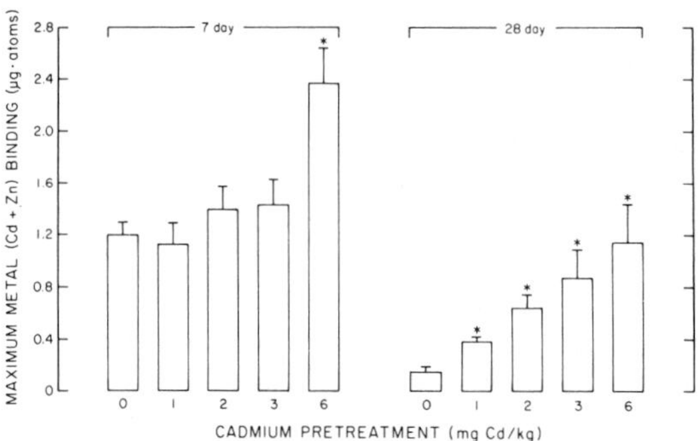

Figure 2. The influence of cadmium administration on hepatic concentrations of metallothionein in 7- and 28-day-old rats. Rats were administered a single subcutaneous injection of cadmium chloride 48 hours prior to killing. Values (mean ± S.D.) represent the metal content of fractions having a relative elution volume (V_e/V_o) of 1.9–2.3 following gel-filtration of a 4.0 ml aliquot of 'cadmium-saturated' cytosol derived from a 20% (w/v) whole homogenate. Asterisks indicate those treatment values which are significantly different ($P < 0.01$) from age-matched controls. (From Bell, 1980, with permission.)

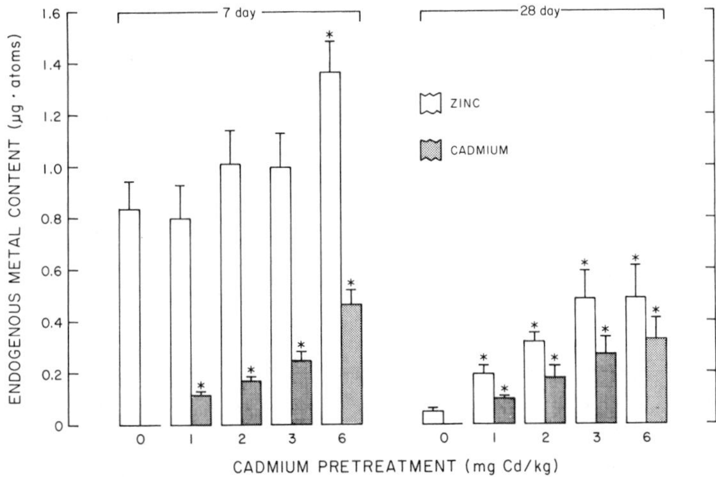

Figure 3. The influence of cadmium exposure on the metal content of hepatic metallothionein in 7- and 28-day-old rats. The cadmium chloride was administered as a single subcutaneous injection 48 hours prior to killing. Values (mean ± S.D.) represent the metal content of fractions having a relative elution volume (V_e/V_o) of 1.9–2.3 following gel-filtration of a 4.0 ml aliquot of 'cadmium-unsaturated' cytosol derived from a 20% (w/v) whole homogenate. Asterisks indicate those treatment values which are significantly different ($P<0.01$) from age-matched controls. (From Bell, 1980, with permission.)

increase in hepatic metallothionein concentrations. That same dose increased metallothionein concentrations in 4-day-old rats by only 10%, yet levels were still 2.5 times higher than in the adults. Wong and Klaassen (1980) also investigated the interaction between metallothionein and cadmium with respect to the age-dependent testicular toxicity produced by that metal. They determined that, following a single cadmium administration at a dose of 1 mg/kg, the testes of 4-day-old rats, which are cadmium-tolerant, had concentrations of the metal 5-fold higher than the testes of 10-week-old adults, which are sensitive to cadmium-induced testicular damage. Although it has been suggested that metallothionein-like proteins are somehow involved in the protection of the testes following repeated exposures to cadmium (Nordberg, 1971), no significant differences were found in testicular metallothionein concentrations when comparing 4- and 70-day-old rats. They concluded that the age-dependent toxicity observed with cadmium was not related to differences in metallothionein levels.

A recent report has implicated metallothionein in an age-dependent effect of cadmium on hepatic mixed-function oxidases in the rat (Asokan et al., 1981). In their study, they confirmed earlier observations (see above) that exposure of 7- and 14-day-old rats to cadmium does not increase hepatic metallothionein levels; however, exposure of 21- and 90-day-old rats to the same dose does. Even though induction was observed in the older animals, the authors reported that it was not sufficient to protect microsomal enzymes from the inhibitory effect of cadmium. The preexisting high levels of metallothionein in the younger rats presumably bound significant amounts of the administered cadmium, reducing the microsomal levels of the metal and thereby protecting against the inhibition.

It should be obvious from the above studies that the role of metallothionein in the neonatal animal, particularly as it relates to cadmium toxicity, needs further clarification.

VI. CADMIUM TOXICITY IN THE NEONATE

1. Neurotoxicity

Experimental studies assessing the effects of cadmium on the nervous system have indicated that the metal can produce neurotoxicity. The administration of large doses of the chloride salt have been reported to cause hemorrhagic lesions in the Gasserian and sensory spinal ganglia of adult rats (Gabbiani, 1966; Gabbiani et al., 1967a,b). In contrast, injection of neonatal rats with a high dose of cadmium produced hemorrhagic suffusions with destruction of cells in the cerebrum and cerebellum (Gabbiani et al., 1967b). In a similar series of experiments, but using lower doses of cadmium, Wong and Klaassen (1982) found lesions in the corpus callosum, caudate putamen and cerebellum 4 days after administration of 4 mg cadmium/kg to 4-day-old rats. A 2 mg/kg dose produced only slight cerebellar damage. 18 days after treatment on day 4 with the 4 mg/kg dose, there was a significant increase in both exploratory and diurnal activity, but not in nocturnal activity. Treatment of adult rats with either 4 or 6 mg cadmium/kg did not produce any morphological signs of brain damage or any significant effects on motor activity. The authors suggested that the increased sensitivity of the newborn rat to the neurotoxic effects of cadmium was probably the result of an immature blood-brain barrier.

In a study conducted in mice, Webster and Valois (1981) administered a single dose of cadmium chloride on postnatal days 1, 8, 15 or 22, with examination 24 hours later. To ensure survival of about 90% of the animals, different doses of cadmium were administered to the different age groups. 1-day-old mice, when exposed to cadmium, displayed a number of petechial hemorrhages throughout the central nervous system. Areas affected included the cerebellum, cerebral cortex, thalamus, olfactory bulbs, pons and medulla. Neurons of the cerebral cortex displayed early degenerative changes. In brains from animals treated on postnatal day 8, hemorrhaging was again observed in the olfactory bulbs, deep layers of the cortex, midbrain, cerebellum and medulla; however, it was less severe than damage observed on day 1. Pycnotic nuclei were seen in the cerebral cortex, olfactory bulbs, basal ganglia and in selected regions of the cerebellum. Mice treated on day 8 and examined at 8 weeks were found to have forebrain destruction, massively dilated lateral ventricles, a very thin cerebral cortex and loss of the basal ganglia. Exposure to cadmium on day 15 again produced cerebellar hemorrhaging within a 24-hour-period. Pycnotic nulei were detected in the deep layers of the cerebral cortex and olfactory bulbs as well as in the internal granular layer of the cerebellum. Upon examination at 8 weeks, there was some thinning of the cerebral cortex and a reduction in the size of the cerebellum. Administration of cadmium (8 mg/kg) on day 22 did not produce any detectable morphological changes in the mouse brain.

Electron microscopic studies indicated that the hemorrhaging was accompanied by capillary vacuolization and also thinning and widening of interendothelial gaps. Damage to nervous tissue appeared to be secondary to capillary effects and was probably caused by edema or anoxia or by physical damage from extruded erythrocytes. A similar capillary effect has been observed in testicular and placental tissue following exposure to cadmium (Parizek, 1964; Aoki and Hoffer, 1978).

Capel et al. (1981) measured metal levels in the hair of dyslexic children, aged 11–15 years, and discovered that the concentrations of a number of elements, including cadmium, were significantly higher than in age-matched control children. The implications and importance of this finding still await clarification.

2. *Pulmonary toxicity*

The subcutaneous administration of cadmium chloride (8 mg/kg) to pregnant rats on days 12–15 of gestation caused a significant increase in fetal death and growth retardation (Daston and Grabowski, 1979). Lung to body weight ratios were reduced following treatment by 20–30%, yet there was no change in the rate of formation of the pulmonary surfactant sphingomyelin. Accumulation of the pulmonary surfactant lecithin occurred at the same rate in cadmium-treated and control fetuses until gestational day 20; however, the dramatic increase in lecithin formation, normally observed in control fetuses between day 20 and 21, never occurred in the treated fetuses. No control neonates developed any respiratory problems, yet 11% of all treated neonates developed signs of respiratory distress, including cyanosis, dyspnea and labored breathing. At necropsy, the lungs were a deep purple-red color and histological examination showed extensive alveolar collapse and the presence of refractile eosinophilic hyaline membranes in the air spaces, indicative of hyaline membrane disease.

The effects of lower doses of cadmium (1, 2 and 4 mg/kg) were investigated in a subsequent study (Daston, 1981). Pregnant female rats were treated on days 12–15 and term fetuses examined on day 21 of gestation. Pulmonary content of sphingomyelin was not affected by cadmium at any of the doses tested; however, the disaturated lecithin content was reduced at even the lowest dose. Although the disaturated lecithin to lung weight ratios of the exposed fetuses were not significantly different from the controls, the author claims that neonatal pulmonary stability is dependent on the absolute amount of lecithin present in the rat lungs. Maternal exposure to cadmium reduced that value and, in the view of the author, may make the neonate more susceptible to respiratory distress.

3. *Other toxic effects*

Chronic oral administration of cadmium to neonatal rats for 45 days at doses of 0.1 and 1.0 mg/kg/day was found to alter significantly hepatic carbohydrate metabolism

(Merali and Singhal, 1980). At both doses of cadmium, blood glucose levels were elevated significantly and hepatic glycogen content was reduced, yet serum insulin levels remained within the normal range. Serum urea levels also were elevated significantly at both treatment levels. Measurement of a number of gluconeogenic enzymes revealed that cadmium exposure had increased the activities of pyruvate carboxylase, fructose-1,6-diphosphatase, glucose-6-phosphatase and phospho*enol*-pyruvate carboxykinase. The authors postulated that the diabetogenic effects they observed following cadmium exposure may be related to an abnormal insulin secretory response of pancreatic beta cells.

One of the many toxic actions attributed to cadmium in adult rats is a marked inhibition of hepatic microsomal mixed-function oxidases (Means et al., 1979). Administration of the metal in vivo has produced decreased concentrations of cytochromes *P*-450 and b_5. A similar effect has been observed after an in vitro addition of cadmium to incubation mixtures. Jahn and Klinger (1982) reported that cadmium, added in vitro, inhibited ethoxycoumarin *O*-deethylation in rats of all ages, including newborns. Maximal inhibition was seen in 15-day-old rats. The application of these findings to the intact neonate is not yet fully understood.

VII. CONCLUSIONS

Although it had been assumed for a number of years that the placenta provided a barrier against maternal to embryo or maternal to fetal passage of cadmium, there now exists evidence which suggests that this barrier is not absolute. The demonstration of placental transfer of this toxic metal in a variety of animal species and its detection in abortion material confirm that low levels of cadmium are able to cross the mammalian placenta. Additionally, cadmium has been measured in human milk and in a number of tissues from the human neonate. Experimental data indicate that at least two systems in the neonate, the blood-brain barrier and the blood-testes barrier, are not developed sufficiently to prevent access of cadmium to these important tissues. Unfortunately, very little is known about the effect of low-level cadmium exposure on development. There is, however, sufficient information available on the toxicity of cadmium in the adult, following occupational exposure, to suggest that the neonate may indeed be at risk. Certainly, the long-term effects of neonatal cadmium exposure on behavior and on reproductive system function and morphology need to be examined more closely.

VIII. REFERENCES

Ahokas, R.A. and Dilts, P.V. (1979) Am. J. Obstet. Gynecol. 135, 219–222.
Aoki, A. and Hoffer, A.P. (1978) Biol. Reprod. 18, 579–591.
Asokan, P., Dixit, R., Mukhtar, H. and Murti, C.R.K. (1981) Biochem. Pharmacol. 30, 3095–3097
Barr, M. (1972) J. Pediatr. 81, 182 (Abstr.).

Barr, M. (1973) Teratology 7, 237–242.
Bell, J.U. (1979a) Toxicol. Appl. Pharmacol. 48, 139–144.
Bell, J.U. (1979b) Toxicol. Appl. Pharmacol. 50, 101–107.
Bell, J.U. (1979c) Toxicol. Lett. 4, 407–411.
Bell, J.U. (1980) Toxicol. Appl. Pharmacol. 54, 148–155.
Berlin, M. and Ullberg, S. (1963) Arch. Environ. Hlth. 7, 686–693.
Brady, F.O. and Webb, M. (1981) J. Biol. Chem. 256, 3931–3935.
Bremner, I., Williams, R.B. and Young, B.W. (1977) Br. J. Nutr. 38, 87–92.
Buchet, J.P., Roels, H., Hubermont, G. and Lauwerys, R. (1978) Environ. Res. 15, 494–503.
Capel, I.D., Pinnock, M.H., Dorrell, H.M., Williams, D.C. and Grant, E.C.G. (1981) Clin. Chem. 27, 879–881.
Chaube, S., Nishimura, H. and Swinyard, C.A. (1973) Arch. Environ. Hlth. 26, 237–240.
Cherian, M.G. and Goyer, R.A. (1978) Life Sci. 23, 1–10.
Chernoff, N. (1973) Teratology 8, 29–32.
Chiquoine, A.D. (1965) J. Reprod. Fertil. 10, 263–265.
Daston, G.P. (1981) Toxicol. Lett. 9, 125–130.
Daston, G.P. and Grabowski, C.T. (1979) J. Toxicol. Environ. Hlth. 5, 973–983.
Ferm, V.H. (1971) Biol. Neonate 19, 101–107.
Ferm, V.H., Hanlon, D.P. and Urban, J. (1969) J. Embryol. Exp. Morphol. 22, 107–113.
Friberg, L., Piscator, M., Nordberg, G.F. and Kjellstrom, T. (1974) Cadmium in the Environment, CRC Press, Cleveland.
Gabbiani, G. (1966) Experientia 22, 261–264.
Gabbiani, G., Gregory, A. and Baic, D. (1967a) Exp. Neurol. 26, 498–506.
Gabbiani, G., Baic, D. and Deziel, C. (1967b) Exp. Neurol. 18, 154–160.
Gale, T. and Ferm, V. (1974) Biol. Neonate 23, 149–160.
Garcia, M. and Lee, M. (1981) Biol. Trace Elem. Res. 3, 149–156.
Gross, S.B., Yeager, D.W. and Middendorf, M.S. (1976) J. Toxicol Environ. Hlth. 2, 153–167.
Hubermont, G., Buchet, J.P., Roels, H. and Lauwerys, R. (1978) Int. Arch. Occup. Environ. Hlth. 41, 117–124.
Jahn, F. and Klinger, W. (1982) Acta Pharmacol. Toxicol. 50, 85–88.
Johnson, W.T. and Evans, G.W. (1980) Biochem. Biophys. Res. Commun. 96, 10–17.
Karp, W.B. and Robertson, A.F. (1977) Environ. Res. 13, 470–477.
Kello, D. and Kostial, K. (1977) Toxicol. Appl. Pharmacol. 40, 277–282.
Kelman, B.J. (1979) Fed. Proc. 38, 2246–2250.
Kelman, B.J. and Walter, B.K. (1977) Proc. Soc. Exp. Biol. Med. 156, 68–71.
Kern, S.R., Smith, H.A., Fontaine, D. and Bryan, S.E. (1981) Toxicol. Appl. Pharmacol. 59, 346–354.
Lauwerys, R., Buchet, J.P., Roels, H. and Hubermont, G. (1978) Environ. Res. 15, 278–289.
Layton, W.M., Jr. and Layton, M.W. (1979) Environ. Res. 19, 229–236.
Leber, A.P. and Miya, T.S. (1976) Toxicol. Appl. Pharmacol. 37, 403–414.
Lucis, O.J., Lucis, R. and Shaikh, Z.A. (1972) Arch. Environ. Hlth. 25, 14–22.
Maruna, H., Maruna, R.F.L. and Eisner, R. (1976) Arztl. Praxis 28, 6–11.
Means, J.R., Carlson, G.P. and Schnell, R.C. (1979) Toxicol. Appl. Pharmacol. 48, 293–304.
Merali, Z. and Singhal, R.L. (1980) Br. J. Pharmacol. 69, 151–157.
Murthy, G.K. and Rhea, U.S. (1971) J. Dairy Sci. 54, 1001–1007.
Nordberg, G.F. (1971) Environ. Physiol. 1, 171–187.
Nordberg, M. and Kojima, Y. (1979) in Metallothionein (Kagi, J.H.R. and Nordberg, M., eds.), pp. 41–116, Birkhauser-Verlag, Basel.
Oh, S.H. and Whanger, P.D. (1979) Am. J. Physiol. 237, E18–E22.
Panemangalore, M., Banerjee, D., Onosaka, S. and Cherian, M.G. (1983) Dev. Biol. 97, 95–102.
Parizek, J. (1964) J. Reprod. Fertil. 7, 263–265.
Pietrzak-Flis, Z., Rehnberg, G.L., Favor, M.J., Cahill, D.F. and Laskey, J.W. (1978) Environ. Res. 16, 9–17.

Probst, A.S., Bousquet, W.F. and Miya, T.S. (1977) Toxicol. Appl. Pharmacol. 39, 61–69.
Riordan, J.R. and Richards, V. (1980) J. Biol. Chem. 255, 5380–5383.
Roels, H., Hubermont, G., Buchet, J.P. and Lauwerys, R. (1978) Environ. Res. 16, 236–247.
Sasser, L.B. and Jarboe, G.E. (1977) Toxicol. Appl. Pharmacol. 41, 423–431.
Schulte-Lobbert, F.J. and Bohn, G. (1977) Arch. Toxicol. 37, 155–157.
Sonawane, B.R., Nordberg, M., Nordberg, G.F. and Lucier, G.W. (1975) Environ. Hlth. Perspect. 12, 97–102.
Tanaka, M., Matsusaka, N., Yuyama, A. and Kobayashi, H. (1972) Radioisotopes 21, 34–36.
Tsuchiya, K. (1969) Keio J. Med. 18, 191–194.
Waalkes, M.P. and Bell, J.U. (1980a) Toxicology 18, 103–110.
Waalkes, M.P. and Bell, J.U. (1980b) Life Sci. 27, 585–593.
Waalkes, M.P., Thomas, J.A. and Bell, J.U. (1982) Toxicol. Appl. Pharmacol. 62, 211–218.
Webb, M. (1970) J. Reprod. Fert. 30, 99–103.
Webb, M. (1972) Biochem. Pharmacol. 21, 2767–2771.
Webb, M. and Cain, K. (1982) Biochem. Pharmacol. 31, 137–142.
Webster, W.S. and Valois, A.A. (1981) J. Neuropathol. Exp. Neurol. 40, 247–257.
Wolkowski, R.M. (1974) Teratology 10, 243–262.
Wong, K. and Klaassen, C.D. (1979) J. Biol. Chem. 254, 12,399–12,403.
Wong, K. and Klaassen, C.D. (1980) Toxicol. Appl. Pharmacol. 53, 343–353.
Wong, K. and Klaassen, C.D. (1982) Toxicol. Appl. Pharmacol. 63, 330–337.

S. Kacew and M.J. Reasor (eds), *Toxicology and the Newborn*
© 1984 Elsevier Science Publishers B.V.

Chapter 10

Critical Periods of Exposure and Developmental Effects of Lead

CAROLE A. KIMMEL*

Perinatal and Postnatal Evaluation Branch, Division of Teratogenesis Research, National Center for Toxicological Research/FDA/DHHS, Jefferson, AR 72079, U.S.A.

CONTENTS

*Present address: US Environmental Protection Agency, RD 689, Reproductive Effects Assessment Group, Washington, DC 20460, U.S.A.

I. INTRODUCTION

The determination of critical age periods during which exposure to an agent causes the greatest toxicity is an important aspect in the identification of the population(s) having the greatest risk to such exposure. In the case of lead, identification of susceptible periods of development is hampered by its pharmacokinetic characteristics. Lead is absorbed poorly from the gut, making it very difficult to achieve significant tissue levels following short-term exposure, and oral absorption varies as a function of age and the form of lead (Barltrop, 1975). Lead also has a long biological half-life, so that once exposure occurs a body burden of lead is maintained for some time, due to lead storage in certain tissues, particularly bone (Keller and Doherty, 1980). Acute high-dose exposure may provide some information on sensitive periods, but often causes other signs of general toxicity and, if given parenterally, may be less relevant to the human exposure situation. In addition, the pharmacokinetic pattern for lead varies, depending on age, nutrition, and other factors (Barltrop, 1975). Therefore, the circulating concentration of lead cannot be predicted simply on the basis of initial lead exposure level. Several recent studies have reported on the bioavailability of orally administered lead to the developing conceptus and neonate at various time points (Bhattacharyya, 1983; Bull et al., 1983; Buchet and Lauwerys, 1981; Miller et al., 1983).

Problems related to the pharmacokinetics of lead are compounded by other factors as well. For example, lead affects multiple endpoints so that defining the sensitive exposure period is a function of the endpoint being evaluated. In addition, the use of the rodent laboratory model, in which comparable developmental periods are extremely short relative to those of man, further complicates the problem of defining periods of greatest susceptibility to lead exposure in man.

Perhaps because of these problems, only a few studies have addressed directly the question of discrete developmental periods and susceptibility to lead exposure in animals. However, there are studies which suggest general ages when the sensitivity of animals to lead is increased, and it is recognized that the young, developing child is more vulnerable to lead exposure (Lin-Fu, 1973). Thus, susceptible periods are likely to be found during prenatal or early postnatal development. This paper focuses on the results of developmental exposure to lead as related to effects on prenatal development, postnatal physical maturation and functional development. The comparisons made are primarily on the basis of time of exposure and endpoint affected. Exposure levels were calculated as noted in the tables to show the amount of lead (in whatever form it was administered), but in the text levels are noted in relative terms. High-level lead refers to those exposure regimens that produced general signs of toxicity, while low levels are the exposure regimens that caused little or no general toxicity at the age and under the specific conditions of the study being discussed.

TABLE 1

SUMMARY OF STUDIES ON THE EMBRYOTOXICITY AND TERATOGENICITY OF LEAD

Route of exposure	Lead form[a]	Exposure period[b]	Daily Pb dose[c] (mg/kg)	Death/ resorption	Malformation	Reference
Rat						
Intravenously	nitrate	8, 9, 10, 11, 12, 13, 14, 15 or 16	23, 33 or 49	+	+	McClain and Becker (1975)
Intravenously	nitrate	9 or 15	16	+	+	Hackett et al. (1982)
Intraperitoneally	acetate	9	13.75	+	+	Zegarska et al. (1974)
Intravenously	nitrate	17	5 or 25	−	+	Minsker et al. (1982)
Intravenously	TriML	8, 9, 10, 11, 12, 13, 14 or 15	14 or 29	+	−	McClain and Becker (1972)
Orally						
Diet	acetate	Continuous	≈666.7	+	−	Stowe and Goyer (1971)
Water	acetate	−6 weeks and continuous thereafter	≈0.05–25	−	−	Kimmel et al. (1980)
Water	nitrate	−3 weeks to weaning	≈0.004–0.42	−	−	Hubermont et al. (1976)
Gavage	acetate	−3 weeks to parturition	50–100	−	−	Miller et al. (1982)
Water	acetate	0–weaning	≈52–457	+	−	Carmichael et al. (1981)
Gavage	acetate	6–16	3.93–393	+	−	Kennedy et al. (1975)
Gavage	acetate	6–18	10–150	+	−	Wardell et al. (1982)
Gavage	TEL	6–16	0.006–6	+	−	Kennedy et al. (1975)
Gavage	TEL	9–11 or 12–14	1.6–6	+	−	McClain and Becker (1972)
Gavage	TML	9–11 or 12–14	10–41	+	−	McClain and Becker (1972)
Gavage	TriML	9–11 or 12–14	3.6–9.3	+	−	McClain and Becker (1972)

Mouse						
Intravenously	chloride	9	≈100	+	−	McLellan et al. (1974)
Orally						
Diet	acetate	0–21	≈833–3333	+	−	Jacquet et al. (1975)
Gavage	acetate	5–15	3.93–393	+	−	Kennedy et al. (1975)
Gavage	TEL	5–15	0.006–6	+	−	Kennedy et al. (1975)
Hamster						
Intravenously	nitrate	8 or 9	16 or 33	+	+	Ferm and Carpenter (1967), Ferm and Ferm (1971)
Monkey						
Intramuscularly	acetate	gestation or gestation and lactation	1 or 5	+ (abortion)	−	Tachon et al. (1983)
Sheep						
Orally						
Diet	metallic	throughout gestation	0.5–16	+	−	Sharma and Buck (1976)
Capsule	acetate	1–59 or 1–106	4.95	+ (abortion)	−	James et al. (1966)
Capsule	acetate	1–45	2.75	−	−	James et al. (1966)

[a]TEL, tetraethyl lead; TriEL, triethyl lead; TML, tetramethyl lead: TriML, trimethyl lead.

[b]Times refer to days of gestation; negative numbers indicate dosing started before mating.

[c]Estimated mg/kg doses of lead are noted by approximation sign. Calculations were based on an average of 20 ml of water or 20 g of diet/day and an average body weight of 300 g for rats and 30 g for mice.

II. PRENATAL EFFECTS OF LEAD

The teratogenicity of lead has been studied by a number of investigators, and several of these studies are summarized in Table 1. The route of exposure and form of lead (i.e., organic or inorganic) appears to be as important in terms of the endpoints affected as is the time of exposure. For example, prenatal inorganic lead exposure results in malformed young in some species if it is administered parenterally in acute high doses during embryogenesis. Inorganic lead injected into rats on day 9 of pregnancy resulted in a variety of developmental defects of the head (Zegarska et al., 1974), urorectocaudal malformations (McClain and Becker, 1975), and gastroschisis (Hackett et al., 1982). In hamsters, sacral-tail malformations were reported in offspring following intravenous injection of dams with lead nitrate on day 8 or 9 of gestation (Ferm and Carpenter, 1967; Ferm and Ferm, 1971). In mice, however, McLellan et al. (1974) did not observe any gross abnormalities following intravenous injection of lead chloride on day 9 of gestation. Tachon et al. (1983) reported that 5 mg/kg/day given intramuscularly to monkeys throughout gestation induced abortions but no malformations, and 1 mg/kg/day had essentially no effect. Following single intravenous doses of inorganic lead to maternal rats on day 15, 16 or 17 of pregnancy, hydrocephalus and/or CNS hemorrhage were reported (McClain and Becker, 1975; Hackett et al., 1982; Minsker et al., 1982). However, organic lead (trimethyl lead chloride) given intravenously to rats during early embryonic development was not teratogenic (McClain and Becker, 1972).

Administration of inorganic or organic lead compounds to animals by the oral route does not appear to produce malformations, but may increase embryotoxicity (growth reduction or death) when given either continuously beginning prior to conception or only during a few days of gestation (Stowe and Goyer, 1971; Carmichael et al., 1981; Kennedy et al., 1975; McClain and Becker, 1972; Wardell et al., 1982; Miller et al., 1982). Low-level chronic exposure (approximately 0.004 to 25 mg/kg/day) in the rat did not significantly alter pregnancy, embryotoxicity or malformation rates (Kimmel et al., 1980; Hubermont et al., 1976; Miller et al., 1982); at higher exposure levels (approximately 200 mg/kg/day and above), reduced fertility and litter size were observed (Carmichael et al., 1981). Oral exposure to high levels of lead also has been reported to result in maternal and embryo/fetal toxicity in mice (Kennedy et al., 1975; Jacquet et al., 1975, 1976), rats (Stowe and Goyer, 1971; McClain and Becker, 1972; Kennedy et al., 1975) and sheep (James et al., 1966; Sharma and Buck, 1976). These toxic signs often were accompanied by general growth retardation and decreased offspring survival rates (Stowe and Goyer, 1971; McClain and Becker, 1972; Jacquet et al., 1975). Pre- and postnatal mortality following lead exposure has been reported in humans for well over a century, and at one time lead was used illegally as an abortifacient (Grandjean, 1975).

A reduction in litter size following lead exposure may be due to interference with implantation. Odenbro and Kihlstrom (1977) demonstrated that oral administration of triethyl lead chloride on days 3–5 of gestation in mice decreased ova implantation and overall pregnancy rates, but not ovulation frequency. In subsequent studies,

Odenbro et al. (1982) demonstrated a reduction in plasma 17β-estradiol and progesterone in lead-exposed mice. Wide and Nilsson (1977, 1979) gave single intravenous doses of lead chloride on days 4–6 of gestation and found that the implantation process was very susceptible to lead treatment, but that lead-exposed blastocysts transferred to control recipients developed normally (Wide, 1983).

In summary, the information available on prenatal development following lead exposure suggests: 1, parenterally administered inorganic lead is teratogenic in rats and hamsters, but not mice (only one study so far with mice); 2, days 8–9 of gestation in the rat and hamster are critical times in development for production of malformations, as are days 15–17 for effects on the developing rat brain; 3, oral exposure to organic or inorganic lead during organogenesis produces embryo and fetal toxicity but does not result in malformations; 4, the effects of lead on embryotoxicity, at least in mice, may be due to disruption of implantation processes.

III. POSTNATAL PHYSICAL MATURATION AND LEAD EFFECTS

The effects of lead on early postnatal physical development have been reported in a few studies. However, most of these studies involved long-term exposure, so that the question of critical periods is almost impossible to address. Little alteration in the appearance of preweaning physical landmarks was reported in rats when low-level lead exposure (approximately 0.05–5 mg/kg/day) in maternal drinking water was begun prior to mating and continued throughout gestation and lactation (Grant et al., 1980). Using a similar experimental design, Reiter et al. (1975) reported a delay in eye opening at approximately 5 mg/kg/day, with no accompanying change in body weight. Overmann et al. (1979) also reported delays in eye opening in pups exposed to lead throughout nursing via the mother's milk, with little or no reduction in pup body weight. In mice exposed to high doses of lead via maternal milk, Silbergeld and Goldberg (1973) reported delayed appearance of body hair and eye opening, in conjunction with growth retardation. Snowdon (1973) also observed 2–3-day delays in eye opening following daily intraperitoneal injections of 80 mg/kg lead acetate to maternal animals, beginning prior to conception.

One aspect of postweaning physical development which appears to be very sensitive to lead exposure is the developing reproductive system. In the female, Der et al. (1974) reported a delay in vaginal opening in Sesco rats given lead acetate injections (100 mg subcutaneously daily, ages 21–61 days) alone or in combination with a low-protein diet. Lead exposure (without growth retardation) or low-protein diet significantly delayed vaginal opening, and the combination completely prevented vaginal opening. Kimmel et al. (1980) showed a dose-related delay in vaginal opening in female albino rats exposed continuously to approximately 2.5, 5 or 25 mg/kg/day lead acetate in drinking water, starting at weaning; growth rates were impaired at the two higher doses only. Once vaginal opening occurred, no effect was noted on the estrous cycle, as judged by vaginal cytology or reproductive function. Offspring were continued on drinking water containing lead at the same levels and exhibited an even greater delay in the day of vaginal opening in the absence of growth retardation than had their mothers (Grant et al., 1980). Gray and Reiter (1977) reported that vaginal opening in CD-1 mice was delayed by continuous lead exposure even when undernutrition was controlled for by pair-feeding. Petrusz et al. (1979) reported that female rats exposed orally beginning at 2 days of age to 40, 100 or 200 mg/kg/day lead acetate showed a suppression in the peak of follicle-stimulating hormone (FSH) at 15 days of age, an event which normally precedes vaginal opening and onset of estrus.

In the male, Wiebe et al. (1982) have recently shown that prenatal and early postnatal exposure to lead at doses that had no effect on gestation or postnatal development produced decreases in Sertoli cell steroidogenesis and FSH binding at 13 or 21 days of age. Further in vitro studies (Wiebe et al., 1983) suggested that the effects of lead may be at multiple sites, including inhibition of steroidogenic enzyme activity and inhibition of the synthesis of steroidogenic enzymes and hormone receptor proteins.

In summary, prenatal exposure to high levels of lead often results in growth retardation if the neonate survives, and this may be accompanied by developmental delays in physical landmarks. In the absence of growth retardation, preweaning physical events are rarely affected, except for a delay in sexual maturation in female rodents. This effect on females increases as exposure continues over two generations, and may be due to an effect on the FSH peak preceding sexual maturation, but can result from lead exposure at the time of and/or shortly before vaginal opening normally occurs. Thus, prenatal or preweaning exposure is not necessary to delay the time of vaginal opening. The effects reported on male sexual development have been at the biochemical level and indicate a likelihood for reduced reproductive function. However, no studies have been reported to confirm an in vivo alteration in male reproductive function.

IV. LEAD EFFECTS ON POSTNATAL FUNCTION

A number of functional alterations have been reported to result from developmental exposure to lead; these include altered thermoregulatory (Fox, 1979), reproductive (Stowe and Goyer, 1971), immune (Luster et al., 1978; Faith et al., 1978), renal (Fowler et al., 1980) and cardiovascular (Williams et al., 1977; Hejtmancik and Williams, 1979) function as well as central nervous system ontogeny and function, the latter having been most thoroughly studied. Only a few of these studies were designed to evaluate the time of lead exposure as it affected the endpoint in question. Selected examples of studies on postnatal function will be discussed here as they relate to critical exposure times.

1. Early functional development

Alterations in the development of some functions which mature early in life have been reported to occur due to lead exposure. Reiter et al. (1975) indicated a delay in the ability of young rats which had normal growth patterns to right in air when exposed chronically via maternal milk from dams consuming 0.5 or 5 mg/kg/day in the drinking water, starting prior to conception. Using a similar dosing regimen, Grant et al. (1980) reported delays in both surface and air righting in animals exposed to 5 or 25 mg/kg/day. In the latter study, the affected pups were smaller than age-matched controls. In neither study were other reflexes, such as auditory startle or visual placing, shown to be affected by lead administration. Overmann et al. (1979) reported delays in air righting in pups exposed to lead via dam's milk throughout lactation.

The development of body temperature regulation has been reported by Fox (1979) to be altered by lead exposure of Long-Evans rat pups via maternal milk on postnatal days 1–21. Lead-exposed pups isolated from their mothers for 1 hour exhibited a significantly greater decrease in body temperature on days 3–14 of age, and were delayed by 2–3 days in their ability to regulate body temperature adequately when away from the dam.

Fox et al. (1977) reported an increase in the latency of the visual-evoked response components throughout the neonatal period and in adult rats exposed only during suckling. Further studies (Fox et al., 1982; Costa and Fox, 1983) showed a supersensitivity to scopolamine in neonatally lead-treated rats and a direct action of lead on visual cortex cholinergic neurons. Fox et al. (1979) also demonstrated preweaning and adult disturbances in seizure responses to maximal electroshock seizure testing in rats exposed from birth to weaning. Bjorklund et al. (1983) reported reduced cerebellar Purkinje neuron discharge in rats injected intraperitoneally with lead acetate from birth to weaning. Pups that were affected were smaller in size, but no differences could be detected in malnourished 'controls'.

Maturation of duodenal calcium absorption has also been shown to be altered by lead exposure, as reported by Toraason et al. (1981). Sprague-Dawley pups exposed in utero and via maternal milk until day 17 postnatally showed a transient reduction in the development of calcium absorption, which returned to control levels by day 24.

In summary, these data indicate that alterations in early development of certain functions may result from lead exposure during the perinatal period. Thermoregulatory control may be affected within 2–3 days after lead exposure to neonates begins. Further information is needed to determine more accurately the critical period(s) of exposure for producing delays in early functional development in the absence of weight reduction. In addition, correlative studies should be conducted to determine whether or not early functional changes are predictive of later alterations, which appears to be the case for the visual-evoked responses and seizure responses (Fox et al., 1977, 1979).

2. *Cardiovascular function*

The effects of lead on cardiovascular function following developmental exposure have been reported recently. Williams et al. (1977) studied the response of the cardiovascular system to norepinephrine in rats that had been exposed to lead via maternal milk from birth to weaning. No effect was seen on the growth rate of offspring, and at 4 months after lead exposure had been discontinued there was no change in blood pressure, but a striking increase in cardiac arrhythmias during norepinephrine infusion was seen in lead-treated versus control animals. Further studies by Hejtmancik and Williams (1979) indicated that exposure during the first 10 days of life is critical for producing these cardiotoxic effects, while exposure from days 11 to 21 had no effect on the same endpoints. The age at evaluation is also critical, in that lead-treated and control animals at less than 70 days of age do not respond differently to the norepinephrine challenge, while at 70 days of age and older the lead-exposed rats exhibited a greater number of premature ventricular contractions during norepinephrine infusion (Williams and Abreu, 1983). Williams and Abreu (1983) also reported studies on the development of the adrenergic innervation of the heart, which occurs during the first 3 weeks postnatally. Several changes, including increased vesicular storage of [^{3}H]norepinephrine and increased steady-state levels of cardiac norepinephrine, were found early postnatally. No changes in β-receptor density or binding were seen, but norepinephrine-stimulated adenylate cyclase activity was decreased at days 15–25. There was an even more pronounced decrease in cyclase activity in animals at 16–19 months of age, suggesting a very persistent effect of early lead exposure. Victery et al. (1982) have reported increased blood pressures in male rats, but not females, continuously exposed to lead from conception; however, the significance of these changes is difficult to determine since animals were being exposed to lead at the time that the blood pressure measurements were taken. Thus, the effect on blood pressure may be transitory in nature, while the arrhythmias appear to reflect a permanent change which may become more apparent as animals age and which can be induced by exposure to lead during the first 10 days postnatally.

3. *Behavioral effects of lead*

A number of studies have reported the effects of lead exposure during development on behavior. This area has been reviewed in detail by Bornschein et al. (1980); therefore, the discussion here will be limited to those studies which provide insight concerning susceptible periods of exposure and altered behavior patterns. Also, since much of the early data on hyperactivity was obtained in animals exhibiting malnutrition, growth retardation and other neurological signs, those studies which report normal growth patterns or some attempt at controlling for undernutrition will be emphasized.

The studies dealing with the effects of lead on behavior have employed a variety of exposure regimens, and some of those which utilized learning paradigms for examining the effects of lead are summarized in Table 2. Exposure of one or both parents beginning prior to conception was studied by Brady et al. (1975). An effect of lead on learning in a water-escape T maze was seen when the male was exposed prior to conception, suggesting the possibility of a gametotoxic effect, or when the female was exposed prior to conception and continuing through pregnancy until weaning. The effect was more pronounced when both parents were exposed, giving further support to the idea that lead effects on postnatal behavior may be mediated through the male parent.

Only one study has investigated the effect of a specific prenatal exposure time on learning. Tesh and Pritchard (1977) administered lead intravenously to pregnant rats on day 17 of gestation and noted an alteration in maze learning in offspring. However, other studies which employed parenteral lead treatment in late gestation (Hackett et al., 1982; Minsker et al., 1982) reported embryotoxicity (see Table 1). Since the work of Tesh and Pritchard (1977) has only been reported in abstract form, it is difficult to discern whether or not the effects reported on learning were associated with other forms of toxicity.

A number of studies have been conducted using lead exposure during the period from birth to weaning (Table 2), with testing of offspring following discontinuation of lead exposure. Sobotka and Cook (1974) and Sobotka et al. (1975) administered lead by gavage to pups postnatally and reported effects on avoidance and operant learning paradigms. Hastings et al. (1977) reported no effect of lead exposure via maternal milk on operant learning while Overmann (1977) reported positive and negative effects of lead, depending on the learning paradigm employed. In an attempt to specify more exactly the critical period of lead exposure, Brown (1975) treated neonatal male rats with lead on days 1–10, 1–20 or 11–20 of postnatal age. Animals were tested at 8–10 weeks of age, by which time the concentration of lead in the blood had returned to normal levels. Those animals treated on days 1–10 or 1–20 showed impaired maze performance, while those treated only on days 11–20 were similar to control rats in performance. These results suggest an age-related difference in sensitivity during the neonatal period, a difference which may be due to maturation of the blood-brain barrier and/or variation in lead kinetics during this time (Momcilovic and Kostial, 1974; Kostial et al., 1973). In addition, morphological (Campbell et al., 1982; Alfano et al., 1983) and functional (McCarren and Eccles, 1983b) alterations in the developing hippocampus have been reported following preweaning exposure, and Petit et al. (1983) have discussed the similarities in behavioral changes, particularly in learning paradigms, resulting from hippocampal damage and lead exposure.

The postweaning period has also been suggested as a time when lead exposure may affect learning. Padich and Zenick (1977) reported significant effects of continuous prenatal, preweaning and postweaning lead exposure on schedule-controlled operant behavior, but no effect of prenatal and preweaning only or postweaning only exposure. These authors suggested that postweaning rats may be sensitive to lead neurotoxicity when there is a history of preweaning exposure. The latter idea was extended by the studies of Cory-Slechta and Thompson (1979) and Angell and Weiss (1982), who reported the effects of lead on operant behavior to be significant with either continuous or postweaning exposure. However, all of these studies include testing of animals during exposure, and may represent only a transitory behavioral toxicity rather than a permanent alteration. Further study is needed to determine the critical nature of the postweaning period for the development of permanent learning disabilities resulting from lead exposure.

Studies of the effects of lead on activity have been grouped according to general

TABLE 2

DEVELOPMENTAL PERIODS OF EXPOSURE TO LEAD AND EFFECTS ON LEARNING IN RATS WITH NORMAL GROWTH RATE

Exposure period	Daily Pb dose[a] (mg/kg)	Route of exposure	Testing age (days)	Exposure during testing?	Learning paradigm	Effect[b]	Reference
Males prior to mating and/or females prior to conception and continuing until weaning	275	orally (gavage)	30	no	maze	+(dual parental exposure greater than single)	Brady et al. (1975)
Day 17 of gestation	13 or 26	intravenously	–	no	maze	+	Tesh and Pritchard (1977)
Birth to weaning	5, 15 or 45	orally (to pups)	24–28	no	avoidance	+	Sobotka and Cook (1974)
	5, 15 or 45	orally (to pups)	60, 150	no	avoidance	+	Sobotka et al. (1975)
			60		operant	+	
+ days 1–10 or 11–20	17.5–35	orally (gavage or water)	50–70	no	maze	+(days 1–10 and 1–20; – on days 11–20)	Brown (1975)
	or 5	intraperitoneally (to pups)					
	≈7 or 35	orally (water)	90	no	operant	–	Hastings et al. (1977)
	6.4, 19.1 or 57.3	orally (water)	26–69	no	avoidance	+	Overmann (1977)
			67–89		operant (response inhibition)	+	
			79–101		maze	–	
			83–105		operant (tactile cues)	+	
			95–117		operant (visual cues)	–	

Prior to conception and continuing until weaning and/or postweaning	478	orally (water)	42–49	yes (for animals exposed postweaning)	operant	+ (continuous from preconception plus postweaning exposure only)	Padich and Zenick (1977)
Postweaning	≈15, 90 or 300 at weaning; 2, 12 or 40 by adulthood	orally (water)	55	yes	operant	+	Cory-Slechta and Thompson (1979)
Preweaning, postweaning or birth through postweaning	≈72 (to dams), ≈485–72 (to pups postweaning)	orally (water)	55–130	yes (for animals exposed postweaning)	operant	+ (postweaning or preweaning plus postweaning exposure)	Angell and Weiss (1982)

[a]Estimated daily mg/kg doses of lead are noted by approximation sign. Calculations were based on an average water consumption of 20 ml/day and average body weight of 300 g for adults or 45 g for weanlings.

[b] + Indicates some change in behavior was observed; − indicates no significant effect.

exposure periods in Table 3. The effects of lead on activity have been variable, especially those in studies employing postnatal exposure but with normal growth patterns. In addition, the activity measurements used in these studies have varied considerably, preventing comparison except in a very general way. As can be seen in Table 3, a change in activity levels was reported in all but three of the studies which employed continuous exposure, whether beginning prior to conception (Reiter et al., 1975; Verlangieri, 1979; Crofton et al., 1980), at conception (Driscoll and Stegner, 1976; Zimering et al., 1982) or at birth (Silbergeld and Goldberg, 1973, 1974; Sauerhoff and Michaelson, 1973), and continuing during testing. This was true whether the animals were retarded in growth or had normal growth patterns. The three exceptions were the studies by Krehbiel et al. (1976), Geist and Praed (1982) and Grant et al. (1980). In the latter study, no change in activity was noted in three different measures of activity.

In the case of exposure from birth to weaning, the results also varied; for example, Kostas et al. (1976) reported a change in activity in animals that were underweight, Hastings et al. (1977), Overmann (1977) and McCarren and Eccles (1983a) reported changes in normal weight animals, while Crofton et al. (1980) and Sobotka et al. (1975) reported no change in activity in normal weight animals. McCarren and Eccles (1983a) reported a slight increase in activity at day 16, but a significant decrease in activity at day 70. Thus, it is unclear what effect lead exposure from birth to weaning may have in altering activity levels. Pharmacological challenge (amphetamine) has proved useful for unmasking the effects of lead even in the absence of baseline activity changes (Sobotka et al., 1975).

The only study which has addressed directly the question of critical periods of exposure and effects on activity was reported by Crofton et al. (1980). Using a home cage with attached exploration area, movement of pups to and from the home cage was monitored and a decrease in activity after postnatal day 16 was found in continuously (preconception through weaning) lead-exposed pups. Further study revealed that pups exposed prenatally and cross-fostered at birth to control mothers were affected, while control pups cross-fostered at birth to lead-treated mothers showed no alterations in activity levels. This study clearly indicated an in utero period of sensitivity for this type of behavior. Another study from this laboratory (McCauley et al., 1982) reported delayed synaptogenesis in cerebral cortex following prenatal exposure.

In summary, the studies discussed indicate a broad time period during which lead exposure can alter behavior patterns; this includes exposure from preconception (paternal or maternal) (Brady et al., 1975) to as late as the postweaning period (Cory-Slechta and Thompson, 1979; Angell and Weiss, 1982). The data of Brown (1975) indicate that the younger the postnatal animal at onset of exposure, the more likely it is to be affected behaviorally in the absence of overt toxic signs, and Crofton et al. (1980) and McCauley et al. (1982) reported a period of prenatal sensitivity to lead exposure. However, the endpoints measured from study to study have varied enough, even when the same general test was used (e.g., open field activity), that it is impossible to make comparisons or to draw sound general conclusions. Only those studies in which comparisons of different exposure times were made within the same

TABLE 3

DEVELOPMENTAL PERIODS OF EXPOSURE TO LEAD IN STUDIES ON ACTIVITY

Exposure period[a]	Daily Pb dose[b] (mg/kg)	Route of exposure[c] (orally)	Species	Exposure during testing?	Testing age (days)	Effect[d]	Growth rate[e]	References
Prior to conception and continuing thereafter (also gestation only and postnatal only)	≈0.5–5	water	rat	yes	120	+	normal	Reiter et al. (1975)
	≈5	water	rat	yes	28–30	+	normal	Verlangieri (1979)
	≈14	water	rat	yes (except for gestation only)	5–21	+ (continuous or gestation only)	normal	Crofton et al. (1980)
	≈0.05–25	water	rat	yes	21–90	−	normal	Grant et al. (1980)
Continuous from conception	≈1.2 or 115	water	rat	yes	31	+	retarded	Driscoll and Stegner (1976)
	≈2123	water	mouse	yes	15–50	+	retarded at birth only	Zimering et al. (1982)
	≈1.3 or 2.5	water	rat	yes	56–61	−	normal	Geist and Praed (1982)
Continuous from birth	≈849–4246	water	mouse	yes	40–60	+	retarded	Silbergeld and Goldberg (1973, 1974)
	≈1697	diet	rat	yes	26–28	+	retarded	Sauerhoff and Michaelson (1973)
	≈529–796	gavage	rat	yes	24–36	−	normal	Krehbiel et al. (1976)
Birth to weaning	≈21–2123	diet	rat	no	90	+	retarded	Kostas et al. (1976)
	5, 15 or 45	to pups	rat	no	30	−	normal	Sobotka et al. (1975)
	≈7 or 35	water	rat	no	30	+	normal	Hastings et al. (1977)
	6.4, 19.1 or 57.3	water	rat	no	22–65	+	normal	Overmann (1977)
	≈36–182	water	rat	yes	12–22	+	normal	McCarren and Eccles (1983a)
				no	70	+	normal	

[a]Exposure periods have been grouped according to the general periods listed.
[b]Estimated daily mg/kg doses of lead are noted by an approximation sign. Calculations were based on an average consumption of 20 ml/day of water or 20 g/day of diet and an average body weight of 300 g for rats or 30 g for mice.
[c]Exposure to dams unless indicated to the pups.
[d]+ indicates <u>some</u> change in activity was observed; − indicates no significant effect.
[e]Indicates growth in pups that were tested but does not indicate any maternal toxicity or increased mortality.

laboratory (e.g., Padich and Zenick, 1977; Angell and Weiss, 1982; Brown, 1975; Crofton et al., 1980; McCauley et al., 1982) can be used to begin to evaluate critical periods of exposure for a particular endpoint. Also, as mentioned several times, growth retardation which may involve temporary or permanent reductions in body weight is often seen following perinatal lead exposure. Weight reduction at the time of functional testing makes interpretation of results very difficult. The role played by temporary weight reduction which has disappeared by testing age has not been evaluated thoroughly. This relationship is important, especially in the study of mechanisms by which functional alterations are produced.

V. SUMMARY AND DISCUSSION

Perinatal exposure to lead can result in a wide variety of toxic effects, ranging from adverse actions on germ cells to subtle alterations in complex behavior. Generally, the earlier lead exposure is initiated, the more serious the consequence for the developing organism.

The form of lead tested, dose used, route of exposure, species tested and endpoint evaluated, as well as the age at treatment, must be considered in any evaluation of the toxic effects. Perusal of the research summarized in the tables indicates there is little similarity in experimental design among the studies on developmental lead toxicity. These differences make it difficult to characterize an effect of lead on a particular endpoint, e.g., activity levels, let alone identify the critical period of exposure for producing such an effect. However, a few statements can be made concerning sensitive periods of lead exposure for particular endpoints and these are summarized in Table 4. Prenatal lead exposure during either organogenesis or the fetal period

TABLE 4

SENSITIVE PERIODS FOR AND EFFECT OF LEAD EXPOSURE ON PARTICULAR END-POINTS

Endpoint	Exposure period
Teratogenicity, embryotoxicity	Organogenesis, fetal period
Delayed vaginal opening	From weaning to the time of vaginal opening, from birth to weaning
Reduced steroidogenesis in the male	Prenatal and early postnatal period
Altered development of thermoregulation	Early postnatal period
Cardiotoxicity	First 10 days postnatal
Altered learning patterns	Preconception, late gestation, birth to weaning (first 10 days), postweaning
Altered activity patterns	Prenatal, birth to weaning
Delayed synaptogenesis	Prenatal

may result in embryotoxicity, teratogenicity with parenteral exposure, altered activity levels and delayed cerebral synaptogenesis. Early postnatal exposure may alter thermoregulatory ability, female sexual development and activity, with exposure during the first 10 days only being sufficient to produce effects on learning ability and cardiovascular function. Prenatal and early postnatal exposure may affect steroidogenesis in the male, and postweaning exposure may affect the timing of puberty in females and cause changes in learning ability when exposure continues through the time of evaluation.

The use of acute and systematic dosing regimens within the same study to identify further critical exposure periods, and procedural designs to investigate the possible correlation between early toxic signs and physical or functional deficits appearing later in life may prove helpful in suggesting the mechanisms by which the toxic effects of lead are produced. In addition, better understanding of the developmental pharmacokinetics of lead and exposure of developing target tissues will aid in the interpretation of the developmental toxicity of lead.

VI. ACKNOWLEDGEMENTS

The assistance of Judy Buelke-Sam in the preparation of the manuscript and tables is greatly appreciated. Rose Huber, Cindy Hartwick and Tina Sykes provided expert typing assistance.

VII. REFERENCES

Alfano, D.P., Petit, T.L. and LeBoutillier, J.C. (1983) Dev. Brain Res. 10, 117–124.
Angell, N.F. and Weiss, B. (1982) Toxicol. Appl. Pharmacol. 63, 62–71.
Barltrop, D. (1975) Postgrad. Med. J. 51, 805–809.
Bhattacharyya, M.H. (1983) Sci. Total Environ. 28, 327–342.
Bjorklund, H., Palmer, M.R., Lind, B., Hoffer, B.J. and Olson, L. (1983) Environ. Res. 31, 448–459.
Bornschein, R., Pearson, D. and Reiter, L. (1980) CRC Crit. Rev. Toxicol. 7, 101–152.
Brady, K., Herrera, Y. and Zenick, H. (1975) Pharmacol. Biochem. Behav. 3, 561–565.
Brown, D.R. (1975) Toxicol. Appl. Pharmacol. 32, 628–637.
Buchet, J.P. and Lauwerys, R. (1981) in Heavy Metals in the Environment, 3rd International Conference, pp. 447–449, CEP Consultants, Edinburgh.
Bull, R.J., McCauley, P.T., Taylor, D.H. and Crofton, K.M. (1983) Neurotoxicology 4, 1–18.
Campbell, J.B., Woolley, D.E., Vijayan, V.K. and Overmann, R. (1982) Dev. Brain Res. 3, 595–612.
Carmichael, N.G., Winder, C. and Lewis, P.D. (1981) Toxicology 21, 117–128.
Cory-Slechta, D.A. and Thompson, T. (1979) Toxicol. Appl. Pharmacol. 47, 151–159.
Costa, L.G. and Fox, D.A. (1983) Brain Res. 276, 259–266.
Crofton, K.M., Taylor, D.H., Bull, R.J., Sivulka, D.J. and Lutkenhoff, S.D. (1980) Life Sci. 26, 823–831.
Der, R., Fahim, Z., Hilderbrand, D. and Fahim, M. (1974) Res. Commun. Chem. Pathol. Pharmacol. 9, 723–738.
Driscoll, J.W. and Stegner, S.E. (1976) Pharmacol. Biochem. Behav. 4, 411–417.
Faith, R.E., Luster, M.I. and Kimmel, C.A. (1978) Clin. Exp. Immunol. 35, 413–420.
Ferm, V.H. and Carpenter, S.J. (1967) Exp. Mol. Pathol. 7, 208–213.

Ferm, V. H. and Ferm, D.W. (1971) Life Sci. 10, 35–39.

Fowler, B.A., Kimmel, C.A., Woods, J.S., McConnell, E.E. and Grant, L.D. (1980) Toxicol. Appl. Pharmacol. 56, 59–77.

Fox, D.A. (1979) Neurobeh. Toxicol. 1 (Suppl. 1), 193–206.

Fox, D.A., Lewkowski, J.P. and Cooper, G.P. (1977) Toxicol. Appl. Pharmacol. 40, 449–461.

Fox, D.A., Overmann, S.R. and Woolley, D.E. (1979) Neurotoxicology 1, 149–170.

Fox, D.A., Wright, A.A. and Costa, L.G. (1982) Neurobeh. Toxicol. Teratol. 4, 689–693.

Geist, C.R. and Praed, J.E. (1982) Percept. Mot. Skills 55, 487–490.

Grandjean, P. (1975) in Lead (Griffin, T.B. and Knelson J.H., eds.), pp. 6–75, Georg Thieme Publishers, Stuttgart.

Grant, L.D., Kimmel, C.A., West, G.L., Martinez-Vargas, C.M. and Howard, J.L. (1980) Toxicol. Appl. Pharmacol. 56, 42–58.

Gray, L.E. Jr. and Reiter, L. (1977) Toxicol. Appl. Pharmacol. 41, 140.

Hackett, P.L., Hess, J.O. and Sikov, M.R. (1982) J. Toxicol. Environ. Hlth. 9, 1021–1032.

Hastings, L., Cooper, G.P., Bornschein, R.L. and Michaelson, I.A. (1977) Pharmacol. Biochem. Behav. 7, 37–42.

Hejtmancik, M. Jr. and Williams, B.J. (1979) Res. Commun. Chem. Pathol. Pharmacol. 24, 367–376.

Hubermont, G., Buchet, J., Roels, H. and Lauwerys, R. (1976) Toxicology 5, 379–384.

Jacquet, P., Leonard, A. and Gerber, G. (1975) Experientia 31, 1312–1313.

Jacquet, P., Leonard, A. and Gerber, G. (1976) Mut. Res. 38, 110.

James, L.F., Lazar, V.A. and Binns, W. (1966) Am. J. Vet. Res. 27, 132–135.

Keller, C.A. and Doherty, R.A. (1980) Toxicol. Appl. Pharmacol. 52, 285–293.

Kennedy, G.L., Arnold D.W. and Calandra, J.C. (1975) Food Cosmet. Toxicol. 13, 629–632.

Kimmel, C.A., Grant, L.D., Sloan, C.S. and Gladen, B.C. (1980) Toxicol. Appl. Pharmacol. 56, 28–41.

Kostas, J., McFarland, D.J. and Drew, W.G. (1976) Pharmacology 14, 435–442.

Kostial, K., Kello, D. and Harrison, G.H. (1973) Int. Arch. Arbeitsmed. 31, 159–161.

Krehbiel, D., Davis, G.A., LeRoy, L.M. and Bowman, R.E. (1976) Environ. Hlth. Perspect. 18, 147–157.

Lin-Fu, J.S. (1973) N. Engl. J. Med. 289, 1129–1233.

Luster, M.I., Faith, R.E. and Kimmel, C.A. (1978) J. Environ. Pathol. Toxicol. 1, 397–402.

McCarren, M. and Eccles, C.U. (1983a) Neurobeh. Toxicol. Teratol. 5, 527–531.

McCarren, M. and Eccles, C.U. (1983b) Neurobeh. Toxicol. Teratol. 5, 533–540.

McCauley, P.T., Bull, R.J., Tonti, A.P., Lutkenhoff, S.D., Meister, M.V., Doerger, J.U. and Stober, J.A. (1982) J. Toxicol. Environ. Hlth. 10, 639–651.

McClain, R.M. and Becker, B.A. (1972) Toxicol. Appl. Pharmacol. 21, 265–274.

McClain, R.M. and Becker, B.A. (1975) Toxicol. Appl. Pharmacol. 31, 72–82.

McLellan, J.S., Von Smolinski, A.W., Bederka, J.P., Jr. and Boulos, B.M. (1974) Fed. Proc. 33, 289.

Miller, C.D., Buck, W.B., Hembrough, F.B. and Cunningham, W.L. (1982) Vet. Hum. Toxicol. 24, 163–166.

Miller, G.D., Massaro, T.F., Granlund, R.W. and Massaro, E.J. (1983) J. Toxicol. Environ. Hlth. 11, 121–128.

Minsker, D.H., Moskalski, N., Peter, C.P., Robertson, R.T. and Bokelman, D.L. (1982) Biol. Neonate 41, 193–203.

Momcilovic, B. and Kostial, K. (1974) Environ. Res. 8, 214–220.

Odenbro, A. and Kihlstrom, J.E. (1977) Toxicol. Appl. Pharmacol. 39, 359–363.

Odenbro, A., Orberg, J. and Lundqvist, E. (1982) Acta Pharmacol. Toxicol. 50, 241–245.

Overmann, S.R. (1977) Toxicol. Appl. Pharmacol. 41, 459–471.

Overmann, S.R., Fox, D.A. and Woolley, D.E. (1979) Neurotoxicology 1, 125–147.

Padich, R. and Zenick, H. (1977) Pharmacol. Biochem. Behav. 6, 371–375.

Petit, T.L., Alfano, D.P. and LeBoutillier, J.C. (1983) Neurotoxicology 4, 79–94.

Petrusz, P., Weaver, C.M., Grant, L.D., Mushak, P. and Krigman, M.R. (1979) Environ. Res. 19, 383–391.

Reiter, L.W., Anderson, G.E., Laskey, J.W. and Cahill, D.F. (1975) Environ. Hlth. Perspect. 12, 119–123.

Sauerhoff, M.W. and Michaelson, I.A. (1973) Science 182, 1022–1024.

Sharma, R.M. and Buck, W.B. (1976) Vet. Toxicol. 18, 186–188.

Silbergeld, E.K. and Goldberg, A.M. (1973) Life Sci. 13, 1275–1283.

Silbergeld, E.K. and Goldberg, A.M. (1974) Exp. Neurol. 42, 146–157.

Snowdon, C.T. (1973) Pharmacol. Biochem. Behav. 1, 599–603.

Sobotka, T.J. and Cook, M.P. (1974) Am. J. Ment. Defic. 79, 5–9.

Sobotka, T.J., Brodie, R.E. and Cook, M.P. (1975) Toxicology 5, 175–191.

Stowe, H.D. and Goyer, R.A. (1971) Fertil. Steril. 22, 755–760.

Tachon, P., Laschi, A., Briffaux, J.P. and Brain, G. (1983) Sci. Total Environ. 30, 221–229.

Tesh, J.M. and Pritchard, A.L. (1977) Teratology 15, 23A.

Toraason, M.A., Barbe, J.S. and Knecht, E.A. (1981) Toxicol. Appl. Pharmacol. 60, 62–65.

Verlangieri, A.J. (1979) Pharmacol. Biochem. Behav. 11, 95–98.

Victery, W., Vander, A.J., Shulak, J.M. Schoeps, P. and Julius, S. (1982) J. Lab. Clin. Med. 99, 354–362.

Wardell, R.E., Seegmiller, R.E. and Bradshaw, W.S. (1982) Teratology 26, 229–237.

Wide, M. (1983) Teratology 28, 293–298.

Wide, M. and Nilsson, B.O. (1979) Teratology 20, 101–114.

Wide, M. and Nilsson, O. (1977) Teratology 16, 273–276.

Wiebe, J.P., Barr K.J. and Buckingham, K.D. (1982) J. Toxicol. Environ. Hlth. 10, 653–666.

Wiebe, J.P., Salhanick, A.I. and Meyers, K.I. (1983) Life Sci. 32, 1997–2005.

Williams, B.J. and Abreu, M.E. (1983) Prog. Clin. Biol. Res. 140, 223–235.

Williams, B.J., Griffith, W.H. III, Albrecht, C.M., Pirch, J.H. and Hejtmancik, M.R. Jr. (1977) Toxicol. Appl. Pharmacol. 40, 407–413.

Zegarska, Z., Kilkowska, K. and Romankiewicz-Wozniczko, G. (1974) Folia. Morphol. (Warsaw) 33, 23–28.

Zimering, R.T., Burright, R.G. and Donovick, P.J. (1982) Neurobeh. Toxicol. Teratol. 4, 9–14.

S. Kacew and M.J. Reasor (eds), *Toxicology and the Newborn*
© 1984 Elsevier Science Publishers B.V.

Chapter 11

Phthalate Acid Esters: Teratogenicity, Fetotoxicity and Effects on Neonates

JOHN A. THOMAS[a], DANIEL WIERDA[b] and MICHAEL J. THOMAS[b]

[a]*Department of Life Sciences, Travenol Laboratories Inc., 6301 Lincoln Avenue, Morton Grove, IL 60053 and* [b]*Department of Pharmacology and Toxicology, West Virginia University Medical Center, Morgantown, WV 26506, U.S.A.*

CONTENTS

I. INTRODUCTION

Phthalate acid esters (PAEs) are linked historically to the use of poly(vinyl chloride)(PVC). PVC was developed in the 1930s and is used in medical devices, furniture, storage bags and food packaging. Pure PVC is a hard glass-like resin which becomes pliable with the addition of compounds called plasticizers. One of the most frequently used plasticizers is the phthalate acid ester, di-2-(ethylhexyl) phthalate (DEHP) (Fig. 1). An estimated 400 million pounds of DEHP are produced annually in the United States (U.S. International Trade Commission, 1978). Because of the widespread presence of DEHP in the environment, humans are exposed to minute quantities of DEHP daily. The risk that this exposure poses to adults is probably minimal; however, little attention has been given to potentially toxic effects of DEHP exposure to the newborn or the neonate. Fortunately, some information is available as to the possible teratogenic actions of certain of the PAEs. Some PAEs appear to be more fetotoxic or embryotoxic than others and there also appear to be age-related differences with respect to certain PAE-induced toxicity, but few studies have focussed specifically upon the effects of these plasticizers on the neonate. Of the large number of commercially available PAEs, DEHP seems to have received the most scientific or toxicologic attention.

A report in 1975 by Hillman et al. demonstrated that the levels of DEHP in post-mortem tissues from infants correlated with the number of transfusions and catheters experienced before death. The mean level of plasticizer in heart residue from these neonates was significantly higher in the study group than in the heart tissues of controls. The authors suggested that DEHP could have contributed to the cause of death in these infants. This clinical observation prompted new investigation into the area of teratogenicity, embryotoxicity and neonatal actions of the PAEs. With the exception of studies pertaining to teratogenicity, considerable research needs to be undertaken on the effects of the PAEs on the neonate. Recently, however, some attention has been devoted to age-related changes in the male gonad and to what extent phthalates cause testicular damage.

II. TERATOLOGY

Table 1 reviews the effects of two PAEs, DEHP and monoethylhexyl phthalate (MEHP), on the reproductive system and the incidence of birth defects in experimental animals. It may be seen that not only did species responsiveness vary to these phthalates, but experimental protocols were quite different (e.g., doses, route of administration, etc.). Earlier reviews by Peakall (1975), Verrett et al. (1969) and Thomas et al. (1978) also discussed the teratogenic effects of some of the phthalates and concluded that while some of the PAEs are clearly more teratogenic than others, all seem to require high doses in order to provoke their embryotoxic actions.

Initial studies by Carpenter et al. (1953) failed to reveal any teratogenic effects. Using DEHP and a comparison of litters born, number of pups born, number of

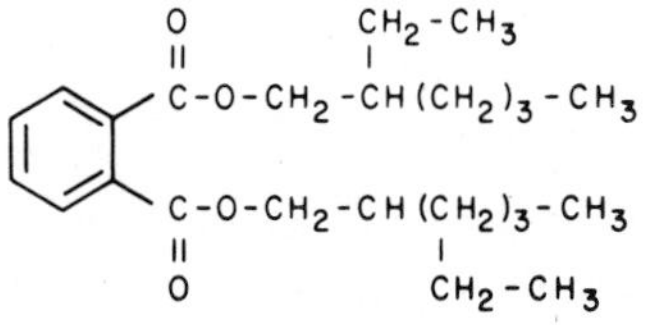

Di(2-ethylhexyl) phthalate (DEHP)

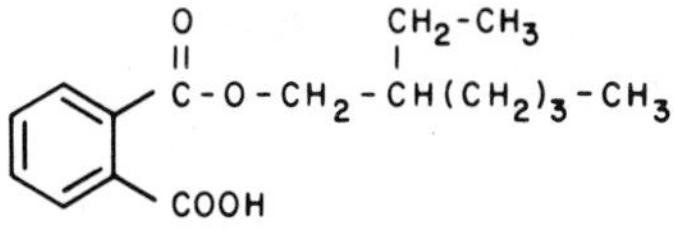

Mono(2-ethylhexyl) phthalate (MEHP)

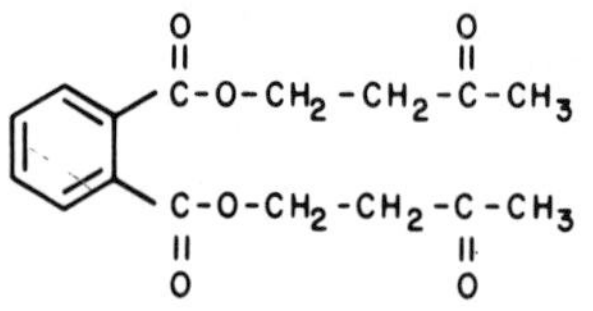

Di(2-methoxyethyl) phthalate (DMEP)

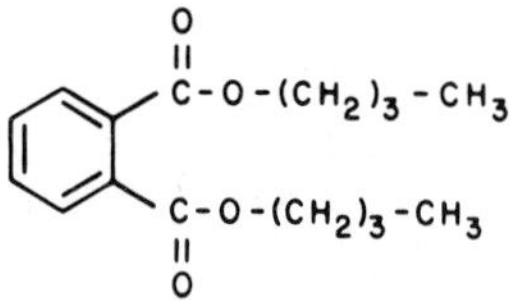

Di(n-butyl) phthalate (DBP)

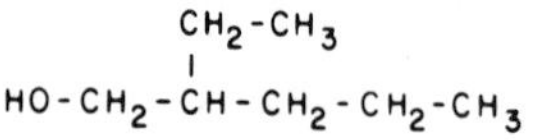

2-Ethylhexanol

Figure 1. Structures of several phthalate acid esters and 2-ethylhexanol.

litters/female, size of litters and incidence of stillborn pups, Carpenter et al. (1953) concluded that this phthalate was not teratogenic in rats. Bower et al. (1970) reported that dibutyloxyethyl phthalate caused congenital malformations in chick embryos.

Studies by Singh et al. (1972) and by Dillingham and Autian (1973), using high doses of DEHP, reported an increased incidence of fetal resorptions. Singh et al. (1972) also examined several different phthalates (dimethyl, dimethoxyethyl, diethyl, dibutyl, diisobutyl, and butyl carbobutoxymethyl phthalate) and reported a higher

TABLE 1

EFFECT OF DEHP/MEHP ON REPRODUCTION/FETAL TOXICITY

Species	Sex	Route of administration[a]	Principal findings	Reference
Rat	F	ip	Fetal resorptions, fetal deaths, and decreased fetal size	Singh et al. (1972)
Mouse	M	ip	Early fetal death and semisterility	Singh et al. (1974)
Rat	F	po	No effect upon fertility	Carpenter et al. (1953)
Rat	F	po	Decreased fetal weight and increased fetal resorptions	Nikonorow et al. (1973)
Rat	F	ip	Reduced conception and increased fetal deaths	Dillingham and Autian (1973)
Rat	M	po	Testicular degeneration	Schaeffer et al. (1945)
Ferret	M	po	Testicular degeneration	Lake et al. (1976)
Rat	F	ip	Adverse effect upon implantation and parturition, and excessive hemorrhaging and fetal retention	Peters and Cook (1973)
Rat	F	iv	No teratogenic or embryonic effects	Garvin et al. (1976)
Rat	F	po	No evidence of teratogenicity	Ruddick et al. (1981)
Mouse	F	po	Embryotoxic	Shiota et al. (1980)
Mouse	F	po	Exencephaly and myeloschisis	Shiota and Nishimura (1982)
Mouse	F	po	Exencephaly, open eyelid, and club foot	Yagi et al. (1980)
Rabbit	F	iv	No evidence of teratogenicity; maternal toxicity at high doses	Thomas et al. (1979)
Rat	F	iv	No evidence of teratogenicity	Lewandowski et al. (1980)
Mouse	F	iv	No gross and skeletal abnormalities	Tomita et al. (1982a)
Aquatic invertebrate			Reduced reproduction	Sanders et al. (1973)

[a] ip, intraperitoneally; iv, intravenously; po, orally.

incidence of fetal skeletal anomalies with these PAEs (20–75%) than with DEHP (0%). Later studies by Singh et al. (1974) revealed that DEHP, when administered intraperitoneally to male mice, caused fetal or embryotoxicity in females subsequently mated to these same males, as evidenced by a higher incidence of resorption compared to those observed in appropriate female controls.

The oral administration of DEHP to rats caused a significant reduction in placental weights (Nikonorow et al., 1973). These authors concluded that the effects of orally administered DEHP on reproduction and fetal development were dose-dependent and were influenced by the duration of phthalate administration.

Garvin et al. (1976) evaluated the teratogenic potential of plasma-soluble extracts of PVC in rats. Examining two different PVC formulations and extracting them with sterile rat plasma led to a plasma concentration of approximately 185 μg/ml of DEHP. Such extracted DEHP solutions, when injected intravenously into pregnant rats, failed to reveal either teratogenic or embryotoxic effects. Garvin et al. (1976) concluded that the concentrations of DEHP leached from plastic posed no teratogenic problem and that only very high doses could cause changes in the reproductive system of laboratory animals.

Female rabbits that had been artificially inseminated and subsequently injected with MEHP at critical intervals during gestation failed to reveal any significant teratogenic effects (Thomas et al., 1979). MEHP administration failed to affect the size of the fetuses, as measured by crown-rump or transumbilical measurements.

Lewandowski et al. (1980) assessed the teratogenic potential of plasma-soluble extracts of DEHP-plasticized PVC in rats. No differences were seen in the growth rates or behavior of the control and DEHP-treated groups. The incidence of gross external, skeletal and visceral defects among offspring was similar between controls and phthalate-treated rats. These authors concluded that plasma extracts of PVC plastics were not teratogenic when administered intravenously to pregnant rats during the so-called critical period of organogenesis.

Yagi et al. (1980) examined the teratogenic potential of both DEHP and MEHP in mice. The oral administration of DEHP in doses representing one-sixth or one-third of the acute LD_{50} on day 7 of gestation led to 100% fatality of all fetuses. Similar toxic effects were observed with MEHP. The gross abnormalities included exencephaly, open eyelid and club foot. Skeletal abnormalities occurred in the skull, cervical and thoracic bones.

When Ruddick et al. (1981) assessed the teratogenic potential of MEHP in the rat, no skeletal defects were observed in the fetuses. Both MEHP-treated and control groups exhibited some disturbances in the placement of the sternebrae plates; no visceral anomalies were observed. These same authors tested MEHP upon five strains of *Salmonella* and failed to demonstrate any mutagenic effect, although lethal responses were observed at high amounts in two of the strains.

DEHP and di-*n*-butyl phthalate (DBP) were administered in the diet to pregnant mice (Shiota et al., 1980; Shiota and Nishimura, 1982). The major teratogenic effect observed was neural tube defects (exencephaly and spina bifida). Either DEHP or DBP caused intrauterine growth retardation and delayed ossification, with an apparent dose-related response. High doses were embryotoxic and possibly teratogenic in mice. These authors concluded that the maximum nonembryotoxic doses of these phthalates in mice were more than 2000 times the estimated level of human intake through the food chain (Shiota and Nishimura, 1982).

A single intraperitoneal injection of dimethoxyethyl phthalate (DMEP) to pregnant rats led to embryopathy, including fetal deaths and fetal resorptions (Parkhie et al., 1982). Fetotoxic effects were expressed by a significant reduction in fetal weights. Hydrocephalus interna, skeletal deformities and appendicular malformations were induced by DMEP. These authors also reported that DMEP caused a significant decrease in fetal zinc levels and suggested that this divalent ion may play a role in PAE-induced teratogenesis in the rat (Parkhie et al., 1982).

A single administration of DEHP on day 7 of gestation caused a reduction in the number and the body weight of live mouse fetuses (Tomita et al., 1982a). There was no significant change in the number of live fetuses and no gross and/or skeletal anomalies at low doses. Higher doses produced some fetotoxicity, a phenomenon that was dose-dependent. The LD_{50} and the non-fetolethal maximum dose of DEHP in a single orally administered bolus were about 600 and 70 mg/kg, respectively.

It should be apparent from the aforementioned teratology literature that most investigations have been undertaken in either the rat or the mouse. When there is evidence of PAE-induced teratogenicity, it occurs only at high doses and in either the skeletal system or the nervous system. Clearly, amounts that humans could potentially be exposed to are not those encountered in the aforementioned laboratory animal experiments.

III. CYTOXICITY AND MUTAGENICITY

Many in vitro studies have shown that DEHP can be cytotoxic to cells in a dose-related fashion (reviewed by Thomas et al., 1978). Jacobson et al. (1974) demonstrated that normal serum which had been stored for 16 weeks in PVC blood bags contained 1.5 mM DEHP. This serum, when added at a concentration of 15% of the total tissue culture medium, inhibited [^{3}H]thymidine incorporation into human fibroblasts by 43% of control. Similar results were obtained by Jones et al. (1975) when they examined the toxicity of DEHP toward the growth of a human diploid cell strain, WI-38. The LD_{50} dose of DEHP for growth inhibition of the fibroblasts was 70 μM. These levels were within the range of concentrations which can be found in blood stored in PVC blood bags. DEHP at a concentration of 0.05 mg/ml was also shown by Lee and Kalmus (1974) to alter the morphology of various embryonic tissues, such as heart, aortic arch and liver cells. Treatment of aortic arch cells for 10 hours with DEHP resulted in a retraction of protoplasmic processes and the formation of various cytoplasmic vacuoles. DeHann (1971) found that aliquots of PVC extracts killed chicken embryo heart cells in culture. In addition, Meyler et al. (1960) found that isolated, perfused rat hearts deteriorated quickly when perfused with certain types of PVC tubing.

Some investigators have reported that DEHP is not cytotoxic in vitro to mouse fibroblasts or chick embryo cells (Fishbein and Albro, 1972; Gesler, 1973). An examination of these reports reveals that very low doses of DEHP were used, so that toxic concentrations were never obtained in culture. This dependency on large quantities of DEHP to produce overt cytotoxicity in vitro is illustrated further by the

TABLE 2

EFFECTS OF DEHP OR MEHP ON THE PRODUCTION OF ANTIBODY-PRODUCING CELLS IN BONE MARROW CULTURES STIMULATED WITH LIPOPOLYSACCHARIDE (10 μg/ml)

DEHP			MEHP		
Dose	Day 5 (% control)	Day 6 (% control)	Dose	Day 5 (% control)	Day 6 (% control)
5 μl[a]	<1	<1	5×10^{-4} M	0	0
High[b]	8	4	1×10^{-4} M	51	98
Medium	99	121	5×10^{-5} M	64	106
Low	94	110	1×10^{-5} M	72	107
			5×10^{-6} M	91	108

Cultures contained 5×10^5 cells in 1 ml of culture medium. Data are from Wierda (1982) and unpublished observations.

[a] Pure DEHP added directly to cultures.

[b] 'Solubilized' DEHP. Medium containing 40 mg/100 ml of DEHP was heated to 90°C for 1 hour, and then 1:10 serial dilutions were made with this solution to give high, medium and low concentrations. This was done since much of the DEHP remains as insoluble droplets in aqueous solution. Thus, cytotoxic bioassays indicate that some DEHP is in solution, but this can only be quantitated chromatographically which was not done in this case. 0.1-ml aliquots of each solution were added to triplicate cultures.

results depicted in Table 2. Pure DEHP, when added at 5 μl to 1-ml cultures, completely inhibited the development of mitogen-induced antibody-producing, mouse bone marrow cells. No antibody-producing cells were found in cultures containing a high concentration of 'solubilized' DEHP. The solubilized phthalate was without effect at lower concentrations. A similar result was obtained with MEHP. At 5×10^{-4} M, MEHP completely eliminated bone marrow antibody-producing cells. At lower concentrations, it appeared that MEHP was significantly toxic to 5-day cultures of mitogen-stimulated cells (5 days is optimal for untreated cultures). However, when cultured another 24 hours (day 6), it was found that all cultures, except at 5×10^{-4} M MEHP, had recovered to control levels. These results showed that exposure to relatively low concentrations of MEHP slowed the development of antibody-producing cells but did not actually kill them. DEHP, on the other hand, produced no changes in the rate of cell growth at low concentrations and was very cytotoxic at high concentrations.

In vivo experiments with DEHP and two metabolites, MEHP and ethylhexanol, have suggested that the body may detoxify significant amounts of these chemicals and prevent bone marrow cell cytotoxicity. Putnam et al. (1983) evaluated orally administered DEHP, MEHP and 2-ethylhexanol for their ability to induce chromosomal damage in the bone marrow cells of male Fischer 344 rats. No significant increase in chromatid and chromosome breaks or structural rearrangements was observed in marrow cells from these rats. Further, the mitotic index was unaffected by DEHP, MEHP or ethylhexanol, which indicated that these chemicals had no apparent effect on bone marrow cell growth.

Mutagenicity studies with DEHP or MEHP have been performed with mice and bacteria. Singh et al. (1974) reported that single, intraperitoneal injections of DEHP into male mice (11.5, 19.2 or 25.3 mg/kg) caused mutations as assessed by a dominant lethal study. Autian (1982) has provided further evidence, with the dominant lethal assay, that the mutagenic index of DEHP increases in a dose-dependent fashion after 1.0–10 ml/kg was administered thrice at 5-day intervals.

In bacterial mutagenicity studies with *Salmonella* organisms, Kozumbo et al. (1982) found that dimethylphthalate and diethylphthalate produced dose-related mutagenic responses with *Salmonella typhimurium* TA100 only in the absence of S-9 liver enzymes. DEHP as well as MEHP were not mutagenic in the presence or absence of S-9 enzymes. Ruddick et al. (1981) also reported that MEHP was not mutagenic when tested in five strains of *Salmonella*. Seed (1982) reported that dimethylphthalate and diethylphthalate were mutagenic and, in addition, found that ethylhexanol was weakly mutagenic. He reported no mutagenicity in bacteria exposed to DEHP. In contrast, Tomita et al. (1982b) found that both DEHP and MEHP were mutagenic to *S. typhimurium* TA100 with and without S-9 enzymes, respectively. The authors explained that mutagenic activity for MEHP is only possible within a high, narrow range (2.5–5 mM) since MEHP was cytotoxic at high doses and was non-mutagenic at low concentrations. The mutagenic activity of MEHP was completely destroyed with S-9 enzymes. DEHP was mutagenic at high doses (5 mg/ml) only with S-9 present. Thus, the mutagenic activity was ascribed to hydrolysis of DEHP to MEHP. The authors concluded that previous research had failed to show mutagenicity in bacteria due to the high, narrow dose range of MEHP for this effect.

In general, MEHP and DEHP appear to be relatively weak cytotoxins and mutagens since these effects are observed only after exposure to high doses either in vivo or in vitro. These detrimental effects can likely be ascribed to the hydrolysis products of DEHP, such as MEHP or 2-ethylhexanol. The mechanism for these toxic effects is unknown, but may involve the disruption of cell membranes. Circumstantial evidence for this hypothesis is provided by reports of increased membrane leakiness in alveolar macrophages exposed to DEHP (Bally et al., 1980), and changes in cell shape and changes in triacylglycerol accumulation in epithelial cell cultures exposed to phthalates (Lee and Kalmus, 1974; Suzuki and Matsumoto, 1980). However, no studies have addressed specifically the question of cellular membrane toxicity caused by exposure to phthalates.

IV. PLACENTAL TRANSFER OF METABOLISM

In an overview by Kluwe (1982), it was remarked that surprisingly little is known about the ability of PAEs to be transferred to offspring. Radioactivity was recovered from fetal tissues following DEHP treatment of maternal rats (Singh et al., 1975).

After injections of MEHP into pregnant rabbits, aqueous homogenates obtained from either the placenta or the uterus contained less than 1 μg/mg tissue (Thomas et al., 1980). Similarly, MEHP levels in rabbit fetuses were found to be less than 1 μg/mg. Very little PAE was detected in the livers of neonatal rats that had been injected previously with MEHP (Thomas et al., 1980). Studies by Bell et al. (1979) suggest that DEHP can cross the placental barrier, as evidenced by inhibition of sterologenesis in the brain and in the liver of fetal and suckling rats from dams previously fed with this phthalate. In another report by Bell (1982), studies indicate that fetuses taken by caesarean section from pregnant rats fed DEHP, beginning 5–10 days after conception, exhibit an impairment of sterologenesis in brain and liver. Further, if dams exposed to DEHP during gestation, and during the postnatal period as well, are permitted to nurse their naturally born offspring, hepatic sterologenesis in pups is reduced (Bell, 1982).

Early studies by Hillman et al. (1975) sought to identify DEHP in human neonatal tissues after umbilical catheterization alone or with administration of blood products. Determination of DEHP levels in neonatal heart and gastrointestinal tissue, using gas chromatography-mass spectroscopy, revealed that those infants which had been previously catheterized or received large amounts of blood products exhibited higher levels of plasticizer than did controls (Hillman et al., 1975).

Parkhie et al. (1982) examined fetoplacental metabolism in the pregnant rat previously injected with DMEP and suggested that there was a rapid transfer of the parent compound to the fetus across the placenta. DMEP caused a significant decrease in the zinc content of the fetus. Other tissues, more specifically the testes, have their zinc metabolism altered by PAEs. Whether zinc metabolism in the neonate is more susceptible to PAE-induced changes than in the adult is not known.

The metabolism and the pharmacokinetics of several different PAEs have been studied in a host of species (Kluwe, 1982). Unfortunately, little attention has been focussed on the neonate with respect to the metabolism of the phthalates. It might be expected that both the developing hepatic and renal metabolic pathways do not possess the same clearance capacities as the adult.

PAEs are distributed widely in the body. The liver is most likely the initial repository organ. Hydrolysis of the PAEs occur prior to intestinal absorption and, as such, is probably not influenced to any great extent by age. Hydrolytic activity is principally enzymatic and not due to enteric microoorganisms.

The liver, kidney and the gastrointestinal tract can sequester temporarily some of the PAEs, but evidence for difference in biodistribution between neonates and adult animals has not been adequately studied. Those PAEs that are relatively more lipid-soluble might be expected to assimilate to a greater extent in the older animal, which possesses larger fat deposits.

It is known that the dialkyl phthalates are metabolized readily to corresponding monoesters in many tissues. In general, most of the monoesters can be excreted by the kidney. Depending upon the particular PAE, and certainly the particular species, most phthalates are cleared quite rapidly by the kidney. Some species, including man and the monkey, form a glucuronide with the phthalate, thereby rendering the metabolite more polar and hence suitable for excretion. In addition, the hamster, guinea pig and mouse form the glucuronide, but the rat does not (Albro et al., 1982). While there are clearly species differences in the metabolism of the various PAEs, there are no studies directed towards elucidating age-related changes.

V. OTHER EFFECTS IN THE NEONATE

The effects of a single injection of MEHP upon different organs in the neonatal rat are depicted in Table 3. It may be seen that, under these experimental conditions, there were no MEHP-induced changes in the gravimetric response in the liver, kidney, cerebral cortex or lung. It is noteworthy that despite the three large-dose regimens employed, there were no significant differences in hepatic weights.

Perhaps, the only other organ that has been examined extensively with respect to PAE-induced changes and age is the testes. Considerable research has been devoted to investigating the effects of different PAEs on the male gonad (Thomas et al., 1979, 1982; Gangolli, 1982; Curto and Thomas, 1982). While no completely systematic study has examined age-related changes clearly, there is some evidence to indicate that the gonad of the younger animal is more susceptible to PAE-induced atrophy. Table 4 reveals the effects of DEHP upon the testes obtained from either immature rats (less than 100 g body weight) or mature rats (greater than 200 g body weight) (Curto, K., unpublished observations). Oral doses of DEHP (1000 or 2000 mg/kg daily × 5) significantly reduced testicular weights in the younger animal compared to the lack of PAE-induced changes in the older animal. While the younger age group does not represent the neonate, it does indicate age-related toxicity in the rodent gonad. Certainly, the blood-testes barrier is less developed in the younger animal, and hence may account for the observed testicular atrophy.

TABLE 3

EFFECTS OF A SINGLE INTRAPERITONEAL INJECTION OF MEHP (IN PEANUT OIL) ADMINISTERED AT 3 DAYS OF AGE TO NEONATAL RATS

Dose	Mean organ weights (mg)			
	Liver	Kidney	Cerebral cortex	Lung
Sham	1722±95	485±33	766±29	502±28
Peanut oil vehicle	1807±95	501±31	780±27	480±27
12.3 mg/kg	1788±95	516±31	788±27	482±27
24.5 mg/kg	1659±95	458±31	768±27	474±27
42.9 mg/kg	1734±95	476±31	771±27	492±27

Animals were killed at weaning (21 days of age). Values are mean±S.D. of at least 10 animals (Thomas and Northup, 1982).

TABLE 4

THE EFFECT OF DEHP (1000 OR 2000 mg/kg ×5 – ORALLY) DAILY ON IMMATURE (<100 g BODY WT.) OR MATURE (>200 g BODY WT.) RATS

Daily dose	Immature	Mature
	Testes weight (% control)	Testes weight (% control)
Control[a]	100	100
1000 mg/kg	58	94
2000 mg/kg	50	91

Data are from K.A. Curto (unpublished observations).
[a]Peanut oil.

VI. SUMMARY

In conclusion, DEHP can cause teratogenic, mutagenic and cytotoxic damage in rodents under the appropriate experimental conditions. Other PAEs, such as dimethylphthalate or diethylphthalate, are more mutagenic than DEHP or are more teratogenic than DEHP, e.g., dimethyloxyphthalate or dibutylphthalate. However, no structure-activity relationships are yet apparent between specific toxicological manifestations and a particular PAE. For the most part, toxic activity toward various biological systems in rodents is only observed within very high dose ranges. One toxic manifestation frequently reported in rats exposed to DEHP is the reduction in testicular weight. This effect is much more pronounced in young, immature animals than in adults, presumably because of the undeveloped excretion mechanisms or enhanced permeability of the blood-testes barrier in very young animals. Future toxicological studies should give priority to characterizing toxicity in neonates exposed to PAEs and to determining whether significant risks exist for human newborns exposed to these chemicals.

VII. REFERENCES

Albro, P.W., Corbett, J.T., Schroeder, J.L., Jordan, S. and Mathews, H.B. (1982) Environ. Hlth. Perspect. 45, 19–25.

Autian, J. (1982) Environ. Hlth. Perspect. 45, 115–118.

Bally, M.B., Opheim, D.J. and Shertzer, H.G. (1980) Toxicology 18, 49–60.

Bell, F.P. (1982) Environ. Hlth. Perspect. 45, 41–50.

Bell, F.P., MaKowske, M., Schneider, D. and Patt, C.S. (1979) Lipids 14, 372–377.

Bower, R.K., Haberman, S. and Minton, P.D. (1970) J. Pharmacol. Exp. Ther. 171, 314–324.

Carpenter, D., Weil, C.S. and Smyth, H.F. (1953) Am. Med. Assoc. Arch. Ind. Hyg. Occup. Med. 8, 219–226.

Curto, K.A. and Thomas, J.A. (1982) Toxicol. Appl. Pharmacol. 62, 121–125.

DeHann, R.L. (1971) Nature New Biol. 231, 85–92.
Dillingham, E.O. and Autian, J. (1973) Environ. Hlth. Perspect. 3, 81–89.
Fishbein, L. and Albro, P.W. (1972) J. Chromatogr. 70, 365–412.
Gangolli, S.D. (1982) Environ. Hlth. Perspect. 45, 77–84.
Garvin, P.J., Lewandowski, M.E. and Wallin, R.F. (1976) Pharmacology 18, 231.
Gesler, R.M. (1973) Environ. Hlth. Perspect. 3, 73–79.
Hillman, L.S., Goodwin, S.L. and Sheehan, W.R. (1975) N. Engl. J. Med. 292, 381–386.
Jacobson, M.S., Parkman, R., Button, L.N., Jaeger, R.J. and Kevy, S.V. (1974) Res. Commun. Chem. Pathol. Pharmacol. 9, 315–323.
Jones, A.E., Kahn, R.A., Groves, J.T. and Napier, E.H. (1975) Toxicol. Appl. Pharmacol. 31, 283–289.
Kluwe, W.M. (1982) Environ. Hlth. Perspect. 45, 3–10.
Kozumbo, W.J., Kroll, R. and Rubin, R.J. (1982) Environ. Hlth. Perspect. 45, 103–110.
Lake, B.G., Branton, P.G., Ganolli, S.D., Butterworth, K.P. and Grasso, P. (1976) Toxicology 6, 341–356.
Lee, H. and Kalmus, G.W. (1974) Experientia 30, 800–801.
Lewandowski, M., Fernandes, J. and Chen, T.S. (1980) Toxicol. Appl. Pharmacol. 54, 141–147.
Meyler, F.L., Willebrands, A.F. and Durrer, D. (1960) Circ. Res. 8, 44–51.
Nikonorow, M., Mazur, H. and Pakacz, H. (1973) Toxicol. Appl. Pharmacol. 26, 253–259.
Parkhie, M.R., Webb, M. and Norcross, M.A. (1982) Environ. Hlth. Perspect. 45, 89–97.
Peakall, D.B. (1975) Res. Rev. 54, 1–41.
Peters, J.W. and Cook, R.M. (1973) Environ. Hlth. Perspect. 3, 91–94.
Putnam, D.L., Moore, W.A., Schechtman, L.M. and Hodgson, J.R. (1983) Environ. Mutag. 5, 227–231.
Ruddick, J.A., Villeneuve, D.C., Chu, I., Nestmann, E. and Miles, D. (1981) Bull. Environ. Contam. Toxicol. 27, 181–186.
Sanders, H.O., Mayer, F.L., Jr. and Walsh, D.F. (1973) Environ. Res. 6, 84–90.
Schaeffer, C.B., Carpenter, C.P. and Smyth, H.F., Jr. (1945) J. Ind. Hyg. Toxicol. 27, 130–135.
Seed, J.L. (1982) Environ. Hlth. Perspect. 45, 111–114.
Shiota, K. and Nishimura, H. (1982) Environ. Hlth. Perspect. 45, 65–70.
Shiota, K., Chou, M.J. and Nishimura, H. (1980) Environ. Res. 22, 245–253.
Singh, A.R., Lawrence, W.H. and Autian, J. (1972) J. Pharm. Sci. 61, 51–55.
Singh, A.R., Lawrence, W.H. and Autian, J. (1974) Toxicol. Appl. Pharmacol. 29, 35–46.
Singh, A.R., Lawrence, W.H. and Autian, J. (1975) J. Pharm. Sci. 64, 1347–1350.
Suzuki, Y. and Matsumoto, M. (1980) Jpn. J. Exp. Med. 50, 253–261.
Thomas, J.A. and Northup, S.J. (1982) J. Toxicol. Environ. Hlth. 9, 141–152.
Thomas, J.A., Darby, T.D., Wallin, R.F., Garvin, P.J. and Martis, L. (1978) Toxicol. Appl. Pharmacol. 45, 1–27.
Thomas, J.A., Schein, L.G., Gupta, P.K., McCafferty, R.E., Felice, P.R. and Donovan, M.P. (1979) Toxicol. Appl. Pharmacol. 51, 523–528.
Thomas, J.A., Martis, L., Giovanetto, S., McCafferty, R.E. and Donovan, M.P. (1980) Fed. Proc. 39, 525.
Thomas, J.A., Curto, K.A. and Thomas, M.J. (1982) Environ. Hlth. Perspect. 45, 85–88.
Tomita, I., Nakamura, Y., Yagi, Y. and Tutikawa, K. (1982a) Environ. Hlth. Perspect. 45, 71–75.
Tomita, I., Nakamura, Y., Aoki, N. and Inui, N. (1982b) Environ. Hlth. Perspect. 45, 119–125.
United States International Trade Commission (1978) Synthetic Organic Chemicals: United States Production and Sales. U.S. Government Printing Office, Washington, DC, 1978, USITC Publication No. 920.
Verrett, M.J., Mutchler, M.K., Scott, W.F., Reynaldo, E.F. and McLaughlin, J. (1969) Ann. N.Y. Acad. Sci. 160, 334–343.
Wierda, D. (1982) The Toxicologist 2, 91.
Yagi, Y., Nakamura, Y., Tomita, I., Tsuchikawa, K. and Shimoi, N. (1980) J. Environ. Pathol. Toxicol. 4, 533–544.

S. Kacew and M.J. Reasor (eds), *Toxicology and the Newborn*
© 1984 Elsevier Science Publishers B.V.

Chapter 12

Pesticides and the Neonate

BRUCE B. VIRGO,

Department of Biology, University of Windsor, Windsor, Ontario, N9B 3P4, Canada

CONTENTS

I. INTRODUCTION

A pesticide is any chemical that is used to cause the death of an organism, the pest, whose activities are undesirable to man. The major pests over which chemical control has been sought include insects, plants, fungi and rodents. These organisms compete with man or his domestic animals for food or space, or are vectors of disease. Interestingly, very large classes of nuisance organisms are excluded rather arbitrarily from the pest category, i.e., bacteria, viruses and endoparasites.

Pesticides have been employed by man for centuries. Reference to them has been made in the writings of Pliny in the first century A.D. Pyrethrum was apparently introduced to Europe by Marco Polo in the late 1200s after centuries of use in Asia. Ground tobacco (for its nicotine) was used as an insecticide by French farmers in the 16th century. However, the widespread and heavy use of pesticidal agents did not begin until the middle of this century.

In 1945 1,1-bis(4-chlorophenyl)-2,2,2-trichloroethane (DDT) and 2,4- dichlorophenoxyacetic acid (2,4-D) were placed on the market and the efficacy of these, the first synthetic organic pesticides, provided the stimulus for the development of the several hundred pesticides now available. The wide-scale employment of these compounds has resulted in the incidental exposure of many non-target species, including man.

That newborns are not simply small adults is worth reiterating, albeit trite. They differ morphologically, physiologically and biochemically from adults. For example, the neonate's CNS is only partially developed and is a site of rapidly differentiating and highly mobile cells. Similarly, the physiology of the hypothalamic/hypophyseal axis is undergoing rapid and permanent change. It is exquisitely sensitive to the negative feedback effects of gonadal steroids, but quickly loses this responsiveness. Other physiological control systems are undergoing similar change. Even the metabolic fuel differs, newborns operate on fat, adults on carbohydrate. Of great toxicological importance is the immaturity of the neonate's hepatic drug-metabolizing enzyme system. The activity of this system is very low in newborns and, in the rat, the various enzymes do not reach adult levels until 30–50 days after birth, i.e., at or after puberty.

Because of such differences, the neonate and the adult frequently respond differently to pesticides and other agents. This difference is not necessarily predictable. It may be quantitative, either greater or lesser in the neonate, or qualitative, and must be determined empirically. The response will depend upon a host of pharmacodynamic factors, which can be conveniently considered as the innate responsiveness of the target tissue(s), and upon pharmacokinetic factors, which determine how much of the agent reaches the responsive tissue and for how long it remains.

Neonates may be exposed to pesticides via three routes, the two most important of which require exposure of the mother. Thus, a very important mode of exposure occurs, while the neonate is in utero, by the transplacental passage of the pesticide from maternal to fetal circulation. Also important is oral exposure to the pesticide residues secreted in the mother's milk. The compounds favoured for such excretion are those that are lipid-soluble and, because milk is more basic than plasma, those that are acidic. One might expect that human neonates could also suffer oral exposure by ingesting insecticidal baits placed on floors or window sills. In practice, this does not occur. An examination of the age distribution of accidental poisoning in children revealed that the earliest case occurred in a 2-month-old male (Rauber, 1975). This age is 30 days after the end of the neonatal period. These authors concluded that accidental, self-inflicted poisoning is positively related to a child's increasing mobility. Human neonates are effectively immobile.

Finally, the neonates of all mammals, including man, may experience direct dermal (and respiratory) exposure from agents that are sprayed, dusted, vapourized or disseminated by other methods that are similarly open to accident and non-specificity of application. There is no evidence that such exposure is important. However, humans and beef cattle may have insecticides deliberately placed on the skin for the control of ectoparasites.

II. ORGANOCHLORINE INSECTICIDES

The organochlorine insecticides are highly lipid-soluble, resistant to environmental degradation and are metabolized into products that frequently retain substantial toxicity and lipophilicity. Consequently, they accumulate in biological tissues and concentrate in organisms at the higher levels of food chains. These agents present a distinct hazard, at present poorly evaluated, to the neonate. The use of these compounds is now severely restricted in most Western nations and the average dietary intake has been declining since the middle 1960s (Edwards, 1973). Consequently, the hazard should be declining. However, restrictions are rare in the Third World and organochlorine residues on foods imported from them may escape detection by regulatory agencies, so that the hazard may be declining more slowly than it should.

1. Acute toxicity

Organochlorine insecticides are CNS stimulants that cause a variety of symptoms, but generally effect death by cardiac and/or respiratory arrest. The early symptoms of intoxication include facial paresthesia, dizziness, tremors and disequilibrium, and, later, clonic and tonic convulsions occur. Cardiac arrest may occur from parasympathetic stimulation. Indeed, dieldrin, and aldrin, its metabolic precursor, appear to act in this manner (Gowdey and Staviaky, 1955). More commonly, the medullary centre for cardiovascular control fails during the postictal depression and thus causes cardiac arrest. Similarly, paralysis of the respiratory muscles may result from either excessive or insufficient cholinergic stimulation from the medullary respiratory centre.

In general, the neonate is considered less susceptible than the adult to CNS stimulation by organochlorine insecticides. Lu et al. (1965) found that for DDT the

LD_{50} in 1-day-old rats exceeded 4000 mg/kg, while in adults it was 194 mg/kg. Similar values were obtained by Harbison (1974). The LD_{50} for 10-day-old rats was found to be 728 mg/kg compared to 250 mg/kg for adults (Henderson and Woolley, 1969). In the case of DDT, the newborn's insensitivity appears to be due partly to the inefficiency of the immature CNS in sequestering the compound from the blood (Henderson and Woolley, 1969). However, these authors observed that the CNS levels of DDT in dead neonates exceeded those in dead adults, suggesting that the newborn's CNS is innately less responsive than that of the adult. On the other hand, DDT causes hyperthermia and convulsions in the adult, responses that are absent in the neonate and which may effect its greater lethality in mature animals (Henderson and Woolley, 1969). Furthermore, the toxicity of DDT in newborns is increased 2-fold by the concomitant administration of phenobarbital (Harbison, 1974), suggesting that the maturation of the hepatic mixed-function oxidase system plays a role in the greater susceptibility of the adult.

Chlordane and heptachlor, both cyclodiene compounds, are also less acutely toxic in the newborn (Harbison, 1974). In contrast, another cyclodiene, dieldrin, is apparently more toxic in the neonate. The LD_{50} in 5-day-old mice is 27 mg/kg, 50% of that for adult females (Costella and Virgo, 1980). In 5- and 10-day-old rats the LD_{50} is 38 and 27 mg/kg, respectively, while in adult males it is 63 mg/kg (Fox and Virgo, 1982). Similarly, Iizuka (1963) found the LD_{50} to be 11 mg/kg in 11-day-old rats. In contrast to these data, Lu et al. (1965) reported an LD_{50} of 168 mg/kg for 1-day-old rats and 37 mg/kg for 60-day-old adults. The reasons for these discrepancies are not clear. The mechanism of the enhanced neonatal toxicity, in the cases where it has been found, is also not clear. However, it does not appear to involve CNS stimulation as dieldrin-treated newborns do not tremor or convulse, or show other symptoms of CNS excitation. Similarly, the dieldrin-induced alterations in carbohydrate metabolism that are seen in adult rats (Kacew and Singhal, 1974) and prenatally treated newborn mice (Costella and Virgo, 1980) do not occur in neonatal rats acutely exposed to a one-LD_{50} dose (Fox and Virgo, 1982).

In humans, the immediate and most important source of organochlorine insecticides is the mother's milk. In turn, the diet is the immediate source of insecticides for most lactating women. The concentration of persistent insecticides in milk is proportional to that in the food, although the exact relationship differs markedly from compound to compound as a function of their physico-chemical properties. Thus, the excretion ratios (ppm in whole milk/dietary ppm) in dairy cattle are: heptachlor epoxide, 0.5; aldrin, 0.39; dieldrin, 0.19–0.39; endrin, 0.07; DDT, 0.04; lindane, 0.038; chlordane, 4×10^{-4}–2×10^{-3} and methoxychlor, 2.3×10^{-4} (Saha, 1969). The levels in human milk vary geographically (see Olszyna-Marzyo (1978) for a review), but in general are substantially higher in the Third World nations compared to the developed countries. In the US the daily dietary intake of DDT, heptachlor epoxide and dieldrin is 0.041, 0.003 and 0.007 mg, respectively (Duggan and Duggan, 1973), while their levels in human milk are 50–200, 8–30 and 1–6 ppm (Rogan et al., 1980). An infant receiving milk containing these levels exceeds the USFDA Maximum Daily Allowance for each compound by 5–8-fold. However, these doses would not cause death, and the immediate and long-term consequences of such exposure are unknown. The possibility of intellectual or emotional impairment requires examination.

It is clear, however, that human neonates can receive lethal doses of organochlorine insecticides through the milk, provided the maternal exposure is high enough. Thus, during 1957, mass poisoning occurred in Turkey due to the consumption of seed grain treated with hexachlorobenzene. Many nursing infants developed pink skin, progressively lost weight, and died (Peters, 1976). Since children in this society receive only breast milk for at least the first 2 years of life, the source of the intoxicant seems evident. The milk is implicated further by the fact that cessation of breast feeding effected a slowing of the development of the toxicity syndrome, the so-called pemba yarda syndrome. Interestingly, the infants of many of the survivors of the 1957 poisoning have also developed pemba yarda, presumably from the hexachlorobenzene stored in the mother during that time (Cripps et al., 1980). Similar neonatal deaths have been reported from India (Khare et al., 1977; Gupta, 1975), as has severe hyperkinesia and mental retardation in the survivors.

Neonates are born with a body burden of organochlorine insecticides that were received in utero via the placenta. The ease with which an agent crosses the placenta varies. Radomski et al. (1971) found that the placental permeability ranged from 0.4 to 0.8 in humans. Thus, in Argentina the blood levels (ppb) of various pesticides in the mother and her neonate were: DDT, 6.9 and 2.8: 2,2-bis(4-chlorophenyl)-1,1-dichloroethylene (DDE), 13.4 and 5.2; dieldrin, 1.6 and 0.7; and lindane, 0.2 and 0.16. The maternal levels are comparable to those found in women in the US. Again, the significance of the neonatal levels is unknown.

The use of lindane against scabies and pediculosis has resulted in the acute intoxication of infants and children (Lee and Groth, 1977). Those afflicted show typical symptoms of CNS hyperexcitability: irritability, restlessness, tremors and, occasionally, convulsions. All affected have recovered and the long-term effects have not been followed. Typically, the proximate cause is a deliberate or accidental prolongation of exposure (Kramer et al. 1980; Shacter 1981). However, absorption may vary with the condition of the skin (Pramanik and Hansen, 1979) and can precipitate toxicity with normal doses. Thus, normal post-therapy blood levels are 5 ng/ml, while in an infant with a severe scabies infection it was 100 ng/ml, and in a child treated only on the rash areas of the body it was 12 ng/ml.

2. *Chronic toxicity*

Organochlorine insecticides are extremely stable and persist in the environment for many years. Moreover, they are very lipophilic. Consequently, they are stored in biological tissues, in proportion to the dose received (Hayes, 1965; Quaiffe et al., 1967), and the highest levels are found in the organisms at the top of food chains.

The possible impairment of mammalian reproductive processes by chronic exposure to residue levels of these insecticides has been evaluated in some 30 studies published since 1948. Typically, the female (and frequently the male) is placed on a diet containing the test insecticide and then mated. The female is then retained on the diet during pregnancy and lactation. Such studies have shown that the insecticides have remarkedly little effect on fertility, litter size, gestation period, etc. (Virgo and Bellward, 1975). However, many produced neonatal mortality (e.g., dieldrin: Murphy and Korschgen (1970), Keplinger et al. (1970), Virgo and Bellward (1975); DDT: Fitzhugh (1948); endrin: Morris (1968); chlordane: Keplinger et al. (1970)).

When caused by dieldrin, the mortality is clearly dose-dependent (Fig. 1). Moreover, either all the pups in a litter die or a normal proportion survive until weaning (Virgo and Bellward, 1975). The reason for this resistance, seen in some litters, is unknown. Only a few of the losses, generally those at high doses, are attributable to abnormal maternal behaviour (Virgo and Bellward, 1975). Of greater significance is the fact that the offspring from dieldrin-treated mice die even when foster-nursed by non-treated females (Fig. 2). Thus, these neonates are congenitally inviable and will die because of the insecticide received in utero. That dieldrin in the milk contributes to these deaths has not been excluded. It is not possible to determine whether the neonatal deaths caused by other insecticides also result from in utero exposure, because fostering studies were not conducted.

The proximate cause of death in the pups exposed in utero is not clear. Dieldrin, at doses that cause inviability, is a potent inducer of the mixed-function oxidase system that metabolizes drugs and steroids. However, exposure of the pregnant female did not lower plasma progesterone levels (Virgo, 1980) and this is the only steroid necessary in the mouse to maintain gestation and permit normal fetal development. The pups show no symptoms of CNS stimulation, but carbohydrate metabolism is

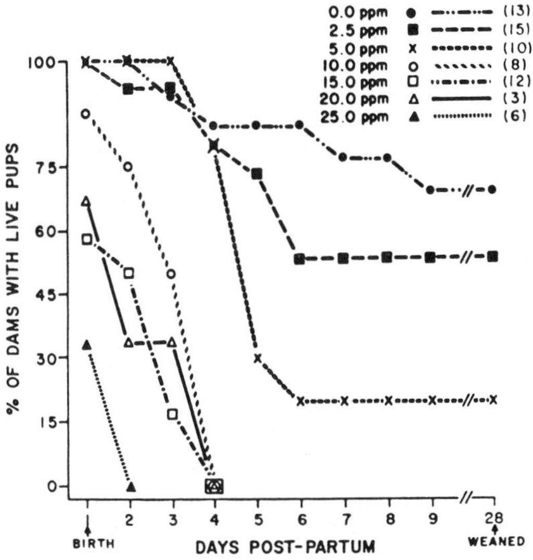

Figure 1. Effect of dietary dieldrin on the proportion of females with one or more living newborns. Number of females in brackets. From Virgo and Bellward (1975), with permission.

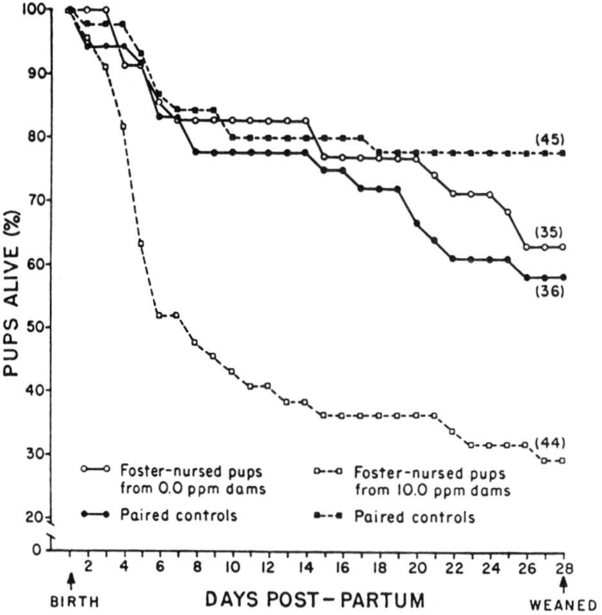

Figure 2. Survival of neonates born to females fed 10 ppm dietary dieldrin and foster nursed by dams fed 0 ppm dieldrin. The foster dams raised some of their own offspring as controls (●, and ■). Fostering per se did not affect survival (i.e. ○ vs. ●, $P<0.10$). Exposure to dieldrin in utero significantly decreased survival (i.e., □ vs. ■, $P<0.005$). From Virgo and Bellward (1977), reproduced with kind permission from PJD Publications Limited, Westbury, NY 11590, U.S.A., from Res. Commun. Chem. Pathol. Pharmacol. (1977) 17, 309–409.

altered (Costella and Virgo, 1980). Thus, blood glucose is decreased at birth and is undetectable 24 hours later; the hepatic, cardiac and muscle stores of glycogen are normal at birth but are reduced markedly 24 hours postpartum (Table 1). It is clear that dieldrin stimulates a rapid utilization of endogenous carbohydrate at a time when the gluconeogenic pathways are essentially inoperative (Girard et al., 1975; Costella and Virgo, 1980) and the processes of lactation and digestion are not yet fully developed. This is a time when energy requirements must be met from the finite reserves laid down during fetal development. There is evidence that dieldrin uncouples oxidative phosphorylation (Bergen, 1971) and it is possible that this may be the key lesion in the inviable neonates. However, it has also been well established that the survival time of anoxic neonates is related directly to the initial glycogen concentrations in the myocardium (Dawes and Shelley, 1968), and their depletion may very well compromise cardiac function.

Some of the changes associated with Mirex-induced neonatal deaths are also known. A prominent feature is marked oedema, the result of decreased plasma protein levels and lowered colloidal osmotic pressure (Grabowski, 1981). This condition may cause cardiovascular insufficiency by lowering venous return. Some 16% of the

TABLE 1

THE CONCENTRATIONS OF PLASMA GLUCOSE AND TISSUE GLYCOGEN IN NEONATES BORN TO DIELDRIN-TREATED MICE

Age of pup (h)	Blood glucose (%)	Liver glycogen (%)	Heart glycogen (%)	Muscle glycogen (%)
0	73±15.6	99± 5.8	94±10.0	94±12.0
19	56±13.4	62±13.0	104±21.0	92± 6.3
24	0*	23± 1.1**	50± 3.7*	40± 0.1*

The dosage was 2 mg/kg/day orally, over days 6–18 of pregnancy. Results are presented as a percentage of control, n = 8–16. Levels of significance are as follows: *$P<0.05$; **$P<0.01$. From Costella and Virgo (1980) Can. J. Physiol. Pharmacol. 58, 635. Reproduced by permission of the National Research Council of Canada from the Canadian Journal of Physiology and Pharmacology, Volume 58, 1980.

offspring are delivered with first- or second-degree heart blocks, while another 4% fail to initiate respiratory activities (Grabowski and Payne, 1983). While the cardiovascular and pulmonary problems seem to be important proximate causes of death, their ultimate causation is unknown.

The effects on the newborn of DDT in the milk have been studied by Fahim et al. (1970), who treated rats with technical DDT from day 2 to day 21 of lactation. A dose of 1 mg/kg/day increased neonatal mortality and decreased the growth of the survivors, while 5 mg/kg/day caused 100% mortality. As in the reproductive studies, most deaths occurred in the first 7 days of life. Of interest is the finding that DDT reduced hepatic calcium and increased hepatic copper in the neonates. The latter may indicate that DDT prevents the transport of copper from its thionein-storage sites, thus reducing its availability for the synthesis of the copper-containing enzymes and other important copper-proteins.

III. ORGANOPHOSPHOROUS AND CARBAMATE INSECTICIDES

The insecticides that inhibit acetylcholinesterase (AchE) have largely replaced the organochlorine compounds because their environmental persistence, days or weeks, is much less, although their acute toxicity is substantially greater. These agents include the phosphate triesters, the phosphorothionates and the carbamate esters.

The mechanism of action is similar for all AchE inhibitors and involves the covalent linkage, via an ester, of the serine residue at the enzyme's esteratic site to the phosphate or carbamyl moiety on the insecticide (Murphy, 1980). The duration of inhibition varies with the insecticide. Carbamates are generally hydrolyzed from the enzyme within a few hours, as are a few of the phosphates, such as trichlorfon. Other phosphates, such as diisopropyl phosphofluoridate (DFP), form complexes with the enzyme that do not dissociate spontaneously.

The consequences of AchE inhibition result from the large number of loci where acetylcholine is used as a neurotransmitter and from its effects on the postsynaptic tissues. Thus, all of these may occur: 1, stimulation of muscarinic end organs; 2, stimulation, followed by inhibition, of nicotinic sites (autonomic ganglia and skeletal muscle); and 3, stimulation, followed by inhibition, of CNS cholinergic areas (mainly muscarinic). In acute poisoning one typically sees: 1, miosis, ciliary spasm, broncho-constriction and -spasm leading to chest tightness and wheezing breathing, gastrointestinal cramps, diarrhoea, nausea, and vomiting; 2, muscle weakness and paralysis. The former are muscarinic effects while the latter are nicotinic responses. In more severe intoxication, salivation, bradycardia, hypotension, lacrimation, urination and defecation may occur. In mild cases of poisoning the CNS effects are ataxia and slurred speech; with increasing doses convulsions, coma, and depression of the medullary vasomotor and respiratory centres occurs.

It is clear that neonates are more susceptible than adults to AchE inhibitors. The triester phosphates and carbamates do not require biotransformation into an active metabolite, but the phosphorothionates do. The required reaction, oxidative desulphuration, yields the active 'oxon' metabolite and is catalyzed by a hepatic cytochrome *P*-450 system which requires NADPH and molecular oxygen. This system is poorly developed in neonates, and in the case of the rat does not reach full activity until 30–50 days of age. Thus, one might expect the adult to be more sensitive than the newborn to the phosphorothionates, but this is not the case: the toxicities of *O*-ethyl-*O*-(4-nitrophenyl) phenylphosphonothioate (EPN), parathion, methylparathion and malathion are 2–5-fold greater in the newborn (Brodeur and DuBois, 1963). Apparently, the in vivo level of active insecticides is limited not by the activation process but rather by detoxification, excretion or redistribution. In the case of malathion, the level of the activating enzyme remains constant for the first 30 days of life and is substantially greater than carboxylic ester hydrolase, the enzyme that degrades malaoxon (Brodeur and DuBois, 1967). The latter enzyme increases during the preweaning period, so that by 30 days of age malaoxon inactivation is equal to its rate of production. Thus, in the newborn the enhanced toxicity reflects, in part, a relatively slow rate of detoxification. However, other enzymatic parameters may also play a role. Mendoza (1976) found that the specific activity of brain AchE is lowest in the 1-day-old rat, and increases for at least the next 3 months. This implies that the number of AchE molecules increases with age and/or that the catalytic activity of the existing molecules increases. In either case, Mass Law predicts that for any concentration of insecticide more AchE will be inhibited in newborns than in adults. Thus, neonatal toxicity will occur at lower doses. Since adult levels of AchE are not attained by the human infant until 4 months of age (Karlsen et al., 1981), one would predict a similar effect in man.

There is also evidence that the enhanced neonatal toxicity of the *O*-arylphosphorothionates (e.g., parathion, EPN) is related to a low rate of detoxification. Their detoxification is effected by hydrolysis of the aryl ester bond, and in the newborn the activity of the enzyme responsible is only 50% of the adult value (Neal and DuBois, 1965).

Thus, the relative immaturity of the detoxification systems of young rats plays an important role in their increased susceptibility to AchE inhibitors. However, the overall metabolic pathways, activating as well as deactivating, are so complicated for most of the agents (Nakatsugawa and Morelli, 1976) that the net effects on toxicity are not easily discernible.

AchE inhibitors are widely used in the beef cattle industry to control ecto- and endoparasites. As in rodents, the toxicity of the agents is greater in calves than in older animals. The magnitude of the difference varies from 30-fold for chlorpyrifos (Palmer et al., 1980) to 2-fold for disulfoton (McCarty et al., 1969). The reasons for these differences have not been investigated.

As discussed above, a potentially important route of neonatal exposure to organochlorine insecticides is the mother's milk. This is not the case with AchE inhibitors. The excretion of carbamate and phosphate insecticides, in milk, either does not occur or is extremely low. Thus, diazinon fed to dairy cows for 6 weeks at dietary doses of 100–500 ppm produced no detectable residues in the milk (Derbyshire and Murphy, 1962). On the other hand, guthion, fed at 35 ppm for 14 days, did not appear in the milk, but its active oxygen analogue did, at a level of 0.17 ppm (Loeffler et al., 1966). The excretion ratio for this compound, 0.006, compares with those for some of the more poorly excreted organochlorines. However, since AchE inhibitors do not accumulate in the tissues any excretion through the milk will cease when exposure of the mother ceases. There are no reports of suckling neonates with symptoms of AchE inhibition.

IV. HERBICIDES

The synthetic organic herbicides have largely replaced the more toxic inorganic compounds used until the release of 2,4-D. In general, the new herbicides are degraded rapidly in the environment and do not accumulate in biological materials. Moreover, their mammalian toxicity ranges from low (g/kg) to moderate (hundreds of mg/kg). Herbicides form a very small proportion of the total pesticide residue in human food. Of 22 organic residues commonly found in food samples taken in 1971 the sole herbicide found was 2,4-D, and it comprised only 0.8% of the total residue by weight (Duggan and Corneliussen, 1972). Thus, these compounds represent little risk to the neonate.

The phenoxyacetic compounds are used more widely than all other herbicides combined (Hassall, 1969). They are moderately toxic, the LD_{50} for the free acid of 2,4-D is 375 mg/kg and for 2,4,5-trichlorophenoxyacetic acid (2,4,5-T) it is 500 mg/kg (Metcalf, 1971), but they degrade in the environment in a few weeks to months.

In rats, however, prenatal exposure to relatively low doses of 2,4-D esters (150 mg/kg) has been reported to cause neonatal mortality both immediately after birth and close to weaning (Schwetz et al., 1971). However, 2,4-D acid was ineffective. Whether the cause of the mortality was effected in utero, or postpartum, or both, is unknown. Similarly, 2,4,5-T acquired notoriety as a teratogen in a variety of species at doses considerably lower than the LD_{50}. However, the teratogenicity was probably caused by the presence of 2,3,7,8-tetrachlorodibenzo-*p*-dioxin (TCDD) in the technical 2,4,5-T formulations that were tested (Courtney et al., 1970). Prenatal exposure to 2,4,5-T containing low amounts of TCDD (0.5 ppm) does not produce terata or postnatal mortality (Moore and Courtney, 1971; Thompson et al., 1971). Several retrospective studies seeking pre- or postnatal effects of 2,4,5-T in man have been conducted and generally have found no relationship between the pesticide and congenital defects. The exception has been an apparent link between 2,4,5-T spraying and an increased frequency of talipes (Hanify et al., 1981).

The dinitrophenol herbicides are uncouplers of oxidative phosphorylation and are highly toxic to many classes of organisms. Thus, they also find use as insecticides and fungicides. The two most commonly used as herbicides, 4,6-dinitrocresol (DNOC) and 2,4-dinitro-*O*-sec-butylphenol (dinoseb), have mammalian LD_{50} values of 30 and 80 mg/kg, respectively. Both accumulate in biological materials because of their lipid solubility and both are weak acids. Thus, excretion in the milk is possible, although there are no reports of neonatal intoxication from such exposure.

The prenatal exposure of mice to these compounds causes hydronephrosis and long-lived (permanent?) changes in kidney function, as indicated by a reduction in *para*-aminohippuric acid (PAH) accumulation in kidney slices from adults (Gibson, 1976). McCormack et al. (1980) have found that hydronephrosis also occurs in rats, but that kidney function is unaltered either at birth or at 42 days of life.

The bipyridylium herbicides include paraquat, of high mammalian toxicity (LD_{50} is 57 mg/kg) and the most common single chemical used in successful suicides in Britain (Fitzgerald et al., 1978). Death is effected by pulmonary fibrosis, leading to respiratory insufficiency, and perhaps by kidney damage. Others in the class, notably diquat, are much less toxic (LD_{50} is 400 mg/kg). All are degraded rapidly in soils by base-exchange with the cations of clay minerals, none accumulate in biological tissues, and thus these agents pose little risk to the newborn. However, Bus and Gibson (1975) have shown in rats that 100 ppm of paraquat in the drinking water, from day 8 of gestation to day 42 of postpartum life, increases neonatal mortality. This occurs as an early peak, due to oxygen toxicity effected by the paraquat sequestered in the lungs prenatally, and as a later peak, at weaning, when the offspring begin to drink the water. The youngest child reported to have been fatally poisoned by paraquat was 18 months old (Burman et al., 1972).

V. FUNGICIDES

The properties of the synthetic organic fungicides are similar to those of the herbicides. Most are rapidly destroyed in the soil, lasting only a few days or weeks. Similarly, most are of low mammalian toxicity and do not accumulate in biological tissues. In general, they present little risk to the neonate; however, some compounds, notably the organomercurials and hexachlorobenzene, potentially are hazardous.

Captan, a broad spectrum fungicide, has been the most widely and extensively used of the fungicidal agents (FAO/WHO, 1970). It is generally considered as one of the safest of all fungicides because of its high LD_{50} (15 g/kg), rapid mammalian detoxification (human half-life is 60 seconds), and complete degradation in the soil within a week of application (FAO/WHO, 1970; Griffiths and Mathews, 1969). Accumulation in biological tissues does not occur and, although it may persist on vegetation, little enters the plant, so that adequate washing will remove it (FAO/WHO, 1970).

Because the compound is a phthalimide derivative, much effort has been directed towards establishing its teratogenic potential. In most species, including rabbits, the compound does not produce terata (Boyd, 1973). However, McLaughlin et al. (1969), using the same dose (75 mg/kg/day) and rabbit strains as others, found that 12% of the fetuses were abnormal in their study. No neonatal deaths have been reported to result from prenatal exposure. Captan is presently a suspected carcinogen (Fairchild, 1978; Decloitre and Martin, 1980) and its continued wide-scale use is in question.

The majority of the organomercurials are of moderate to high acute toxicity (e.g., ethylmercuric chloride, 30 mg/kg; methoxyethylmercuric chloride, 570 mg/kg). However, the chronic toxicity of these compounds greatly exceeds their acute toxicity. For example, the LD_{50} for phenylmercuric acetate is 2100 mg/kg, but consuming a dietary concentration of 0.5 ppm for 90 days causes serious kidney damage (Metcalf, 1971). This propensity for chronic toxicity is of serious concern since these agents are lipid-soluble and contain Hg^{2+}, and thus accumulate in biological tissues.

The neurotoxicity of the organomercurials has been well established in man (Bakir et al., 1980) and animals (Reuhl et al., 1981) of all ages. Since the toxicology of methylmercury is covered in chapter 8 of this volume, it suffices to say: 1, that the damage inflicted by organomercurials is inversely related to age, with prenatal exposure being most hazardous (Spyker and Spyker, 1977; Amin-Zaki et al., 1979); and 2, impairment of behaviour occurs at doses that do not cause biochemical or morphological lesions in the CNS (Weis and Spyker, 1974).

Hexachlorobenzene is used as a fungicidal seed dressing as well as an insecticide and, as discussed above, large-scale poisonings of human neonates have occurred on several occasions in the Third World due to the eating of foods made from treated grain and the subsequent contamination of breast milk.

VI. RODENTICIDES

Historically, the inorganic compounds arsenic, barium, thallium and phosphorous and the plant toxins strychnine and Red Squill have been employed in baits to control rodents. More recently, these have been replaced by the synthetic compounds sodium fluoroacetate (compound 1080) and warfarin.

Compound 1080 is extremely toxic, its LD_{50} is 0.5 mg/kg, and is used on wild carnivores as well as on rodents. Its mechanism of action is inhibition of the trichloroacetic acid cycle, leading to a deficiency of ATP: fluoroacetic acid, formed in vivo by the condensation of fluoroacetate and oxaloacetic acid, is a potent inhibitor of the enzyme aconitase. In most jurisdictions, its acute toxicity has restricted its use to licensed pest-control operators and government personnel. Thus, the hazard it poses to neonates is limited. In the recent literature there is but one report of a child being poisoned — an 8-month-old, who recovered upon treatment (Reigart et al., 1975).

Warfarin is an anticoagulant, and in the rat several days exposure to 1 mg/kg/day effectively inhibits prothrombin formation by antagonizing the effects of vitamin K. Death results from hemorrhage. When employed as a rodenticide, warfarin offers little risk to neonates. Of 38 children who ingested warfarin baits all were 9 months of age or older, and none developed toxicity symptoms (Gehlbach and Williams, 1977). However, warfarin is also employed therapeutically and it is believed generally that its use in the first trimester of pregnancy causes a cluster of teratogenic defects (Stevenson et al., 1980; Pauli and Hall, 1979), although Warkany (1976) has pointed out that all of the presumed cases are confounded by the mothers' simultaneous use of other drugs and/or exposure to environmental chemicals.

VII. SUMMARY

The newborn differs morphologically, physiologically and biochemically from the mature organism. Of particular toxicological significance are differences in the hepatic monooxygenases and in the CNS. The former affect the levels of pharmacologically active pesticides in vivo, because of differences in the rates of activation and detoxification, and this largely explains the greater toxicity of acetylcholinesterase inhibitors in neonates. The latter is expressed as an innate difference in the responsiveness of the CNS to a compound and appears to explain the lesser toxicity of most organachlorine insecticides in newborns.

Exposure of the newborn to pesticides may occur via dermal or respiratory contact to sprays, dusts, etc., via the mother's milk or via the placenta during in utero development. Direct contact is not an important exposure route. Exposure via the placenta or milk is proportional to the degree of maternal exposure and is especially significant for lipid-soluble compounds that accumulate in the mother's tissues.

The organochlorine insecticides remain the agents with the greatest potential impact on newborns. This is true even in the Western world, where their use and human intake has been reduced markedly over the past 15 years. The hazard is largely due to their longevity in the environment, their lipophilicity and their bioaccumulation in tissues. Even humans are born with ppb levels in their plasma, although the significance of these are unknown. DDT, heptachlor epoxide and chlordane are less acutely toxic to newborns than to adults, perhaps because lower amounts are taken into the CNS and perhaps because the CNS is unresponsive. Dieldrin is more toxic to neonates. Chronic exposure to residue levels of most organochlorines produces neonatal mortality. Dieldrin causes mortality by exposure in utero; the ultimate cause may be energy deficiency due to the rapid depletion of tissue glycogen that occurs postpartum. Mirex causes cardiac defects and respiratory malfunction. Human neonates have died from hexachlorobenzene in their mother's milk; indeed, the offspring of surviving females have also developed intoxication symptoms due to the agent being mobilized from body tissues and excreted in the milk.

Organophosphate and carbamate insecticides, herbicides, fungicides and rodenticides present less hazard to the newborn. In general, these compounds degrade rapidly in the environment, are relatively hydrophilic and are excreted rapidly. Hence, there is little accumulation in tissues and they impact the fetus/newborn only when the female is directly exposed. All classes contain exceptions to these generalizations, e.g., dinitrophenol herbicides, organomercurial fungicides.

The organophosphate insecticides are of greater toxicity to neonates than to adults because they detoxify the agent more slowly. Also, there is less acetylcholinesterase in the newborn's brain and significant inhibition would be produced by lower doses of insecticide.

Esters of 2,4-D cause neonatal mortality by unknown means, but the free acid does not. The dinitrophenols when given to the fetus cause hydronephrosis in newborns and perhaps alter the mechanisms of nephron secretion in adults. Paraquat exposure in utero precipitates oxygen toxicity and death in the neonate.

The organomercurials are the fungicides of greatest concern. They are lipid-soluble and are stored in tissues. Their chronic toxicities occur at doses much lower than the acute LD_{50}. Damage to the CNS is of most concern and is inversely proportional to the age at exposure; in utero exposure is most damaging. Of current concern is the possible carcinogenicity of Captan, the most widely used fungicide.

The rodenticides, warfarin and sodium fluoroacetate, present little hazard to newborns because of the controls on their use.

In conclusion: 1, the newborn generally is less responsive to organochlorine insecticides than the adult and more responsive to organophosphates; 2, age-dependent toxicity data is not available for the other pesticides; 3, except for the acetylcholinesterase inhibitors, the mechanisms of pesticide toxicity in neonates are poorly understood.

VIII. REFERENCES

Amin-Zaki, L., Majeed, M.A., Elhassani, S.B., Clarkson, T. W., Greenwood, M.R. and Doherty, R.A. (1979) Am. J. Dis. Child. 133, 172–177.

Bakir, F., Rustam, H., Tikriti, S., Al-Dambyi, S.F. and Shidristani, H. (1980) Postgrad. Med. J. 56, 1–10.

Bergen, W. (1971) Proc. Soc. Exp. Biol. Med. 136, 732–735.

Boyd, E.M. (1973) in Pesticides and The Environment (Deichmann, W. B., ed.), Vol. 2, pp. 277–305, Intercontinental Medical Book Corp., New York.

Brodeur, J. and DuBois, K.P. (1963) Proc. Soc. Exp. Biol. Med. 114, 509–511.

Brodeur, J. and DuBois, K.P. (1967) Can. J. Physiol. Pharmacol. 45, 621–631.

Burman, D., Hodson, A.K. and Mott, M.G. (1972) Lancet 1, 201.

Bus, T.S. and Gibson, J.E. (1975) Toxicol. Appl. Pharmacol. 33, 461–470.

Costella, J.C. and Virgo, B.B. (1980) Can. J. Physiol. Pharmacol. 58, 633–637.

Courtney, K.D., Gaylor, D.W., Hogan, M.D., Falk, H.L., Bates, R.R. and Mitchell, I. (1970) Science 168, 864–866.

Cripps, D.J., Gormen, A. and Peters, H.A. (1980) Arch. Dermatol. 116, 46–50.

Dawes, G.S. and Shelley, H.J. (1968) in Carbohydrate Metabolism and Its Disorders (Dickens, R., Randle, R.J. and Whelan, W.J., eds.), pp. 87–121, Academic Press, London.

Decloitre, F. and Martin, M. (1980) Carcinogensis 1, 329–336.

Derbyshire, J.C. and Murphy, R.T. (1962) J. Agric. Food Chem. 10, 384–386.

Duggan, R.E. and Corneliussen, P.E. (1972) Pestic. Monit. J. 5, 331–341.

Duggan, R.E. and Duggan, M.B. (1973) in Environmental Pollution by Pesticides (Edwards, C.A., ed.), pp. 334–364, Plenum Press, New York.

Edwards, C.A. (1973) Persistent Pesticides in the Environment, pp. 99–124, CRC Press, Cleveland, OH.

Fahim, M.S., Bennett, R. and Hall, D.G. (1970) Nature 228, 1222–1223.

Fairchild, E.J. (1978) Suspected Carcinogens, National Institute of Occupational Safety and Health, Castle House Publishing, Philadelphia, PA.

FAO/WHO (1970) The Monographs. FAO/PL:1969/M/17/1, WHO/Food Add. /70.38. FAO and WHO, United Nations, Rome.

Fitzgerald, G.R., Earniville, G., Flanagan, M., Silke, B. and Carmody, M. (1978) J. Ir. Med. Assoc. 71, 103–108.

Fitzhugh, O.G. (1948) Ind. Eng. Chem. Ind. Ed. 704–705.

Fox, G.R. and Virgo, B.B. (1982) Proc. Can. Fed. Biol. Soc. 25, 47.

Gehlbach, S.H. and Williams, W.A. (1977) South Med. J. 70, 12–24.

Gibson, J.E. (1976) Environ. Hlth. Perspect. 15, 2121–2130.

Girard, J.R., Cuendet, G.S., Maruss, E.B., Keruran, A., Rientort, M. and Assan, R. (1975) Am. J. Physiol. 229, 446–473.

Gowdey, C.W. and Staviaky, G.W. (1955) Can. J. Biochem. Physiol. 33, 272–282.

Grabowski, C.T. (1981) J. Toxicol. Environ. Hlth. 7, 705–714.

Grabowski, C.T. and Payne, P.B. (1983) J. Toxicol. Environ. Hlth. 11, 301–315.

Griffiths, R.L. and Mathews, S. (1969) Ann. Appl. Biol. 64, 113–118.

Gupta, P.C. (1975) Indian J. Med. Res. 63, 601–606.

Hanify, J.A., Metcalf, P., Nobbs, C.L. and Worsley, K.J. (1981) Science 212, 349–351.

Harbison, R.D. (1974) Toxicol. Appl. Pharmacol. 32, 443–446.

Hassall, K.E. (1969) World Crop Protection, Vol. 2, pp. 154–208, Iliffe Books, London.

Hayes, W.J. (1965) Annu. Rev. Pharmacol. 5, 27–52.

Henderson, G.L. and Woolley, D.E. (1969) J. Pharmacol. Exp. Ther. 170, 173–180.

Iizuka, Y. (1963) Sangyoigaku 5, 746–756.

Kacew, S. and Singhal, R.L. (1974) J. Pharmacol. Exp. Ther. 188, 265–276.

Karlsen, R.L., Stern, S., Lyngaas, S. and Fonnum, F. (1981) Scand. J. Clin. Lab. Invest. 41, 301–302.

Keplinger, M.L., Deichmann, W.B. and Sala, F. (1970) in Pesticide Symposium (Deichmann, W.B., ed.), p. 125, Halos, Miami, FL.

Khare, S.B., Rizvi, A.G., Shukla, O.P., Singh, R.R., Perkash, C., Misra, V.D., Gupta, J.P. and Sethi, P.K. (1977) J. Assoc. Physic. India 25, 215–222.

Kramer, M., Hutchinson, T.A., Rudnik, S.A. and Leventhal, J.M. (1980) Clin. Pharmacol. Therap. 27, 149–155.

Lee, B. and Groth, P. (1977) Pediatrics 59, 643.

Loeffler, W.W., Trimberger, G.W., Fox, F.H., Ridgeway, R.L., Lisk, D.J. and Gyrisco, G.G. (1966) J. Agric. Food Chem. 14, 46–47.

Lu, F.C., Jessup, D.C. and Lavallee, A. (1965) Food Cosmet. Toxicol. 3, 591–596.

McCarty, R.T., Haufler, M., Osborn, M.G. and McBeth, C.A. (1969) Am. J. Vet. Res. 30, 1149–1153.

McCormack, K.M., Abuelgasim, A., Sanger, V.L. and Hook, J.B. (1980) J. Toxicol. Environ. Hlth. 6, 633–643.

McLaughlin, J., Reynaldo, E.F., Lamar, J.K. and Marliac, J.-P. (1969) Toxicol. Appl. Pharmacol. 14, 641.

Mendoza, C.E. (1976) Toxicol. Appl. Pharmacol. 35, 229–238.
Metcalf, R.L. (1971) in Pesticides in the Environment (White-Stevens, R., ed.), Vol. 1, Part 1, pp. 1–144, Marcel Dekker, New York.
Moore, J.A. and Courtney, K.D. (1971) Teratology 4, 236.
Morris, R.D. (1968) Can. J. Zool. 46, 951–958.
Murphy, D.A. and Korshgen, L.J. (1970) J. Wildl. Manage. 34, 887–903.
Murphy, S.D. (1980) in Toxicology: The Basic Science of Poisons (Doull, J., Klaassen, C.D. and Amdur, M.O., eds.), 2nd edn., pp. 357–408, Macmillan, New York.
Nakatsugawa, T. and Morelli, M.A. (1976) in Insecticide Biochemistry and Physiology (Wilkinson, C.F., ed.), pp. 61–114, Plenum Press, New York.
Neal, R.A. and DuBois, K.P. (1965) J. Pharmacol. Exp. Ther. 148, 185–199.
Olszyna-Marzyo, A.E. (1978) Acta Paediatr. Scand. 67, 571–576.
Palmer, J.S., Rowe, L.D. and Crookshank, H.R. (1980) Am. J. Vet. Res. 41, 1320–1323.
Pauli, R.M. and Hall, J.G. (1979) Lancet 2, 144.
Peters, H.A. (1976) Fed. Proc. Am. Soc. Exp. Biol. 35, 2400–2403.
Pramanik, A.K. and Hansen, R.C. (1979) Arch. Dermatol. 115, 1224–1225.
Quaiffe, M., Winbush, W. and Fitzhugh, O.G. (1967) Food Cosmet. Toxicol. 5, 39–50.
Radomski, J.L., Astolfi, E., Deichmann, W.B. and Rey, A.A. (1971) Toxicol. Appl. Pharmacol. 20, 186–193.
Rauber, A. (1975) Clin. Toxicol. 8, 391–397.
Reigart, J.R., Brueggeman, J.L. and Keil, J.E. (1975) Am. J. Dis. Child. 129, 1224–1226.
Reuhl, K.R., Chang, L.W. and Townsend, J.W. (1981) Environ. Res. 26, 281–306.
Rogan, W.J., Bagniewska, A. and Damstra, T. (1980) N. Engl. J. Med. 302, 1450–1453.
Saha, J.G. (1969) Residue Rev. 26, 89–126.
Schwetz, B.A., Sparschu, G.L. and Gehring, P.J. (1971) Food Cosmet. Toxicol. 9, 801–817.
Shacter, B. (1981) J. Am. Acad. Dermatol. 5, 517–527.
Spyker, D.A. and Spyker, J.M. (1977) Toxicol. Appl. Pharmacol. 40, 511–527.
Stevenson, R.E., Burton, O.M., Ferlanto, G.J. and Taylor, H.A. (1980) J. Am. Med. Assoc. 243, 1549–1551.
Thompson, D.J., Emerson, J.L. and Sparschu, G.L. (1971) Teratology 4, 243.
Virgo, B.B. (1980) Can. J. Physiol. Pharmacol. 58, 638–642.
Virgo, B.B. and Bellward, G.D. (1975) Environ. Physiol. Biochem. 5, 440–450.
Virgo, B.B. and Bellward, G.D. (1977) Res. Commun. Chem. Pathol. Pharmacol. 17, 399–409.
Warkany, J. (1976) Teratology 14, 205–209.
Weis, B. and Spyker, J.M. (1974) Pediatrics 53, 851–859.

S. Kacew and M.J. Reasor (eds), *Toxicology and the Newborn*
© 1984 Elsevier Science Publishers B.V.

Chapter 13

Reproductive and Developmental Toxicology of Selected Epoxides

CAROLE A. KIMMEL[a,*], JAMES B. LaBORDE[a] and BRYAN D. HARDIN[b]

[a]*Perinatal and Postnatal Evaluation Branch, Division of Teratogenesis Research, National Center for Toxicological Research, FDA Department of Health and Human Services, Jefferson, AR 72079,* [b]*Experimental Toxicology Branch, Division of Biomedical and Behavioral Science, National Institute of Occupational Safety and Health, Centers for Disease Control, Department of Health and Human Services, Cincinnati, OH 45226, U.S.A.*

CONTENTS

*Present address: US Environmental Protection Agency, RD 689, Reproductive Effects Assessment Group, Washington, DC 20460, U.S.A.

I. INTRODUCTION

The proximate, or directly active, form of a number of carcinogens and mutagens is known to be an epoxide metabolite. Epoxides have also been proposed as the active form of certain teratogenic agents (Martz et al., 1977; Kankaapaa et al., 1979; Gordon et al., 1981). Due to their strained three-member ring, epoxides are chemically reactive electrophilic compounds that readily attack nucleophilic centers in an alkylation reaction. It is largely this reactivity that makes the epoxides valuable in industrial processes.

The toxic effects of four industrially important 1,2-monoepoxides are reviewed here, with particular emphasis on the mutagenic, reproductive and developmental effects. These four epoxides are ethylene oxide (EO, oxirane, Chemical Abstracts Service (CAS) 75-21-8), propylene oxide (PO, methyl oxirane, CAS 75-56-9), butylene oxide (BO, ethyl oxirane, CAS 106-88-7) and styrene oxide (SO, phenyl oxirane, CAS 96-09-3) (see Figure 1 for structural formulae). As a class, epoxy compounds are irritating to the skin and respiratory system, and these four epoxides can be severe irritants. Local effects may be intensified where the epoxide is confined, e.g., in skin folds, under nails, or by prolonged close contact with incompletely cured epoxy resins or with EO-sterilized products that have not been allowed adequate 'off-gassing'. All four of these epoxides can be serious fire and explosion hazards (Hine et al., 1981). The American Conference of Governmental Industrial Hygienists (ACGIH) has recommended Threshold Limit Values and the Occupational Safety and Health Administration (OSHA) has set Permissible Exposure Limits for EO and PO as follows: for EO, ACGIH: 10 ppm, OSHA: 50 ppm (both are currently considering a reduction to 1 ppm); for PO, ACGIH: 20 ppm, OSHA: 100 ppm. There are no exposure limits set for BO or SO.

Several extensive reviews of the mutagenic and carcinogenic potential of epoxides have been published recently. Hine et al. (1981) postulated "that low-molecular-weight diepoxides should be considered as possibly carcinogenic until proven

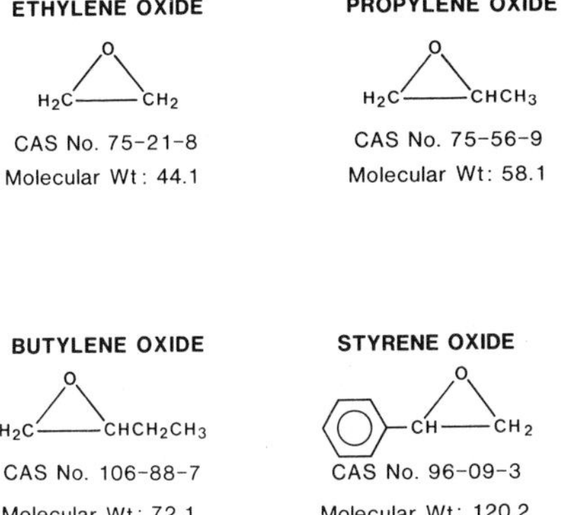

Figure 1. Structural formulae, CAS numbers and molecular weights of four industrially important epoxides.

otherwise and that most monoepoxides, though mutagenic, should not be considered oncogenic until shown to be". However, after evaluating the statistical power of negative carcinogenicity tests, Ehrenberg and Hussain (1981) concluded that the probability of false negative results was too high to draw such a conclusion. For ethylene oxide, the question of carcinogenicity has recently come to the fore with two as yet unpublished studies demonstrating unequivocal carcinogenicity in rats (OSHA, 1982, 1983). In addition, a number of new studies on the teratogenicity, fertility and reproductive effects of ethylene oxide have generated concern about workplace exposure and OSHA is considering a reduction of the occupational exposure limit to 1 ppm (OSHA, 1983). A recently completed chronic toxicity study of propylene oxide, conducted by the National Toxicology Program (NTP), disclosed evidence of carcinogenicity in rats and mice (NTP, 1984). The carcinogenicity of styrene oxide has also been suggested by preliminary evidence from several studies (Maltoni, 1982; Huff, 1984; data from Ponomarkov et al., cited in Huff, 1984).

II. USAGE, EXPOSURE AND MUTAGENICITY

1. Ethylene oxide

With an estimated annual production in 1982 of 4.9×10^9 pounds, EO ranked 26th in US production of organic chemicals. Approximately 99% of the EO produced is consumed in chemical synthesis: ethylene glycol, ethylene glycol alkyl ethers, polyester resins, poly(ethylene glycols), etc. (Hine et al., 1981). Only a small fraction of a percent of the total production is used for medical sterilization and fumigation of furs and certain foods. Based on the National Occupational Hazard Survey (NOHS), conducted in 1972–1974, the National Institute for Occupational Safety and Health (NIOSH, 1977) estimated that about 145,000 American workers are occupationally exposed to EO. Glaser (1978), in his detailed report on the conditions of exposure in hospitals, estimated that approximately 75,000 workers were potentially exposed to EO in the health-related occupations.

The mutagenicity of epoxides has long been recognized, as reflected in the excellent review by Ehrenberg and Hussain (1981). In fact, EO has been used by plant breeders to generate desirable mutant strains (Wolman, 1979; Ehrenberg and Hussain, 1981). These reviews also summarize reports of EO mutagenicity in various in vitro test systems utilizing *Salmonella, Klebsiella, Escherichia coli, Neurospora* and *Aspergillus.* EO reaction products, 2-haloethanols, found in fumigated foodstuffs have also been mutagenic in bacteria (Pfeiffer and Dunkelberg, 1980). Germ line mutations induced by EO were first demonstrated in the *Drosophila* sex-linked recessive lethal test (Rapoport, 1948; Bird, 1952). More recently, dominant lethal mutations have been demonstrated in rats (Embree et al., 1977) and mice (Cumming and Michaud, 1979; Generoso et al., 1980, 1983), although Appelgren et al. (1977) failed to detect dominant lethal mutations in mice. Generoso et al. (1980) observed a dose-related induction of heritable translocations in EO-treated mice.

Evidence has been accumulating that humans are subject to somatic cytogenetic damage as a result of occupational exposure to EO. An increased frequency of sister chromatid exchanges has been reported (Garry et al., 1979; Lambert and Lindblad, 1980; Yager et al., 1983) in lymphocytes of workers exposed to fugitive emissions of EO used for gas sterilization. Hogstedt et al. (1983) reported no increase in sister chromatid exchanges among workers exposed to EO at factories where medical supplies were packaged and sterilized, but there was a significant increase in lymphocyte chromosome aberrations and in micronuclei in polychromatic erythrocytes. A causal role of EO exposure in these observations is supported by recent studies in which rats (Kligerman et al., 1983), rabbits (Yager and Benz, 1982) and monkeys (D. Lynch, NIOSH, personal communication) showed significant concentration-related increases in sister chromatid exchanges following inhalation exposure to EO. Lynch et al. (1982) also observed reduced sperm counts and motility in EO-exposed monkeys, but no increase in abnormal sperm head morphology. Pero et al. (1981, 1982) suggested a reduced capacity to repair DNA lesions by demonstrating that human lymphocytes exposed to EO, both in vitro (1981) and in vivo (1981, 1982), exhibit reduced unscheduled DNA synthesis. Chromosome aberrations were induced in human cells exposed to EO in vitro (Poirier and Papadopoulo, 1982).

2. Propylene oxide

Approximately 1.8 $\times$ 10^9 pounds of PO are produced annually in the US, of which over 90% is used in chemical synthesis (propylene glycol, poly(propylene glycols), mixed polyglycols, and propylene glycol ethers) (Hine et al., 1981). The balance is used in miscellaneous applications, including fumigation of some foodstuffs. Based on NOHS data, NIOSH (1977) estimated that about 270,000 workers are occupationally exposed to PO in the United States.

Data are far more limited than for EO, but PO is clearly mutagenic in several in vitro bacterial assays, including *Salmonella* and *E. coli* (Bootman et al., 1979; Pfeiffer and Dunkelberg, 1980; Wade et al., 1978). Halopropanol reaction products found in PO-fumigated foodstuffs are also mutagenic in bacteria (Pfeiffer and Dunkelberg, 1980). Similarly, there is limited evidence for PO-induced germ line mutations. Sex-linked recessive lethal mutations were detected when male *Drosophila* were exposed to PO vapor (Hardin et al., 1983b). However, neither vapor (Hardin et al., 1983b) nor oral (Bootman et al., 1979) exposure of rats and mice, respectively, induced detectable dominant lethal mutations. As was the case with EO, Lynch et al. (1983) reported that monkeys chronically exposed to PO had reduced sperm counts and motility, but no increase in the frequency of abnormal sperm head morphology.

Chromosome damage had been detected following in vitro PO treatment of human lymphocytes, but orally dosed mice did not have a detectable increase in the frequency of micronuclei in polychromatic erythrocytes (Bootman et al., 1979). As was the case with EO, Pero et al. (1982) reported that unscheduled DNA synthesis was impaired in peripheral lymphocytes from workers exposed to PO. There is a single report (Theiss et al., 1981) of chromosome aberrations among chemical workers exposed to a variety of potential mutagens, including ethylene, propylene and butylene oxides, among others.

3. *Butylene oxide*

Annual production of BO in the US is estimated to be less than 10^7 pounds. The major use of BO (about 75% of production) is as a stabilizer in chlorinated hydrocarbon solvents. Approximately 20% is used in chemical synthesis (glycol ethers, poly(butylene glycols), etc.) (Hine et al., 1981), with the balance exported or used in miscellaneous applications. NIOSH (1977) estimated that about 37,000 workers are occupationally exposed to BO. This excludes exposure to trace amounts present in chlorinated hydrocarbon solvents.

Relatively little information is available on the mutagenicity of BO. Mutagenic activity has been reported in vitro in *Salmonella* (Wade et al., 1978), *Klebsiella* (Knaap et al., 1982), and in a mammalian cell point mutation assay (Knaap et al., 1982). McGregor (1981a) detected no unscheduled DNA synthesis in human cells exposed to BO in vitro. BO was mutagenic in the *Drosophila* sex-linked recessive lethal test by abdominal injection (Knaap et al., 1982), but McGregor (1981a) detected no induced mutations when *Drosophila* were exposed to BO vapor. Similarly, McGregor (1981a) detected no induction of dominant lethal mutations in rats, no increase in abnormal sperm head morphology in mice, and no increase in chromosomal aberrations in rat bone marrow cells following exposure to BO vapor.

4. *Styrene oxide*

No production estimates are available for SO, most of which is used in chemical synthesis. Some SO is used as a diluent in epoxy resin systems. NIOSH (1977) estimated that about 40,000 workers are exposed to SO occupationally. However, SO is the initial product of styrene metabolism, which is produced in an annual volume of 6.6×10^9 pounds, with an estimated exposure population of about 330,000 workers (NIOSH, 1977).

Because of its role in styrene metabolism, there have been a number of investigations of the mutagenic potential of SO. Loprieno et al. (1978) summarized a series of in vitro tests, utilizing bacterial, yeast and mammalian cells in culture, in all of which SO was active. Chromosomal aberrations and sister chromatid exchanges have been detected in primary cultures of human lymphocytes treated with SO (Linnainmaa et al., 1978; Norppa et al., 1981). Although McGregor (1981b), employing inhalation exposures, failed to detect mutagenic activity in a rat bone marrow cytogenetics assay, Loprieno et al. (1978) observed chromosomal aberrations in the bone marrow of mice orally dosed with SO. Donner et al. (1979) observed significant induction of sex-linked recessive lethal mutations in *Drosophila* exposed to SO either by feeding or as the vapor. McGregor (1981b) exposed *Drosophila* to SO vapor at a lower concentration and detected no induction of sex-linked recessive lethal mutations.

No reports are available on the effects in humans of exposure to SO, but workers exposed to styrene and other chemicals in the manufacture of polystyrene products have been reported to have increased frequencies of chromosomal aberrations in peripheral lymphocytes (Meretoja et al., 1977; Fleig and Theiss, 1978).

5. *Summary*

All the epoxides considered here have been mutagenic in several test systems (see Table 1), including tests for point mutations as well as for blastogenic effects. All induce germinal mutations in *Drosophila*, but germ line mutations have been detected in mammals only after exposure to EO. Although some of these epoxides have had no detectable activity in the hands of some investigators or in certain systems, the fact remains that all have been mutagenic in more than one test system. In individual cases, activity is dependent on the reactivity of the specific epoxide and on the dose of epoxide reaching the cellular target (Ehrenberg and Hussain, 1981). Therefore, all four of these epoxides warrant restricted exposure and care in handling.

III. REPRODUCTIVE AND DEVELOPMENTAL TOXICITY

1. *Ethylene oxide*

The concern over exposure of hospital workers to EO associated with the use of gas-sterilization equipment as well as leaching of EO from medical devices when improperly aerated has led to several studies on the developmental toxicity of EO and its reaction product, ethylene chlorohydrin (EC).

A series of studies has been completed recently on the teratogenicity of EO and EC when administered intravenously to mice and rabbits during gestation. LaBorde and Kimmel (1980) administered EO in doses of 0 (vehicle, 5% dextrose), 75 or 150 mg/kg to CD-1 mice on days 4–6, 6–8, 8–10 or 10–12 of gestation. Maternal mortality was increased significantly and maternal weight gain was decreased significantly in the groups treated on days 4–6, 8–10 and 10–12 of gestation with 150 mg/kg. However, no signs of maternal toxicity were apparent in the high-dose group treated on days 6–8, or in the 0 and 75 mg/kg group treated at any gestation interval. The incidence of malformations was increased significantly in the 150 mg/kg dose group treated on days 6–8 or 10–12. The types of malformations included craniofacial defects and fusions or absence of skeletal vertebral elements, primarily in the cervical and upper thoracic regions. Fetal weights were reduced significantly in all four groups treated with the high dose, and resorptions were increased significantly in the groups treated with 150 mg/kg on days 8–10 or 10–12 of gestation. No increase in malformations or in other types of fetotoxicity was noted in any group treated with 75 mg/kg.

The results of the study on EO in mice suggested a teratogenic potential for EO, albeit at extremely high dose levels. In order to explore this potential further, similar studies were carried out in rabbits. When EO was administered intravenously to New

TABLE 1

SUMMARY OF MUTAGENICITY STUDIES

	EO	PO	BO	SO
Prokaryotic systems	+ Ehrenberg and Hussain (1981) (review) + Pfeiffer and Dunkelberg (1980)	+ Bootman et al. (1979) + Pfeiffer and Dunkelberg (1980) + Wade et al. (1978)	+ Knaap et al. (1982) + Wade et al. (1978)	+ Loprieno et al. (1978) + Wade et al. (1978)
Mammalian cells in vitro			+ Knaap et al. (1982)	+ Loprieno et al. (1978)
Human cells in vitro	+ Pero et al. (1981) + Poirier and Papadopoulo (1982)	+ Bootman et al. (1979)	− McGregor (1981a)	− McGregor (1981b) + Linnainmaa et al. (1978) + Loprieno et al. (1978) + Norppa et al. (1981)
Drosophila sex-linked recessive lethal	+ Bird (1952) + Rapoport (1948)	+ Hardin et al. (1983b)	− McGregor (1981a) + Knaap et al. (1982)	− McGregor (1981b) + Donner et al. (1979)

Mouse sperm head morphology		– Hardin et al. (1983b)	– McGregor (1981a)	± McGregor (1981b)
Rodent dominant lethal	+ Cumming and Michaud (1979) + Embree et al. (1977) + Generoso et al. (1980, 1983) – Applegren et al. (1977)	– Bootman et al. (1979) – Hardin et al. (1983b)	– McGregor (1981a)	– McGregor (1981b)
Mammalian cytogenetics in vivo	+ Generoso et al. (1980) + Yager and Benz (1982) + Kligerman et al. (1983)	± Bootman et al. (1979)	± McGregor (1981a)	– McGregor (1981b) + Loprieno et al. (1978)
Human cytogenetics in vivo	+ Garry et al. (1979) + Hogstedt et al. (1983) + Pero et al. (1981, 1982) + Theiss et al. (1981) + Yager et al. (1983) + Lambert and Lindblad (1980)	+ Pero et al. (1982) + Theiss et al. (1981)	+ Theiss et al. (1981)	+ Fleig and Theiss (1978)[a] + Meretoja et al. (1977)[a]

–, No mutagenic activity detected; +, mutagenic activity reported; ±, inconclusive results, or mixed results on multiple tests.
[a] Exposures were in styrene and polystrene industries.

Zealand White rabbits on days 6–9 of gestation at 0, 18 or 36 mg/kg or on days 6–14 of gestation at 0, 9, 18 or 36 mg/kg, no indication of teratogenic effect was seen (Jones-Price et al., 1983a). Maternal toxicity was pronounced at all doses in the animals treated on days 6–14, and the incidence of resorptions also was increased. Dosing on days 6–9 resulted in minimal maternal toxicity and no evidence of fetotoxicity. Thus, EO did not show evidence of teratogenic potential but was fetotoxic at doses that were also toxic to the maternal rabbit.

Further studies with EC were done using protocols in mice and rabbits similar to those used for EO. In rabbits treated intravenously with 0, 9, 18 or 36 mg/kg on days 6–15 of gestation, no indication of maternal or fetal toxicity was reported (Jones-Price et al., 1983b). Mice were treated with 0, 60 or 120 mg/kg EC on days 4–6, 6–8, 8–10 or 10–12 of gestation (Jones-Price et al., 1983c). Dose-related increases in maternal and fetal toxicity following treatment at all periods were seen, as well as a marginal increase in the incidence of malformations following the high-dose treatment on days 8–10. Although the increase was minimal, the types of defects seen were similar to those in the EO mouse study, i.e., craniofacial defects and skeletal fusions and dysplasias. These defects were found only in the presence of significant maternal toxicity.

Only one other study has dealt with the effects of EC. Courtney et al. (1982) dosed CD-1 mice orally with EC by gavage (0, 50, 100, 150 mg/kg) or in drinking water (0, 16, 43, 77, 227 mg/kg) on days 6–16 of gestation. The highest dose by gavage resulted in 100% mortality of pregnant animals, while the 100 mg/kg dose caused maternal and fetal toxicity, including a slight increase in the incidence of 14th ribs. In the drinking water study, no treatment-related effects were noted, even though the highest dose was more than twice the 100 mg/kg dose in the gavage study. However, intake via drinking water is less stressful than gavage and probably does not allow as high a peak concentration to be reached in the animals.

The developmental effects of inhalation exposure to EO also have been studied. Hackett et al. (1982) exposed rabbits for 7 hours per day on days 1–19 or 7–19 of gestation to 150 ppm EO (see Hardin et al. (1983a) for a summary). No maternal or fetal toxic effects were noted. Rats were exposed similarly to 150 ppm EO from 3 weeks prior to mating through gestation day 16 or only on days 1–16 or 7–16 of gestation. Maternal toxicity, an increased incidence of resorptions and reduced fetal weight were observed, but no increase in the incidence of malformations was noted.

Snellings et al. (1982a) also studied the effects of inhalation exposure of EO to Fischer 344 rats during pregnancy. Animals were exposed 6 hours per day to 0, 10, 33 or 100 ppm on days 6–15 of gestation. No maternal toxicity was apparent, although body weights were not obtained. The only fetal effect observed was a significant reduction in body weight at the highest exposure level (100 ppm).

In a further one-generation study, Snellings et al. (1982b) exposed male and female Fischer 344 rats for 12 weeks (6 hours/day, 5 days/week) to 0, 10, 33 or 100 ppm EO. Animals were then mated, and females were continued on the exposure during days 0–19 of gestation (6 hours/day, 7 days/week). Significantly fewer pups were born per litter in the highest exposure level group. In addition, there was a reduction in the number of implantation sites and a smaller ratio of number of fetuses born per number of implantation sites in the 100 ppm group. Also, more animals had a gestation length greater than 22 days in this group. No other signs of maternal toxicity, such as changes in body weight, were noted and no other effects on offspring were observed postnatally to day 21, even when the mothers were exposed during lactation. Thus, EO appeared to cause several types of reproductive and developmental effects in Fischer 344 rats when exposure began several weeks prior to gestation and included paternal exposure. Whether the effect is on the male, female or both is not clear from the studies conducted so far.

The results of the reproductive studies of Snellings et al. (1982b) are interesting in light of a recent study by Hemminki et al. (1982, 1983) in which an increased incidence of spontaneous abortions was reported in hospital workers who used chemical sterilizing equipment during pregnancy; the highest incidence was found in the group exposed to EO. Exposure information on these workers is sparse, but the authors reported that 20-minute measurements of 5–10 ppm were found on opening the sterilizing chamber, and that peak concentrations as high as 250 ppm were sometimes measured. Although these data are suggestive of a reproductive effect for EO, the exposure information is not sufficient to ensure a direct causal relationship. An earlier report by Yakubova et al. (1976) (cited by Snellings et al., 1982b) also indicated an increased incidence of miscarriages in workers in an EO production plant, but the authors stated that these women were also exposed to rapid temperature rises and to high-frequency noise.

In summary, there appears to be a potential for EO to cause teratogenic effects, but perhaps only when exposure results in acutely high levels, e.g., via intravenous injections. EO is a highly reactive chemical (biological half-life of approximately 9 minutes, Ehrenberg and Hussain, 1981) and probably does not reach the target site in high enough concentrations when administered by other than the intravenous route. The effects of EC, the major breakdown product, are less clear, but appear to occur at doses that cause overt maternal toxicity. The effects of EO on other reproductive indices such as reduced fertility and reduced offspring viability are more striking and these types of effects should be of greater concern. If the exposure levels assumed by Hemminki et al. (1982) in hospital workers are correct, it would indicate a higher level of sensitivity in humans to EO than in laboratory animals.

2. *Propylene oxide*

Extensive information on the acute and subacute toxicity of propylene oxide (PO) in several species of laboratory animals exposed by intubation or inhalation is readily available in the literature (Rowe et al., 1956; Smyth et al., 1969; Hine et al., 1981; Kirk and Dempsey, 1982). Only a limited number of studies have been designed and conducted to determine the possible risk of reproductive and developmental toxicity after exposure to PO.

Recently, Hackett et al. (1982) completed inhalation toxicity studies (summarized by Hardin et al., 1983a) designed to evaluate the reproductive and developmental toxicity of PO in Sprague-Dawley rats and in New Zealand White rabbits. Rabbits and rats were exposed by inhalation to 500 ppm PO. Pregnant rabbits were exposed to PO for 7 hours/day, 7 days/week, on gestation days 1–19 or 7–19, and killed on day 30. In contrast, rats were pregestationally exposed to PO for 7 hours/day, 5 days/week for 3 weeks. Following mating, the animals were exposed daily (7 hours/day) on gestation days 1–16 and killed on day 21. Other animals were similarly exposed only on gestation days 1–16 or 7–16. Maternal rabbits showed a decrease in food consumption following PO exposure in the days 1–19 and 7–19 groups, and a slight but significant decrease in body weight in the days 7–19 group. An increase in the number of resorptions in rabbit litters that had resorptions was the only evidence of embryotoxicity reported, and this was observed only in the rabbits exposed to PO on gestation days 1–19. No evidence of fetal toxicity or of developmental defects was noted in the rabbits exposed during either period of gestation. In rats, a decrease in food consumption and in maternal body weight were evident in those animals exposed to PO prior to mating and during both periods of gestation. A significant reduction in the number of corpora lutea, implantation sites and live fetuses was reported in the rats exposed during the pregestational period. Some degree of fetal toxicity was observed in all PO-exposed groups, as reflected by a significant reduction in fetal body weight and in crown-rump length. Except for a significant increase in wavy ribs and reduced ossification in fetal vertebrae and ribs in the days 1–16 exposure group, no other significant alterations in fetal development were noted. These data indicate the potential for adverse effects of PO on fertility and survival of offspring as well as other forms of fetal toxicity. It is unclear whether or not these alterations were due to maternal toxicity or were manifestations of direct developmental effects.

3. Butylene oxide

A review of the literature revealed a paucity of published toxicological and teratological studies on butylene oxide (BO). Most of the toxicological data available have been derived from studies on the mixed isomers of BO (80–90%, 1,2-butylene oxide and 10–20% 2,3-butylene oxide) and have been summarized by Hine et al. (1981).

The recently completed studies by Sikov et al. (1981) (reported by Hardin et al., 1981, 1983a) are the only studies, to our knowledge, to have evaluated the developmental and reproductive toxicity of BO in laboratory animals. Wistar rats and New Zealand White rabbits were exposed to 250 or 1000 ppm vapor concentrations of butylene oxide. Some rats were exposed for 7 hours/day, 5 days/week for 3 weeks before breeding, then mated and gestational exposure continued for 7 hours/day, 7 days/week through day 19. Other rats were exposed only during gestation. Rabbits were not exposed to BO during pregestation but were exposed following mating to 250 or 1000 ppm BO on days 1–24 and killed on day 30 of gestation.

Rat maternal toxicity was evident by a significant reduction in body weight at

1000 ppm during the pregestation exposure period and at both concentrations during pregnancy. However, no statistically significant changes were observed in any measure of reproductive success, embryo/fetal survival or development. Maternal rabbits were affected more severely than rats, as noted by a significant increase in maternal mortality at both exposure concentrations. Despite this increase in mortality, no significant change in maternal body weight or other reproductive parameters in surviving rabbits was observed. Although significant maternal toxicity in rabbits was noted at the 250 ppm exposure level, there was no evidence of toxicity in any embryo/fetal developmental parameters examined. Suggestive evidence, although not statistically significant, of rabbit embryo/fetal toxicity was observed in the 1000 ppm exposure group. Thus, BO did not produce any significant developmental toxicity in rats or rabbits in these inhalation studies (Hardin et al., 1983a).

4. Styrene oxide

The possible impact of styrene oxide (SO) for increasing the incidence of congenital defects in pregnant women in the work force has led several investigators to evaluate the potential embryo/fetal toxicity and teratogenicity of this epoxide. Vainio et al. (1977) reported SO to be embryotoxic and teratogenic in chick embryos during the early stages of embryonic development at concentrations of 0.5–5 μmol/egg. Malformations that were observed included deformities of the eyelid, skull, upper bill and lower extremities as well as exencephaly and brain hemorrhage. Kankaapaa et al. (1979) observed similar embryotoxic and teratogenic properties of styrene oxide in chick embryos exposed on the 3rd day of embryogenesis. In addition, these investigations indicated that SO is a more potent and reactive compound than its parent compound, styrene, and that the embryotoxicity of both could be potentiated by the administration of the epoxide hydrase inhibitor, trichloropropylene oxide.

Sikov et al. (1981) (as summarized by Hardin et al., 1981, 1983a) also tested SO in a study similar to that employed for BO. Rats were exposed to 100 ppm SO 7 hours/day, 5 days/week for 3 weeks before breeding and on gestation days 1–19, or only on gestation days 1–19. Rabbits were exposed to 15 or 50 ppm SO on gestation days 1–24. Significant maternal mortality and reduced body weight gain were noted in SO-exposed rats. There also was a significant reduction in the proportion of sperm-positive females exposed from day 1 that were pregnant at term. Differences were not statistically significant, but exposure to SO before breeding appeared to reduce the number of corpora lutea. The only evidence of fetal toxicity was reduced body weight and crown-rump length of fetuses from SO-exposed rats. In rabbits exposed to 50 ppm SO, significant maternal mortality and reduced body weight gain were observed. In contrast to the observation in rats, there was no reduction in the number of artificially inseminated rabbits that were pregnant at term. No evidence of teratogenicity was seen in either species. In summary, although no evidence of teratogenicity was observed, styrene oxide was maternally toxic to both species. Increased fetal mortality was noted only in the rats at 100 ppm.

TABLE 2

COMPARATIVE REPRODUCTIVE AND DEVELOPMENTAL TOXICITY OF SELECTED EXPOXIDES

Agent	Route and exposure time[a]	Species	Exposure levels	Teratogenicity	Fetal/postnatal toxicity	Fertility/ reproductive toxicity	References
Ethylene oxide	iv, gd 4–6, 6–8, 8–10, 10–12	mouse	75, 150[b] mg/kg	increased malformations — 150 mg/kg (days 6–8, 10–12)	increased resorptions — 150 mg/kg (days 8–10, 10–12); reduced fetal weight — 150 mg/kg (all groups)	–	LaBorde and Kimmel (1980)
	iv, gd 6–9, 6–14	rabbit	9[b], 18[b], 36[b] mg/kg	–	increased resorptions, reduced fetal weight — 36 mg/kg (days 6–14)	–	Jones-Price et al. (1983a)
	inhal., 3 weeks pregest. + gd 1–16, gd 1–16, gd 7–16	rat	150[b] ppm	–	increased resorptions (pregest. + gd 1–16); reduced fetal weight (all groups)	–	Hackett et al. (1982) (see Hardin et al., 1983a)
	inhal., gd 1–19, gd 7–19	rabbit	150 ppm	–	–	–	Hackett et al. (1982) (see Hardin et al., 1983a)
	inhal., gd 6–15	rat	0, 10, 33, 100 ppm	–	reduced fetal wt. — 100 ppm	–	Snellings et al. (1982a)
	inhal., 12 weeks premating (males and females) + gd 0–19 (females)	rat	0, 10, 33, 100 ppm	–	reduced litter size — 100 ppm	reduced no. implantations, increased gest. length — 100 ppm	Snellings et al. (1982b)
	inhal., during pregnancy (assumed)	human	? (5–10 ppm)	–	–	increased spontaneous abortions	Hemminki et al. (1982)
	inhal., during pregnancy (assumed)	human	? (5–10 ppm)	–	–	increased spontaneous abortions	Yakubova et al. (1976)

Propylene oxide	inhal., 3 weeks pregest. + gd 1–16, gd 1–16, gd 7–16	rat	500^b ppm	–	reduced No. live fetuses (pregest. + gd 1–16); reduced fetal weight (all groups)	reduced No. corpora lutea, implantation sites (pregest. + gd 1–16)	Hackett et al. (1982) (see Hardin et al., 1983a)
	inhal., gd 1–19, gd 7–19	rabbit	500^b ppm	–	increased resorptions in litters with resorptions (gd 1–19)	–	Hackett et al. (1982) (see Hardin et al., 1983a)
Butylene oxide	inhal., 3 wks. pregest. + gd 1–19, gd 1–19	rat	250^b, 1000^b ppm	–	–	–	Sikov et al. (1981) (see Hardin et al., 1983a)
	inhal., gd 1–24	rabbit	250^b, 1000^b ppm	–	–	–	Sikov et al., (1981) (see Hardin et al., 1983a)
Styrene oxide	inhal., 3 wks. pregest. + gd 1–19, gd 1–19	rat	100^b ppm	–	reduced fetal weight (pregest. + gd 1–19)	reduced pregnancy rate (gd 1–19); marginal reduction in No. corpora lutea (pregest. + gd. 1–19)	Sikov et al. (1981) (see Hardin et al., 1983a)
	inhal., gd 1–24	rabbit	15, 50^b ppm	–	–	–	Sikov et al. (1981) (see Hardin et al., 1983a)
	in ovo, day 3 of incubation	chick	0.5–5 μmol/egg	increased malformations	reduced survival — 2–5 μmol/egg	–	Vainio et al. (1977)
	in ovo, day 3 of incubation	chick	0.8 μmol/egg	increased malformations	reduced survival	–	Kankaapaa et al. (1979)

[a] iv, intravenously; gd, gestation days; inhal., inhalation; pregest., pregestation.
[b] Significant maternal toxicity.

IV. SUMMARY AND DISCUSSION

The mutagenic and carcinogenic potential of epoxides provides a strong impetus for studying the reproductive and developmental effects of these agents. Chromosomal aberrations are associated with a number of malformation syndromes, and at least two known human teratogens, diphenylhydantoin (Martz et al., 1977) and thalidomide (Gordon et al., 1981), have been proposed to act via the formation of an arene oxide (epoxide) metabolite. In addition, Kankaapaa et al. (1979) suggested a similar mechanism for styrene and stryene oxide teratogenicity in the chick embryo.

In the case of the four epoxides reviewed here, only EO was clearly teratogenic in in vivo mammalian systems (see Table 2), and then only in the mouse following intravenous dosing during certain periods of organogenesis (LaBorde and Kimmel, 1980). The teratogenic effects of EO in the mouse and SO in the chick may be due to the acute administration of a large enough dose of the epoxide to allow delivery of a critical level to the site of action. None of the studies employing intravenous administration of lower doses of EO to rabbits (Jones-Price et al., 1983a) or inhalation exposure of any of the four epoxides to rabbits or rats (Hardin et al., 1983a) indicated a teratogenic effect. The intravenous administration of EC to mice (Jones-Price et al., 1983b) resulted in a slight increase in malformations which possibly could be related to the in vivo formation of an epoxide, as suggested by Ehrenberg and Hussain (1981).

Fetal toxicity in the form of increased resorptions or reduced fetal weight was always associated with a dose that also produced maternal toxicity (Table 2), except perhaps in the case of the rat EO-inhalation exposure studies by Snellings et al. (1982a,b). Thus, although a direct fetotoxic effect cannot be ruled out, it is likely that much of the fetotoxicity noted was secondary to the maternal toxicity, including effects on fertility and reproductive function.

In the inhalation exposure studies on these four epoxides reported by Hardin et al. (1983a), the highest maternal exposure level chosen was one that would induce some minimal maternal toxicity. If one compares the relative effects of inhalation exposure to these four compounds, maternal toxicity increased as molecular size increased, except for SO, which was toxic at or below the toxic levels for EO. This relative order of toxicity appears to be similar to the mutagenic potency on a molar basis in the Ames assay (Wade et al., 1978; Bootman et al., 1979; Ehrenberg and Hussain, 1981); i.e., SO > EO = PO > BO. The same trend may be present in the effects of these epoxides on fertility, with EO, PO and SO all causing some reduction in numbers of implantation sites, corpora lutea or pregnancy rate, while BO did not alter fertility at exposure levels which were much higher (Table 2). The fact that reduced fertility occurred primarily in animals in which exposure began prior to gestation suggests the possibility for gametotoxic effects of these epoxides. Mattison and coworkers (1980, 1983) have provided evidence to support the importance of an epoxide metabolite in reducing fertility and increasing oocyte toxicity in mice following exposure to benzo(*a*)pyrene. However, other possible mechanisms of reproductive toxicity should not be overlooked.

In summary, the teratogenicity of these four epoxides is likely dependent on delivery of large acute levels of the agent proximal to the site of action. However, the potential for mutagenicity, carcinogenicity and reduced fertility as suggested by the studies reviewed here strongly indicates the need for care in handling and monitoring for such effects in occupational exposure situations. The fact that EO and EC may be encountered in medical devices also emphasizes the need for reducing potential exposure by adequate degassing procedures. Since EO and SO appear to have a relatively higher potency for producing various forms of toxicity, occupational situations in which exposure to these two epoxides occurs may require the most careful surveillance of exposure concentrations and worker health. Further delineation of structure-activity relationships would be helpful in determining the developmental and reproductive hazards of exposure to epoxide compounds.

V. ACKNOWLEDGEMENTS

The authors would like to express their gratitude to Rose Huber, Cynthia Hartwick and Sandra Clark, who aided in the preparation of this manuscript.

VI. REFERENCES

Appelgren, L.-E., Everoth, G. and Grant, C. (1977) Proc. Eur. Soc. Toxicol. 18, 315–317.
Bird, M.J. (1952) J. Genet. 50, 480–485.
Bootman, J., Lodge, D.C. and Whalley, H.E. (1979) Mut. Res. 67, 101–112.
Courtney, K.D., Andrews, J.E. and Grady, M. (1982) J. Environ. Sci. Hlth. B17(4), 381–391.
Cumming, R.B. and Michaud, T.A. (1979) Environ. Mutagen. 1, 166–167 (Abstract).
Donner, M., Sorsa, M. and Vainio, H. (1979) Mut. Res. 67, 373–376.
Ehrenberg, L. and Hussain, S. (1981) Mut. Res. 86, 1–113.
Embree, J.W., Lyon, J.P. and Hine, C.P. (1977) Toxicol. Appl. Pharmacol. 40, 261–267.
Fleig, I. and Theiss, A.M. (1978) Scand. J. Work. Environ. Hlth. 4 (Suppl. 2), 254–258.
Garry, V.F., Hozier, J., Jacobs, D., Wade, R.L. and Gray, D.G. (1979) Environ. Mutagen. 1, 375–382.
Generoso, W.M., Cain, K.T., Krishna, M., Sheu, C.W. and Gryder, R. M. (1980) Mut. Res. 73, 133–142.
Generoso, W.M., Cumming, R.B., Bandy, J.A. and Cain, K.T. (1983) Mut. Res. 119, 377–379.
Glaser, Z.R. (1978) J. Environ. Pathol. Toxicol. 2, 173–208.
Gordon, G.B., Spielberg, S.P., Blake, D.A. and Balasubramanian, V. (1981) Proc. Natl. Acad. Sci. U.S.A. 78, 2545–2548.
Hackett, P.L., Brown, M.G., Buschbom, R.L., Clark, M.L., Miller, R.A., Music, R.L., Rowe, S.E., Schirmer, R.E. and Sikov, M.R. (1982) Battelle Pacific Northwest Laboratories, Richland, WA (Final report to DHHS (NIOSH), Contract No. 210–80–0013).
Hardin, B.D., Bond, G.P., Sikov, M.R., Andrew, F.D., Beliles, R.P. and Niemeier, R.W. (1981) Scand. J. Work. Environ. Hlth. 7 (Suppl. 4), 66–75.
Hardin, B.D., Niemeier, R.W., Sikov, M.R. and Hackett, P.L. (1983a) Scand. J. Work Environ. Hlth. 9, 94–102.
Hardin, B.D., Schuler, R.L., McGinnis, P.M., Niemeier, R.W. and Smith R.W. (1983b) Mut. Res. 117, 337–344.
Hemminki, K., Mutanen, P., Saloniemi, I., Niemi, M.-L. and Vainio, H. (1982) Br. Med. J. 285, 1461–1463.

Hemminki, K., Mutanen, P. and Niemi, M.-L. (1983) Br. Med. J. 286, 1976–1977.
Hine, C.H., Rowe, V.K., White, E.R., Darmer, Jr., K.I. and Youngblood, G.T. (1981) Patty's Industrial Hygiene and Toxicology, 3rd edn., pp. 2141–2257, Wiley Interscience, New York.
Hogstedt, B., Gullberg, B., Hedner, K., Kolnig, A.-M., Mitelman, F., Skerfving, S. and Widegren, B. (1983) Hereditas 98, 105–113.
Huff, J.E. (1984) in Industrial Hazards of Plastics and Synthetic Elastomers (Jarvisalo, J., Pfaffli, P. and Vainio, H., eds.), pp. 227–238, Alan R. Liss Inc., New York.
Jones-Price, C., Kimmel, C.A., Marks, T.A., LeDoux, T.A., Reel, J. R., Fisher, P.W., Langhoff-Paschke, L. and Marr, M. (1983a) Final Report (Rb80-EO), NIEHS Contract NO1-ES-2127.
Jones-Price, C., Kimmel, C.A., Marks, T.A., LeDoux, T.A., Reel, J. R., Fisher, P.W., Langhoff-Paschke, L. and Marr. M. (1983b) Final Report (Rb79-EC), NIEHS Contract NO1-ES-6-2127.
Jones-Price, C., Kimmel, C.A., Marks, T.A., LeDoux, T.A., Reel, J. R., Fisher, P.W., Langhoff-Paschke, L. and Marr, M. (1983c) Final Report (Mi79-EC), NIEHS Contract NO1-ES-2127.
Kankaapaa, J.T.J., Hemminki, K. and Vainio, H. (1979) Acta. Pharmacol. Toxicol. 45, 399–402.
Kirk, R.O. and Dempsey, T.J. (1982) Encyclopedia of Chemical Technology, 3rd edn., pp. 247–274, Wiley Interscience, New York.
Kligerman, A.D., Erexson, G.L., Phelps, M.E. and Wilmer, J.L. (1983) Mut. Res. 120, 37–44.
Knaap, A.G.A.C., Voogd, C.E. and Kramers, P.G.N. (1982) Mut. Res. 101, 199–208.
LaBorde, J.B. and Kimmel, C.A. (1980) Toxicol. Appl. Pharmacol. 56, 1622.
Lambert, B. and Lindblad, A. (1980) J. Toxicol. Environ. Hlth. 6, 1237–1243.
Linnainmaa, K., Meretoja, T., Sorsa, M. and Vainio, H. (1978) Mut. Res. 58, 277–286.
Loprieno, N., Presciuttini, S., Sbrana, I., Stretti, G., Zaccaro, L., Abbondandolo, A., Bonatti, S., Fiorio, R. and Mazzaccaro, A. (1978) Scand. J. Work Environ. Hlth. 4 (Suppl. 2), 169–178.
Lynch, D.W., Lewis, T.R., Moorman, W.J., Sabharwal, P.S. and Burg, J.A. (1983) The Toxicologist 3, 60 (Abstract).
Maltoni, C. (1982) in Occupational Health Hazards of Solvents (England, A., Ringer, K. and Mehlman, M., eds.), pp. 97–110, Princeton Science Publishers Inc., Princeton, NJ.
Martz, F., Failinger, C. III and Blake, D.A. (1977) J. Pharmacol. Exptl. Therap. 203, 231–239.
Mattison, D.R., White, N.B. and Nightingale, M.R. (1980) Pediatr. Pharmacol. 1, 143–151.
Mattison, D.R., Shiromizu, K. and Nightingale, M.S. (1983) Prog. Clin. Biol. Res. 117, 191–202.
McGregor, D.B. (1981a) Report 28, NIOSH Contract 210-78-0026, 187 pp.
McGregor, D.B. (1981b) Report 29, NIOSH Contract 210-78-0026, 172 pp.
Meretoja, T., Vainio, H., Sorsa, M. and Harkonen, H. (1977) Mut. Res. 56, 193–197.
NIOSH (1977) National Occupational Hazard Survey, Vol. III, Survey Analysis and Supplemental Tables, USDHEW, PHS, DHEW (NIOSH) Publication No. 78-114, 792 pp.
Norppa, H., Hemminki, K., Sorsa, M. and Vainio, H. (1981) Mut. Res. 91, 243–250.
NTP (1984) Technical Report on the Toxicology and Carcinogenesis Studies of Propylene Oxide (CAS No. 75-56-9) in F344/N Rats and B6C3F1 Mice (Inhalation Studies), TR No. 267, National Toxicology Program, Research Triangle Park, NC, 165 pp.
Occupational Safety and Health Administration (1982) Federal Register 47 (17), 3566–3571.
Occupational Safety and Health Administration (1983) Federal Register 48 (78), 17284–17319.
Pero, R.W., Widegren, B., Hogstedt, B. and Mitelman, F. (1981) Mut. Res. 83, 271–289.
Pero, R.W., Bryngelsson, T., Widegren, B., Hogstedt, B. and Welinder, H. (1982) Mut. Res. 104, 193–200.
Pfeiffer, E.H. and Dunkelberg, H. (1980) Food Cosmet. Toxicol. 18, 115–118.
Poirier, V. and Papadopoulo, D. (1982) Mut. Res. 104, 255–260.
Rapoport, I.A. (1948) Dokl. Akad. Nauk. USSR 60, 469–472 (in Russian).
Rowe, V.K., Hollingsworth, R.L., Oyen, F., McCollister, D.D. and Spencer, H.C. (1956) A.M.A. Arch. Indust. Health 13, 228–236.
Sikov, M.R., Cannon, W.C., Carr, D.B., Miller, R.A., Montgomery, L. F. and Phelps, D.W. (1981) DHHS (NIOSH) Publications No. 81-124, 76 pp.
Smyth, Jr., H.F., Carpenter, C.P., Weil, C.S., Pozzani, U.C., Striegel, J.A. and Nycum, J.S. (1969) Am. Indust. Hyg. Assoc. J. 30, 470–476.

Snellings, W.M., Maronpot, R.R., Zelanak, J.P. and Lafoon, C.P. (1982a) Toxicol. Appl. Pharmacol. 64, 476–481.
Snellings, W.M., Zelenak, J.P. and Weil, C.S. (1982b) Toxicol. Appl. Pharmacol. 63, 382–388.
Theiss, A.M., Schwegler, H., Fleig, I. and Stocker, W.G. (1981) J. Occup. Med. 23, 343–347.
Vainio, H., Hemminki, K. and Elovaara, E. (1977) Toxicology 8, 319–325.
Wade, D.E., Airy, S.C. and Sinsheimer, J.E. (1978) Mut. Res. 58, 217–223.
Wolman, S.R. (1979) J. Environ. Pathol. Toxicol. 2, 1289–1303.
Yager, J.W. and Benz, R.D. (1982) Environ. Mutagen. 4, 121–134.
Yager, J.W., Hines, C.J. and Spear, R.C. (1983) Science 219, 1221–1223.
Yakubova, Z.N., Shamova, N.A., Miftakhova, F.A. and Shilova, L.F. (1976) Med. Zh. 57, 558–560 (in Russian).

Subject Index